Critical Thinking in Nursing:
An Interactive Approach
Second Edition

M. Gaie Rubenfeld, RN, MS
Associate Professor
Department of Nursing
Eastern Michigan University
Ypsilanti, Michigan

Barbara K. Scheffer, RN, MS
Associate Professor
Department of Nursing
Eastern Michigan University
Ypsilanti, Michigan

Illustrations by Mark Steele

Lippincott
Philadelphia • New York • Baltimore

Acquisitions Editor: Ilze Rader
Assistant Editor: Dale Thuesen
Project Editor: Tom Gibbons
Senior Production Manager: Helen Ewan
Production Coordinator: Michael Carcel
Design Coordinator: Brett Mac Naughton
Indexer: Victoria Boyle
Interior Design: Christine Cantera
Cover Design: Melissa Olson

2nd edition

Library of Congress Cataloging in Publications Data

Rubenfeld, M. Gaie.
    Critical thinking in nursing : an interactive approach / M. Gaie
Rubenfeld, Barbara K. Scheffer. — 2nd ed.
        p. cm.
    Includes bibliographical references and index.
    ISBN 0-7817-1634-9 (paper : alk. paper)
    1. Nursing—Philosophy. 2. Critical thinking. 3. Nursing—
Problems, exercises, etc. I. Scheffer, Barbara K. II. Title.
    [DNLM: 1. Nursing Process. 2. Problem Solving nurses'
instruction. 3. Nursing problems. WY 100 R895c 1999]
RT84.5.R83 1999
610.73—dc21
DNLM/DLC
for Library of Congress   98-46410
                                                                CIP

Care has been taken to confirm the accuracy of the information presented and to describe generally accepted practices. However, the authors, editors, and publisher are not responsible for errors or omissions or for any consequences from application of the information in
this book and make no warranty, express or implied, with respect to
the contents of the publication.
The authors, editors and publisher have exerted every effort to ensure
that drug selection and dosage set forth in this text are in accordance
with current recommendations and practice at the time of publication.
However, in view of ongoing research, changes in government regulations, and the constant flow of information relating to drug therapy
and drug reactions, the reader is urged to check the package insert for
each drug for any change in indications and dosage and for added
warnings and precautions. This is particularly important when the
recommended agent is a new or infrequently employed drug.
Some drugs and medical devices presented in this publication have
Food and Drug Administration (FDA) clearance for limited use in restricted research settings. It is the responsibility of the health care
provider to ascertain the FDA status of each drug or device planned
for use in their clinical practice.

9 8 7 6 5 4 3 2 1

This book is dedicated to all of our undergraduate
nursing students, whose diverse thinking styles
and abilities constantly inspire us.

Contributor to Chapter 12

Barbara G. Walton, RN, MS, CCRN
President, CEO
Nurse Notes Inc.
Milan, Michigan

Reviewer

Gail Keenan, RN, PhD
Assistant Professor
University of Michigan School of Nursing
Ann Arbor, Michigan

Foreword

I began my teaching career 30 years ago as an instructor in a foundations of nursing practice course. We spent a lot of time in the lab teaching skills. Most of the skills were physician-delegated assessment and treatment procedures. Doing a complete physical assessment was taught as well as doing many procedures—giving medications, trach care, chest tube care, IV therapy, and so on. Although we did introduce the nursing process and had students write long care plans for particular patients, there was a lack of emphasis on decision making. Nurses collected physical and other data mostly to pass on to the physician, and they did procedures when they were directed to do so by the physician. Teaching foundations at that time was easier than it is today because the role of the nurse was limited.

However, as a nurse and instructor, I was frustrated by the limitations imposed on the nurse, and I wished that nurses were able to do more and get more credit for what they could do. The wish is coming true. I remember the first time I heard someone talk about making a nursing diagnosis at a continuing education conference sometime in the mid-70s. Hearing about the concept of a nursing diagnosis was a liberating experience for me—for the first time in my nursing career I understood that nursing had something unique to contribute to patient care. I don't want to overstate it, but prior to this I felt there was a good deal of confusion in the profession about what nursing was and what a nurse did (other than assist the physician). It was like being in a dark tunnel; the light that came with nursing diagnosis and its components of autonomy and accountability provided some direction for the way out. The last three decades have been an exciting time for nursing, with the nurse's role expanding rapidly. Nurses are now accountable health professionals who make diagnoses and deliver interventions, both independently and collaboratively. We have not yet achieved full participation in the health care policy-making arena, but we are getting closer. This goal will be reached when we have data that demonstrate our worth; the data will be based on the documentation of care delivered by thinking nurses.

Critical Thinking in Nursing provides a good beginning for nurses who must learn how to do and how to think in today's complex health care world. It takes the new student through the incredibly complicated and confusing maze of thinking about what a nurse does. At each stage of the nursing process the authors help the novice nurse to focus on the judgments that need to be made. The writing is clear, yet the text is sophisticated and comprehensive, referencing and including the learnings of related works. When there are confusions within the profession, these are acknowledged and dealt with as best as possible. The authors use several learning devices—the THINK Inventory, case studies, action learning assignments—that require the student to get involved, and yes, do some critical thinking.

Critical thinking in nursing is about making good clinical judgments. What are the patient's diagnoses? What are the desired outcomes? What interventions should be used to achieve the outcomes? Were the outcomes achieved? A nurse's judgments or decisions in the areas of diagnoses, interventions, and outcomes are documented using standardized language (NANDA diagnoses, NIC interventions, NOC outcomes). When we use standardized language to document our care decisions, then we can aggregate data across similar patients and study both the cost and the effectiveness of nursing care.

Having data to demonstrate our worth is very important if nurses are to be included in the various health care policy-making arenas. This book, which teaches a new nurse how to make decisions, is complementary to the work on nursing classification that began with the NANDA work in the 1970s. My own work has been as the Principal Investigator of a large research team at the University of Iowa to develop a comprehensive classification of treatments that nurses perform. The research to develop the Nursing Interventions Classification (NIC) began in 1987, with the first edition published in 1992 and the second in 1996. NIC includes all interventions that all nurses do, no matter the specialty or setting. It is now being used in many educational and practice settings to communicate the treatments nurses perform. I have also been a consultant to another research team at Iowa that has developed a classification of patient outcomes sensitive to nursing interventions. The Nursing Outcomes Classification (NOC), published in 1997, completes the trilogy of comprehensive classifications needed to document a patient encounter. *Critical Thinking in Nursing* discusses the NANDA, NIC, and NOC classifications; the authors help the new nurse understand how critical thinking leads to decisions about diagnoses, interventions, and outcomes and documentation of these decisions with the languages of NANDA, NIC, and NOC.

Although much work remains to be done to define the practice base of nursing, much has been accomplished and the light at the end of the tunnel is becoming clearer. Those who are entering the profession today will continue to define the nursing role and the nurse's impact on the quality of patient care. This book will help you find your way and help you add to the collective knowledge base of nursing.

Joanne Comi McCloskey
Distinguished Professor
Director, Center for Nursing Classification
College of Nursing
The University of Iowa

Foreword to the First Edition

Like two gardeners who planted seeds long ago, we continue to smile with pleasure as we observe the growth and development of ideas about the *nursing process*!

Our work on the *nursing process* began in 1965. We produced the first edition of *The Nursing Process* in 1967, which culminated in four subsequent editions. The framework for the intellectual, interpersonal, and technical skills that are required for its use had been established. Many of the ideas that were presented to the listening professional public 30 years ago have been elaborated by Rubenfeld and Scheffer. With an emphasis on critical thinking, they have taken the framework of the *nursing process* including the three types of skills and have developed all of them explicitly for the nurse and for the consumer of nursing and health care. They have advanced the thinking and doing dimensions of the *nursing process* and have specified the way the consumer can experience "Great Nursing." Since the mid-60s, there have been dialogues, seminars, classes, formal, and informal discussions, as well as oral and written reactions, reports and responses to ideas about the *nursing process*. In the decade of the 70s, more intensive work about *nursing diagnosis* began. The 80s saw the incorporation of the *nursing process, nursing diagnosis* and *nursing theory* into daily practice. As the end of the 20th century draws near, it is obvious that the armamentarium of the nurse is more adequate than it was 30 years ago, mainly because the *nursing process* has been clearly identified and accepted as the system that defines and encompasses *nursing.*

As nursing nears the end of the third decade of relying on the *nursing process*, it is with sheer delight that we witness this production by Rubenfeld and Scheffer. They have taken the planted seed of the *nursing process* and have nurtured the growth and development of this significant idea in a way that makes the two original gardeners very proud. The focus on critical thinking places the appropriate emphasis on the *nursing process* and enablees the use of intellectual, interpersonal, and technical skills to succeed in nursing.

Rubenfeld and Scheffer have described effectively how nursing has grown and developed over the past three decades. The *nursing process* continues in its traditional form with expansion of its components according to the expertise of the nurse. The use of *nursing diagnosis* has grown and developed, and its application in patient care poses a significant challenge to the nurse who strives for accuracy in defining the patient's needs. Finally, learners are encouraged to select and/or translate theoretical concepts to enable more effective use of the *nursing process* when providing nursing care. Throughout the learning activities of the nurse, the focus of the text is on thinking. Not only will the beginning student benefit from the content and experiences designed in the text, but the experienced nurses who may need to refine their thinking and recapture lost aspects in their practice of the *nursing process* will benefit as well. Most of all, the thinking and doing aspects of the *nursing process* will benefit the consumer of the *nursing proceses*. The text clearly shows to the consumers and their families and significant others, that great nursing is possible, desirable, and should be demanded.

Having been associated with the *nursing process* in a number of ways, over the years, this production about critical thinking by Rubenfeld and Scheffer provokes a warm, enthusiastic, excited feeling as one reads the presentations. It is a very user-friendly and learner-focused book. In no way does it "speak down" to the reader or to the learner. On the contrary, it seems to hit the level of learner for which it was meant—beginning students. The examples throughout the text are not only interesting but are so well-suited to the context of the *nursing process* and the point the authors wish to achieve that readers will have the "aha" reaction.

The authors have managed to do in this text what all teachers of nursing try to do in planning and implementing learning experiences for nursing students—build on what the student brings to the learning experience, personalize the approach to teaching and learning, enhance the self-esteem of the beginning students, and ease into the diversity of ideas and outcomes when applying the *nursing process* with well and ill consumers of nursing.

A picture is worth a thousand words and so is a good example. Consistent with the sound educational principle of moving from simple to complex learning, less complex situations are used in the early part of the book to illustrate critical thinking. The final situation that is presented as a learning opportunity is a more complex one that employs a greater number of critical thinking skills, more detailed challenges, and requirements for greater depth of knowledge.

Kudos are in order for the authors of this text, for several reasons. They present specific patient situations to illustrate how thinking can enable the use of *nursing process* when providing quality patient care. They include the use of mind-catching terms and phrases such as the Thinking-Learning Checks that make the content a realistic and intimate part of each reader/user's repertoire. The authors encourage using record diaries and logs to enhance thinking and learning. The eye-catching sketches and illustrations designed by Mark Steele make the text more meaningful. The use of selected references completes the picture of the nurse caring for and about how patients in any setting through the knowledgable use of the *nursing process*. Throughout the text, students can hear the voice of the built-in mentor urging, supporting, clarifying, and commending them along the way. There are references to a multitude of resources for students that are not overwhelming. There is a positive reinforcement at strategic points along the way, and there is a helpful distinction between independent and interdependent nursing practice throughout the text.

Teachers are always seeking learning materials to enable top-notch learning among students. Conscientious and concerned students maintain a vigilance for new publications that will help them improve their understanding of what is essential for their professional knowledge. A happy and joyful declaration is now being sent to teachers and to students: this is IT! This is the text, the new publication that you have been waiting for! This is the book that will make the *nursing process* an even more meaningful part of your professional life. The authors have designed a nursing text that explicates how and why "the *nursing process* is a dynamic entity of multiple processes within a larger process all working in harmony to achieve *great* nursing care." They show with compelling clarity the significance of the intellectual, interpersonal, and technical skills required to become and to be "the *great nurse.*"

To those of you who have entertained dreams, ambitions, new ideas and creative ways of approaching the usual, or the well-known—here is the answer! Here is a friendly text that guides, directs, chides, and urges the reader and the learner to reach for new heights and to seek new levels of understanding. Beyond nudging the learner, direction and guidance are provided for which the novice is grateful, and the better-informed student is appreciative. Ultimately, both the novice and the better-informed learner will reap the benefits from using this text.

The legal and ethical bases of practice are inherent in all the presentations. They are portrayed as a natural expectation of critical thinking in following the *nursing process* as nursing care is provided. Lawyers, ethicists, physicians, nutritionists, and the varied health care therapists associated with the nurse and consumer can readily see what it takes to achieve great nursing (in contrast to "okay" nursing or "good enough" nursing).

As old-timers in the business of *nursing process,* we have relied heavily on components of this orderly system of nursing for many years. As users of this text peruse its printed pages, it will become evident that Rubenfeld and Scheffer are comfortable and well-acquainted with the *nursing process.* This book is evidence that they are valuable teachers who have respect and concern for the learner, and have a ready grasp of what the nursing students need in order to provide nursing. Their presentation communicates a respect for learners, as well as a warmth and genuine concern for people—whether student, colleague, or patient. Most of all, they exemplify a true belief in the essential nature of the *nursing process* and an understanding of the merits of the *nursing process* in the care of patients.

Helen Yura-Petro
Mary B. Walsh

Preface

This is not a typical textbook. It is an active learning book designed to help beginning students of nursing develop the thinking skills necessary to provide great care. If you, the reader and user of this book, are used to passively reading with no writing implement in your hand, you will find this book to be a change of scene. If you are a margin-scribbler, you will appreciate that there is more than the usual margin space to write as you read.

Content Focus of the Book

This book focuses on critical thinking as it is used with the nursing process. Thinking is conceptualized into five modes, which, collectively, represent the broad definition of critical thinking. The five modes, *Total Recall, Habits, Inquiry, New Ideas and Creativity,* and *Knowing How You Think,* are explored from both a personal and nursing perspective. The readers are helped to build on their existing thinking styles to incorporate the nursing focus.

The nursing process is presented in its traditional four-part format of assessing, planning, implementing, and evaluating, as described by Yura and Walsh (1988). Specific discussions of nursing diagnoses as part of the nursing process follow the guidelines of the North American Nursing Diagnosis Association (NANDA, 1996). To keep the content of this book applicable to the majority of potential users, no specific theoretical framework of nursing is advocated. Although the classic nursing process and nursing diagnosis approaches are usable with any theoretical framework, some users of this book may want to translate specific terminology to their theoretical language for ease of student learning.

Because *Critical Thinking in Nursing* is intended for use by beginning students, most of the nursing situations in early chapters, although "real," are not overly complex. The nursing knowledge needed to understand the situations is commonly learned early in nursing programs. At the same time, as students progress through the book, their knowledge will be increasing; therefore, in the last section of the book, a more complex case study is used as a learning opportunity.

Structure of the Book

Readers will note that there are two forewords in this book. The foreword to the first edition was written by Helen Yura-Petro and Mary Walsh, who conceptualized the nursing process as it is still used today. Their insight and vision almost three decades ago formalized thinking as a key component of the nursing process and provided the foundation for the system of problem solving that underlies professional nursing. The foreword to this second edition was written by Joanne Mc-Closkey, Director of the Center for Nursing Classification, whose work represents the thinking of professional nursing as it moves into a new century. The contributions of these three nursing leaders have been incorporated into this text in a variety of ways to help beginning nursing students appreciate the roots as well as the future of professional nursing.

This book is divided into four parts and 17 chapters. Part I provides an overview of thinking, doing, and the nursing process. Part II povides details of the nursing process, with a focus on the thinking that occurs while using the nursing process. Part III focuses on communicating the thinking and the nursing process. Part IV pulls all of the book's content back together and, using a complex patient situation, applies the thinking concepts.

Although there is a building of content throughout the book, readers who so desire can feel free to study Part IV, or any part before the others. Each person's brain works in unique ways. Learning occurs best when those natural tendencies are not stifled. Each chapter begins with *learning outcomes* that provide direction for the reader. The outcomes can be used as a learning check at the end of each chapter. If the reader can meet those outcomes, then the desired learning has occurred.

This book has a combination of information to read and **Action Learning** exercises to complete. The exercises are numbered consecutively throughout the book. Action Learning exercises provide a way for readers to use several senses as they learn. Multisensory learning increases retention of information because more of the brain's capacity is used.

Following each Action Learning exercise is a discussion section called **Think about this**. . . . The questions and issues raised can be used for class discussions or as a stimulus for additional thinking.

Because of the unique nature of this book, especially when Action Learning exercises are introduced, there are frequent uses of the word "you." In those places the reader is asked to relate what is being said to a personal perspective.

Another learning enhancer is the use of mnemonics. These are phrases or abbreviations that are easy to remember. Mnemonic devices trigger the brain's memory programs and allow a learner to retain large sets of information more easily. An example of mnemonic devices used throughout the book is the world *T.H.I.N.K.*, which represents the five modes of thinking used in nursing.

Each chapter also has periodic **Thinking-Learning Checks.** These are summaries of information presented to that point. Frequent reviews help to check and clarify learning and enhance retention of information. They also give one's brain a chance to sort the new information and plug it into relevant places for future use. They are used more in early chapters where new information is presented. Later chapters that focus on application of previously learned material have fewer Thinking-Learning Checks.

Similar to Thinking-Learning Checks are the **Thinking Logs** at the end of each chapter. These logs are designed for learners to keep a diary of thinking. Specific instructions for each thinking log give directions for what should be included. The reader should not feel held back by the directions, however; if something is discovered about personal thinking, each person should feel free to add it to the log.

At the end of the book, each learner should be able to go back and see how personal thinking has evolved.

Last-Minute Remarks to Users of This Book

It is the authors' intent in this book to help you to recognize your existing thinking skills, to build on your current thinking skills, and to enhance your skills so you can apply them to nursing situations. Throughout all the chapters you will be consistently reading, thinking, and doing to achieve this goal. Grab a pen or pencil, find a comfortable place to study, and begin this exciting journey into your mind and into great nursing.

REFERENCES

North American Nursing Diagnosis Association (1996). *NANDA nursing diagnoses: Definitions and classification 1997–1998*. Philadelphia: NANDA.

Yura, N., & Walsh, M. B. (1988). *The nursing process: Assessing, planning, implementing, evaluating* (5th ed.). Norwalk, CT: Appleton & Lange.

Acknowledgments

Many people have been supportive of our efforts on this project. Professor Mary Walsh's mentorship planted the seeds for this project over two decades ago. We would like to express our gratitude to her and to Helen Yura-Petro, whose work with Walsh was the original inspiration for this book. We want to thank Dr. Joanne McCloskey for her efforts in writing the second foreword to this book and acknowledging it as a contribution for beginning students. We also want to thank Dr. Gail Keenan for her review and guidance in helping to achieve an accurate report of the use of Nursing Interventions Classifications (NIC) and Nursing Outcomes Classifications (NOC). We are grateful to Mark Steele for his ability to capture the quintessential meaning of concepts with his illustrations and for his new illustrations of equal quality in the second edition. We want to extend special thanks to the staff at Lippincott Williams & Wilkins: Susan Keneally, whose caring attention to the project made the work easier; Ilze Rader, Acquisitions Editor; Dale Thuesen, Assistant Editor; and Tom Gibbons, Project Editor. Most of all we thank Donna Hilton, whose vision nurtured the seeds of this project almost a decade ago when the first edition was still just "a great idea." Thanks also to Sasha Gobeski from the EMU Nursing Class of 1999, whose excellent Mind-Map provided the example for Appendix G. Finally, we offer a huge thank you to our families—Rich, Jesse, Tyler, Kenn, Dan and Amanda, who have survived the labors of the second edition and continued to support us.

Contents

Part II
Details of Thinking and the Nursing Process   127

Part III
Communicating Thinking and the Nursing Process   229

11 Written and Verbal Communication of Thinking and Doing   231

12 Consequences of Thinking and Not Thinking When Documenting   261

Part IV
Thinking Through a Complex Patient Situation   285

13 Assessing a Complex Patient Situation   287

Action Learning Exercises

Overview of Thinking, Doing, and the Nursing Process

Thinking

This chapter begins (or continues) your journey of learning about your thinking in nursing. In addition to lots of thinking the journey includes intrigue, fun, and hopefully, some "ahas" along the way. Welcome to this thinking profession—nursing.

Exploring one's thinking may not be an expected part of learning about nursing—a profession that is often associated with lots of "doing" things. However, all of the things that nurses do require high-level thinking; no action is performed without critical thinking.

This chapter, and each succeeding one, will begin with learning outcomes. These short descriptions tell you what you will have accomplished after completing the chapter.

✳ *Learning Outcomes*

After reading and doing the exercises in this chapter, you will be able to:

Draw your thinking cap.

Describe a model of critical thinking in nursing.

Explore obstacles to your thinking.

Identify what makes your thinking unique.

Examine the impact of thinking on learning and the practice of nursing.

Embrace new ways of thinking about your thinking.

⊃Action Learning #1: Draw Your Thinking Cap

Before you read anything, consider how you think right now. Draw a picture of your personal "Thinking Cap." Get something to draw with and be adventurous!

Pretend you have your thinking cap on. Describe in a sentence or two how you *feel* when you are thinking.

Explain your thinking cap drawing to a classmate.

THINK ABOUT THIS ■ Now, why do you **think** you were asked to do these three things at the beginning of the book—draw your personal thinking cap, describe your **feelings** when **thinking**, and explain the picture? Here are some reasons. How do they compare with your reasons?

- Having a picture and written description provides a concrete reminder of how you think today. Periodically, you can return to your drawing and description to see if or when your thinking has changed.
- Some people process and understand information best when they see it. They are visual learners, and drawing pictures helps them process information visually.
- Some people process and understand information best when they hear it. They are auditory learners, and speaking and listening help them process information.
- Processing and understanding information is a key part of thinking.
- How you feel has a strong influence on how you think.
- Feedback from another person can help clarify your thoughts.

WAYS OF THINKING

Based on the above activity with your thinking cap, what conclusion have you drawn about your style of processing information? Are you auditory? Are you visual? Are you both? Are you neither? What does this all mean? It means that people are not alike in the way that they process information, nor are they alike in the way that they think about the information; it is not easy to categorize human processes like thinking into neat boxes.

Thinking is not a static process; it may change daily or even hourly. Because *thinking* is so dynamic (constantly changing) and because all nursing actions require thinking, it is important to understand *thinking* in general. It is also important to figure out one's own unique styles and patterns and to identify what helps one *think* better.

In the 10 minutes before you began reading this text, you might have thought, "Should I read now or watch TV?" "Should I lie on the bed or sit in the chair?" "Should I use a highlighter or just read?" For each of those questions you thought of an answer. How did you think of that answer? Did you recall a teacher telling you that it improves concentration if you sit at a desk? Are you lying on the bed because you always lie on the bed when you study? Did you consider all of your options and think about their pros and cons before choosing your mode of studying?

Each of these options or their combinations required different modes of thinking. You may have relied on past habits or approached the studying situation as a problem to solve. Perhaps you decided to do something new or different such as reading while you pedalled your exercise bicycle and listened to music. Just about everything you do requires some thinking, but not all thinking is the same. If you are like most people, you have not spent lots of time thinking about the different ways of thinking. You may not even think such delving is important. We believe it is important. The better you understand your thinking the easier it is to develop and nurture your thinking in nursing.

A Definition of Critical Thinking in Nursing

Several years ago we decided that critical thinking in nursing needed to be explored. There existed in the literature a few definitions of critical thinking, but very few that specifically defined critical thinking in nursing. In 1997 and 1998, a research study to define critical thinking in nursing was completed. In that study an international panel of nurses was asked several sets of questions to find the essence of critical thinking in nursing (Scheffer & Rubenfeld, in press). That study is described more fully in the last chapter of this book under a discussion on research. The resulting consensus statement is this:

> Critical thinking in nursing is an essential component of professional accountability and quality nursing care. Critical thinkers in nursing exhibit these habits of the mind: confidence, contextual perspective, creativity, flexibility, inquisitiveness, intellectual integrity, intuition, open-mindedness, perseverance, and reflection. Critical thinkers in nursing practice the cognitive skills of analyzing, applying standards, discriminating, information seeking, logical reasoning, predicting, and transforming knowledge.

As you can see, there are many descriptors of the ideal critical thinker in that statement. Learning to develop those characteristics and skills is a challenge for a beginner in nursing—one that you will rise to as you learn about nursing.

A Model of Critical Thinking in Nursing

Before conducting the study that resulted in that definition, we tried to find a way to help beginning-level students learn about critical thinking and consequently we developed the model of critical thinking in nursing that became the underlying theme of this book. The definition presented above, therefore, was not originally a part of this model of critical thinking. Because critical thinking is being studied more and more in nursing, you, the reader, will want to critically study this recent definition and others that you find in your readings.

The nursing critical thinking model for this book grew out of this question: Just what types of thinking make up critical thinking in nursing? Many classifications of thinking can be found in the literature, especially in the field of education. One example is the system used by Costa and colleagues (1985), "The Six Rs"—remembering, repeating, reasoning, reorganizing, relating, and reflecting. Although the six Rs are useful, they do not directly match the thinking that occurs in nursing. We developed descriptions of five modes of thinking that, collectively, represent critical thinking in nursing. The five modes are TOTAL RECALL, HABITS, INQUIRY, NEW IDEAS AND CREATIVITY, and KNOWING HOW YOU THINK (Fig. 1-1). To help you remember the five modes of thinking for nursing in this book, each letter of the word *think* is used to represent a mode (Display 1-1). T.H.I.N.K., therefore, becomes a mnemonic device, a catchy word or phrase to help you remember something important. (Authors' note: mnemonic devices are used several times in this book to enhance the reader's retention of important information. You may recall other mnemonic devices that you have used before, such as the saying that goes with the twelve cranial nerves: "On Old Olympus' Towering Top, A Frog And Groundhog Vaulted A Hedge.")

The best thinkers, and certainly the best nurses, are able to use all of these modes all of the time. The phrase "all of the time" is purposefully used to show that these modes are not used individually so much as in combination with each other. As you will discover, nursing has few aspects that fit into clearly delineated, mutually exclusive categories. T.H.I.N.K. is no exception to that rule. The goal of this book is to help you use all of these modes well. You already use some very well; others probably could use some polish.

FIGURE 1–1   Modes of T.H.I.N.K.

DISPLAY 1–1. **Five Modes of Thinking**

T   =   Total Recall
H   =   Habits
I   =   Inquiry
N   =   New Ideas and Creativity
K   =   Knowing How You Think

Before examining the details of the T.H.I.N.K. model, it may be helpful for you to study the assumptions underlying this approach.

T.H.I.N.K. Assumptions

The first assumption is that thinking, feeling, and doing are all essential components of nursing expertise that work together with synergy. Thinking without doing is an academic exercise in futility. Doing without thinking is downright dangerous. And thinking or doing without feeling is essentially impossible unless you are a Vulcan-like Mr. Spock. Feelings, also known as affective states, have an influence on both thinking and doing and must be considered when examining both thinking and conclusions of thinking. Acknowledging the valuable contributions of all three (thinking, feeling, and doing) is a beginning step toward professional practice.

The second assumption recognizes that although thinking, feeling, and doing are inseparable in real-life nursing practice, they can be artificially separated for discussion in texts and in the classroom. This allows the learner to identify, value, and further develop his or her strengths in thinking, feeling, and doing as they relate to nursing practice.

The third assumption is that nurses and students of nursing are not blank slates; they come to nursing with a variety of thinking skills. The modes that make up critical thinking in nursing, therefore, are not foreign entities; they are the same modes that are used in everyday life. It is the context of using those modes—namely, nursing—that is unique. You will be encouraged throughout this book to look at your current thinking processes and see how they fit with those thinking processes needed in nursing, and also how to enhance them so that they work even better.

The fourth assumption is that enhancing thinking is a deliberate act that can be taught and learned; it does not occur through osmosis. Because this is a textbook on critical thinking, it might stand to reason that we think our readers can learn to enhance their thinking. However, some believe that critical thinking is something you either can or cannot do well—that your ability to think critically is your lot in life and that's that. Years ago, critical thinking was not something that was specifically taught in nursing curricula. Somehow students were expected to just think like nurses after they were given nursing knowledge. Today, however, we realize that teaching that excessive urination is accompanied by the risk of lowered potassium in the body does not necessarily mean that a nurse will look at very pale, dilute urine and question its meaning relative to potassium levels. The ability to question beyond the obvious is a part of critical thinking; one can learn and be taught how to make links among knowledge and practice through such questions. In short, one can learn how to think critically.

The fifth assumption is that most students and nurses find it difficult to describe their thinking skills. Most people are rarely asked to describe *how* they think; usually they are asked *what* they think. The two are not the same. Because we are rarely asked to describe how we think, we do not have an adequate vocabulary to describe those processes. Therefore, any model of critical thinking that starts with valuing the existing thinking abilities of its readers/learners needs a method for learners to describe what they already have.

The sixth assumption is that critical thinking in nursing is a composite of several thinking activities that are linked to the context of the situation in which thinking occurs. It is a complex process that is far from being linear. Although it can be broken apart for study, its components must be "reattached" for optimum use in nursing situations.

It is with this last assumption fresh in your mind that you can now look at the five modes of critical thinking individually.

T.H.I.N.K. Modes

Total Recall (T)

Total recall means remembering facts or remembering where and how to find them when they are needed. Nursing "facts" come from many sources—the content taught in classes, information in books, those things told to the nurse by a patient or significant other, patient data collected through the senses, instruments, and so forth. Some examples of facts include the date the Crimean War ended; normal values for hematocrit; a specific patient's hematocrit; who Florence Nightingale was; the second disassociation constant of maleic acid; a patient's statement, "I'm so tired all the time"; the correct way to don sterile gloves; and so forth. These facts are stored in memory, for either short or long periods of time. Total recall is comparable to having the ingredients and equipment for a cake. Having the ingredients is the first step; there is no cake yet because nothing has been done with the ingredients, but they are a necessary prerequisite.

Total recall also is the ability to access knowledge, with knowledge being something learned and kept in the mind. Each person has a variety of knowledge clusters in his or her mind. Some clusters are very large—these represent things about which a person is very knowledgeable. Other clusters are small. Beginners in nursing have a small cluster of nursing knowledge that rapidly expands during the school years.

How total one's recall is depends on memory. Memory is a complex process. Some people can remember many seemingly isolated facts effortlessly; others struggle. If you are a struggler, don't despair. There are ways to help you remember. Putting facts into patterns is one way. The T.H.I.N.K. mnemonic is an example—a pattern to help you remember the five modes of thinking. Often, however, patterns are not quite so obvious. You have to make or find the patterns in your brain and use them. Look at this set of numbers: 5555068527. Now, look at the same set written this way: (555) 506-8527. As you can see, it is a telephone number. The numbers are easier to remember because there is a familiar pattern to them. Look at another list. See if you can remember this after reading it: car, train, fork, orange, plate, apple, spoon, airplane, cup, banana, bicycle, watermelon. Now look at the same list arranged in a pattern. There are four items in each of three categories.

car	fork	orange
train	plate	apple
airplane	spoon	banana
bicycle	cup	watermelon

The way people receive information also affects their ability to recognize patterns. Test this out with a friend. Create a list of items that you know can be categorized, mix up the items, and read them to a friend to see if he or she can remember them. Then show the friend the written words in the order that you originally read them and see if he or she can remember them. Which way was easier? Could the friend recognize the patterns more quickly when hearing or when seeing? Have the friend do the same for you. Learn how your mind processes information to get it into your memory. The experience will also give you some clues on how to study and learn the mountains of "facts" you need to remember in nursing school.

Another process for remembering is the association of a fact with some experience. Most forty-ish people can remember exactly what they were doing the day President John Kennedy was shot. Other associations may be less dramatic. You may remember something you heard in a lecture because the teacher supported the fact with a funny story. You may remember something else because you had to perform some action to or with it. For example, if someone told you how to use jumper cables to start your car, you might remember it. But you would remember it better if you actually got stuck and had to jump start your car with cables?

⊃ACTION LEARNING #2: Can You Remember?

Answer the following TOTAL RECALL questions:

What is your Social Security number?
What is a normal oral body temperature?
How many days are in September?
What medications would a physician most likely request rapidly during a cardiac arrest?

Where would you look for the normal lab values for red blood cells (RBC)?
How do you memorize long lists such as the 12 cranial nerves?

THINK ABOUT THIS ■ Which of the answers do you know instantly? Which are OK to take the time to look up? How many facts can you memorize? What patterns do you use to increase your memory ability?

Habits (H)

Habits are thinking approaches that are repeated so often they become second nature. They result in accepted ways of doing things that work, save time, or are necessary. People often describe things that they do habitually as "things I do without thinking." It's not that habit actions are done without thought; it's just that the thought processes have become so ingrained that they seem to be, or actually may be, subconscious.

Habits allow one to do things without having to figure out a new method each time. Riding a bicycle and driving a car are habits for people who do them on a regular basis. Have you ever driven several miles and then realized you could not remember what you saw or what streets you passed? Hopefully, you did not cause any accidents as you got from point A to point B with no recollection of the trip. You could do this "mindless" driving because you had already mastered the basic mechanics of driving and could do it without conscious effort. (This *is not* a recommended way of driving a car, but it does demonstrate how habits work.)

Cardiopulmonary resuscitation (CPR) is a very useful habit in nursing. When someone is lying at your feet looking dead, there is no time to come up with a creative way to bring him or her back to life. A quick solution is needed here. Nursing has many other procedures comparable to CPR—the proper way to give an injection, take a temperature, insert a catheter, and many more such activities. When these actions are first learned, they obviously are not yet habits, but as they are used repeatedly, they become second nature; they become habits. You will appreciate how many of these habits will be formed by the time you graduate.

Sometimes habits can be traced back to thinking sources easily. CPR, for example, if practiced repeatedly, can become second nature; however, most nurses can remember their first experience with that process and explain how it became a habit with time.

There are other habits whose thinking roots are not as obvious. These are intuitive processes. Intuition is often described as a "gut level reaction." Polanyi (1964) described a similar phenomenon, which he called "tacit knowing," in which the steps of the discovery cannot be identified. Nurses use expressions such as, "I just had a feeling something was wrong," to describe their thinking that led to their "feeling" in certain situations. Usually these situations are ones with which the nurse is familiar. It is very difficult to put those thought processes into words because they seem to be instantaneous or "thought-less." Intuition, which used to be seen as "unscientific" and invalid, has recently received more attention in nursing. During their research, Benner, Tanner and Chesla (1996) have asked nurses to describe their thoughts, including those that are intuitive. They found that there are specific thought processes at work in intuitive situations and have boldly concluded that reason *requires* intuition.

⊃**ACTION LEARNING #3: Your Personal Habits**

Identify three things in your life that you would call habits.

Describe to a friend or classmate your ability to recognize your intuition and how you use your intuition.

THINK ABOUT THIS ■ How did these things become habits? Why are these activities useful? What is the best way for *you* to develop habits?

Inquiry (I)

Inquiry means examining issues in depth and questioning those that may seem immediately obvious. If you did this level of questioning in a social situation, you would be called "really pushy." It involves digging and questioning everything—especially one's own assumptions in a given situation. It means not taking anything at face value, looking for the less-evident factors, doubting all first impressions, and checking out everything, no matter how seemingly insignificant.

Inquiry is the primary kind of thinking used to reach conclusions. Conclusions can be reached without using inquiry, but conclusions are better (more accurate) if inquiry is used. For example, one day, while sitting at her desk, Sue glanced up at the window and saw that it was wet. Her immediate conclusion was, "It's raining and I won't be able to go to the beach when I'm finished studying." On a closer look, Sue saw that there was no water on the grass, the sun was shining, there were no clouds, and there was a ladder visible on the side of the window. Sue really wanted it to be sunny because she wanted to go to the beach after she finished her studying, so she stopped for a moment to make sure her mind was not playing tricks.

She considered that a lawn sprinkler might be spraying the window. She stood up to look at a different angle (inquire), and there was a window washer on the ladder with a squeegee. Relieved, Sue came to the most accurate conclusion—the windows were being washed.

In this story, Sue used inquiry when she did the following:

- saw something (received information)
- came to an immediate conclusion
- recognized some gaps in her knowledge
- collected additional information to rule in or rule out the first idea (immediate conclusion)
- compared new information to what was already known about situations like this by using past experience
- questioned any biases
- considered one or more alternative conclusions, and
- validated the original or the alternative conclusion with more information

This process of collecting and analyzing information to confirm or to make additional conclusions beyond the obvious ones is the essence of inquiry. Conclusion-making will be discussed in much greater detail in later chapters, but, for this discussion of inquiry, it is important to consider the pitfalls to making accurate conclusions. It is very easy to jump to a conclusion based on insufficient information or on one's own assumptions. It is also tempting to jump to conclusions without inquiry because it is a faster process. Inquiry, especially when it is first being practiced, can be a slow, cumbersome, even a scary process. Take the consideration of missing information, for example. A beginning nurse might need to find a book and look up facts to know that more information is needed. The ability to recognize what is missing and to fill in those gaps is essential to counteract premature conclusion-making and well worth the time.

The ability to self-critique also is essential to inquiry-based conclusions. Everyone has assumptions about all kinds of things. These assumptions may be so ingrained that we are unaware of them. However, most of the time, if we stop and question ourselves, we can see our assumptions. The stopping and questioning must be cultivated; it doesn't just happen. Interactions with other students and nurses, especially those with backgrounds different from one's own, will help in recognizing one's assumptions.

Another questioning part of inquiry is considering consequences, or asking "what if" questions. What will happen if . . . (I do this) (I make this conclusion) (the patient thinks this)? Projecting future actions or reactions helps verify and justify the conclusions one makes.

In this window-washer situation, the final conclusion is probably quite accurate and fairly simple. Obviously, not all situations in nursing are quite this simple. Most situations in nursing practice require inquiry. Sometimes a single validated conclusion emerges; at other times, several conclusions may seem equally valid. In those cases, the nurse needs to repeat the inquiry until the one conclusion that is *most accurate* is found. This sounds very time consuming, and sometimes it is, but in most cases the process occurs in microseconds, especially for experienced nurses. Many textbooks refer to this process when they describe diagnostic reasoning. In Chapters 5 to 8 you will see why this thinking is used for diagnostic reasoning.

Examine this example of a fairly simple nursing situation:

It's 3 AM in the hospital and Ms. Avon, the nurse, sees a patient's overhead room light on.

She walks into the room and says, "Hi, Mr. Trent, I noticed your light on. How are you doing?"

The patient smiles and says, "I'm fine."

The nurse observes that there are wads of used tissues on the floor; the sheets are all twisted; Mr. Trent's eyes are puffy and red.

Inquiry is called for here. The nurse must make a preliminary conclusion about something that is not readily apparent. The patient is smiling and saying nothing is wrong. Would Ms. Avon accept his response and conclude that he is fine? Not if she were using Inquiry. She would have to put several pieces of information together to make some sense out of the situation. She would recognize that there may be no simple answer, but several possible conclusions.

Using inquiry allows Ms. Avon to consider at least the following four conclusions:

• The patient is fine, is normally awake at this hour, and may have been rubbing his eyes because of his allergies.
• The patient is fine but can't sleep because he napped all day because of boredom. His eyes are always red and puffy.
• The patient is not fine but doesn't want to talk about it or bother anyone.
• The patient is not fine but doesn't know how to ask for help.

To say with any degree of certainty that one of these four conclusions is better than the others, the nurse needs to validate her conclusion, to put together as much information as possible, and to ask Mr. Trent directly if he agrees with the final conclusion. (She might say, "Mr. Trent, you said you were fine, but it seems to me you might be upset.") To get the necessary information, the nurse must ask questions and observe reactions and the surroundings. She would need to analyze the information by looking for patterns and determining what was significant. Determining significance is dependent upon the nurse's ability to think about how the information about the patient compares with the nursing knowledge she has learned. For example, she compares the patient's red, puffy eyes with her knowledge about what "normal" eyes look like. This comparison leads her to conclude that red, puffy eyes are significant (relevant) information.

Note that the knowledge (Total Recall thinking) is not enough. A nice, neat package or "answer" to many real world situations cannot always be found in a book. Books help nurses see patterns by providing factual information, such as typical behavior patterns or the appearance of eyes, but the nurse has to put that information together with the information found in each unique situation. Books describe the *usual* ways to interpret information and the *usual* rules, but not everyone or every situation fits into these usual patterns (norms). For example, most people are asleep at 3 AM, but not all; most people's eyes are not red and puffy, but some people's eyes are. You have to use inquiry to collect key information and put the pieces together in meaningful patterns. No books can do this for you. Only your thinking can do the job!

Based on the descriptions of inquiry thus far, how would you judge your present ability to use inquiry on a scale of 0 to 10, with 10 being outstanding? Be sure to write this number down so you can compare it with your inquiry ability at the end of the book.

My ability to use Inquiry on _____ (date)
0‒‒‒1‒‒‒2‒‒‒3‒‒‒4‒‒‒5‒‒‒6‒‒‒7‒‒‒8‒‒‒9‒‒‒10
(poor)   (outstanding)

Compare your answer with that of a classmate. Is there a difference? Talk about the reasons behind each of your decisions and about your inquiry skills.

⊃ACTION LEARNING #4: Inquiry into Bertha's Body

Answer the following questions about Bertha and then compare your answers with those of a classmate. Bertha is a 31-year-old woman who is 5′2″. She recently gained weight and weighs 150 pounds. She is wearing a baggy sweatsuit.

What conclusions are most obvious?

What are your biases about weight? Women? People who wear baggy sweat suits? People named Bertha? Thirty-one-year-old women?

What are some less-obvious possible conclusions?

What information would you need to validate your conclusions?

THINK ABOUT THIS ■ Do you think you thought of all the possible answers to these questions? When you compare your answers with those of a classmate, do you find many differences?

(Authors' note: You will be asked to share your work with a classmate many times. The purpose of this sharing is NOT to see if one of you did better than the other, *but* to start a lifelong process of collaboration with peers. Peer *thinking* is a valuable resource that frequently gets ignored in the nursing profession.)

New Ideas and Creativity (N)

New ideas and creativity comprise a thinking mode that is very special to you. This individualized thinking goes beyond the usual to reconfigure the norm. Like inquiry, this mode allows you to go beyond textbook ideas. Creative thinking is at the opposite end of the spectrum from the HABIT mode. Instead of saying, "This is the way things have always been done," the creative thinker says, "Let's try this new way." Creative thinking is not for the faint-hearted; one must be willing to risk looking foolish occasionally and not fitting the mold. A creative thinker appreciates mistakes for their learning value. (This can be uncomfortable if you have been told all of your life to avoid mistakes.) Chances are, if you are like most people, you have not been encouraged to be creative to the point of being "different from the rest of the crowd"; however, everybody is creative under certain circumstances.

New ideas and creativity are very important in nursing because they are at the root of customized or individualized care. Many things nurses learn have to be mixed, matched, and reworked to fit each unique patient situation. Nursing has many standard approaches to care that save time and generally work well, but they do not work the same way for everyone. Take, for example, Ethel (not her real name), who lived in a nursing home and spent her days wheeling her wheelchair up and down and up and down the same hall. She spoke to no one despite repeated verbal prompting by very caring nurses who knew the importance of communication.

When thinking of communication, most people think of talking to somebody; that is the standard way to encourage people to communicate. So that is what most nurses did, except for Maria (her real name). One day Maria knelt down next to Ethel's wheelchair, gave her a big hug, looked Ethel straight in the eye and, with a big smile, said, "Let's sing." Guess what happened? Ethel sang. Not only could she sing, but she had the voice of an Irish folk singer.

Now what is the thinking lesson in this story? Other nurses knew recipes (standards) for therapeutic communication that they learned in the textbooks. They used them with the best intentions. Standard verbal approaches to therapeutic communication work with most patients. Maria, however, expanded the definition of communication to include singing and touching, thus creating an individualized approach for Ethel that was not in any textbook.

From that point on, Ethel always responded to Maria by smiling. She even gave one- or two-word responses to Maria's questions and, on occasion, sang with the other nurses. One small, creative approach that individualizes care often has a way of mushrooming into bigger and better things.

⊃**ACTION LEARNING #5: Your New Ideas and Creativity**

Describe a situation in which you were creative or had a new idea. (It doesn't have to be related to nursing.)

THINK ABOUT THIS ■ How did you feel when you were creative or had a new idea? How many times a day are you creative? How many times a week? A month? How much energy does it take to be creative? What are some of the dangers of being creative?

Knowing How You Think (K)

Knowing how you think, the last, but not the least, of the T.H.I.N.K. modes, means thinking about one's thinking. Thinking about thinking is called "metacognition," a word composed of the prefix, "meta," which means "among or in the midst of," and "cognition," which means "the process of knowing." If you get in the midst of your process of knowing, you will get to know how you think.

⊃**ACTION LEARNING #6: How You Think**

Write down and explain to someone how you think. Be careful to focus on *how* you think, not what you think.

THINK ABOUT THIS ■ Was this difficult to do? (It is for most people.) Why do you think it is hard to do? One reason why it is difficult is that a special vocabulary of analytical terms is needed to describe HOW one thinks. Typically, few people (except for philosophers and some teachers) routinely learn or use such a vocabulary.

Display 1-2 provides a vocabulary that is useful in describing how one thinks. As you think about your thinking, you may use these words as cues. Ask yourself, for example, what *assumptions* you tend to make, what your *point of view* and *biases* are, and how you *elaborate* on ideas. Think about what *evidence* means to you and how you deal with *contradictions*. Continue in this way until you have considered all the words on the list.

Knowing how you think is not as simple as it may sound. Most of us "just think"; we do not spend a great amount of time pondering how we think. Nursing, however, requires that we be critical thinkers. Part of critical thinking is the constant striving to makes one's thinking better or to "know how you think." Making one's thinking better is impossible if one doesn't know where one is to begin with. One of the ways to identify where you are now and to begin exploring how you think is with the use of self-reflection.

Schon (1983), a well-known educator, wrote what is now a classic work for practitioners who want to be more reflective. He advocated a reflection-in-action approach for professionals, especially those in fields where problems and solutions are not easily found in textbooks. Certainly, nursing fits into what Schon calls the "swampy lowlands," or areas of practice where situations are messy and often not conducive to clear-cut, technical solutions offered by textbooks. The best nurses use this reflective process (knowing how you think) to constantly adapt their thinking to the ever-changing contexts of patient needs and the health care arena.

So, what is a good way to identify your skills in reflection and begin to nurture them? It is often easier to describe something abstract (such as knowing how you think) by linking it to a specific situation, rather than trying to talk about it in general terms (Brookfield, 1987). Reflective nurses take time to think over specific sit-

DISPLAY **1–2. Vocabulary for Thinking About Thinking**

Ambiguous (ambiguity): unclear; having multiple meanings

Assume (assumption): take for granted

Bias: a neutral, negative, or positive inclination

Conclude (conclusion): make a judgment or decision based on reasoning

Contextual (context): situational; environmental; having to do with background

Contradict (contradiction): state an opposing view; deny

Creative (creativity): inventive; bringing into existence

Credible (credibility): worthy of belief or trust

Discriminate (discrimination): to observe differences between; make fine distinctions; discerning

Distinguish: recognize plainly by the senses; to separate and classify

Elaborate (elaboration): expand on

Empathetic (empathy): intellectual identification of oneself with another to increase understanding

Evidence: data that support conclusions

Infer (inference): a strong or weak, justified or unjustified conclusion based on information and assumptions

Interpret (interpretation): explain the meaning of; make understandable

Intuitive (intuition): immediate knowing or learning without conscious use of reasoning

Justify (justification): to show to be just, right, or in accord with reason

Kinesthetic (kinesthesia): having to do with motion; felt through nerves, muscles, tendons, or joints

Logical (logic): using reason; following a sequence of principles of reasoning

Point of view: perspective; one's personal way of looking at the world based on background and experiences

Relevance: importance; significant relationships

Spatial (space): relating to distance within or among things

Validate (validation): to verify; to search for evidence to support a conclusion

uations while they are in those situations and afterward. They mull things over in their minds and try to improve how they think and what they do by focusing on what they thought, felt, and did in that particular situation. They ask themselves questions such as these: "Why did I feel comfortable (or uncomfortable) in that situation?" "How could I have missed that?" "What did I assume and why?" "What would have helped?" "Is the patient's thinking similar to mine?" There are many such questions that change from situation to situation. As more and more situations are reflected upon, the nurse grows in the Knowing How You Think mode.

The following is an example of a nurse who exhibits the Knowing How You Think mode as he describes his thinking style:

I know I have a tendency to jump to conclusions because I need to keep things neat. Not being able to figure out what's going on right away makes me anxious. When I'm anxious I tend to focus on the negative part of things, like not having enough time to do everything, and that adds to my premature conclusion-making. What I do now, because I know that, is to think aloud more when I'm in patient situations. I let them know what I'm thinking so they can validate or correct my conclusions. I also say to myself, do I have evidence to support my inference here? I also don't have a very good memory for specific things like lab values, so I have trouble determining the relevance of those things. Therefore, I always keep reference books handy so I can look things up easily. I used to be afraid to say "I don't know," thinking that I should know everything a patient asks me, but now I take those uncertain opportunities and turn them into learning situations for the patient and me. I say things like, "Well, let's see if we can figure this out together." I also know that I have biases against people who do not take an active role in their care. Thinking out loud with all patients helps me overcome that bias because it puts partnership into the forefront.

For more examples of this kind of expert nursing thinking you may want to check out a book by Benner, Tanner, and Chesla (1996) called *Expertise in Nursing Practice: Caring, Clinical Judgment, and Ethics.* In this book the authors present many direct quotations from nurses as they describe their thinking in the real-life, "swampy lowlands" of nursing.

Thinking in Context

Critical thinking in nursing does not occur in isolation. Nurses work in many kinds of health settings and with many kinds of thinkers (other health care professionals) as well as thinking patients. All of these factors constitute the *context* in which thinking occurs, that is, the circumstances surrounding the situation.

Knowing how you think helps you select the kind of health care setting that maximizes your thinking or helps you find ways to cope with environments that hinder your thinking. If you think best in quiet, structured environments, you may not want to seek a job in a trauma center where noise, confusion, and split-second decisions are the norm.

Knowing how you think can also help as you are working collaboratively with other health care professionals. If, for example, you know that you get intimidated when people are confrontational and direct, you may want to set up a cue for yourself. Such a cue might be to take a deep breath and count to three whenever those situations occur. Or you may want to practice responses such as, "I need some time to think about this; I can't answer you immediately." If you know that you think quickly on your feet and get impatient with those around you who do not, you might want to work on increasing your patience.

One of the most important aspects of knowing how you think has to do with reflecting on how your thinking and the patient's thinking are working together.

Critical thinking in nursing is a partnership process. Patients have their own thinking styles. They have the ultimate control over their health care and have a right to be a part of all decision making relative to their health care. Sometimes there is a natural alliance between the nurse's and the patient's thinking; sometimes there is not. Because nurses can be seen as being in power, some patients are reluctant to share their thinking with nurses. They may hold back, thinking they don't want to be viewed as pushy. The best nurse critical thinkers make sure their patients know their thinking is a valued part of the process. They live by the saying "two heads are better than one." There are situations, however, in which that saying is not true. Two heads actually make things seem "worse" when there is a wide gap between what and how the nurse is thinking and what and how the patient is thinking. It is tempting for a nurse to actually see those situations as "worse," or negative, and consequently take control of the decision-making process. However, that can't be done for many reasons, not the least of which are those related to the moral and ethical nature of professional nursing.

Before reading further, it is time for a quick summary. One of the best ways to learn is to break things into manageable parts and review them periodically before adding more information. Quite a bit of information has been presented in this chapter, so this is a good time for a thinking-learning check.

✔ *Thinking-Learning Check*

You should be able to elaborate on these ideas:
- ✔ Your thinking cap and how it works
- ✔ The T.H.I.N.K. model and its underlying assumptions
- ✔ Details of each part of T.H.I.N.K.: TOTAL RECALL, HABITS, INQUIRY, NEW IDEAS AND CREATIVITY, KNOWING HOW YOU THINK
- ✔ The challenges of describing how you think
- ✔ What it means to think about the context of thinking

OBSTACLES TO HIGH-QUALITY THINKING

Habits and Ruts

One of the biggest obstacles to *thinking* is getting into a rut, and the most common way of getting into a rut is to overuse the HABIT mode. Novices do not have many nursing habits, but they develop them quickly. Habits provide security and comfort, so they have definite value. Nurses need habits. Beginning nurses need to follow recipes at first to provide safe, basic nursing care; otherwise they are a menace to patients.

Problems occur, however, when nurses stop *thinking* after they have developed some comfortable, secure, and safe habits of patient care. Habits not only feel good, they discourage the use of inquiry and new ideas. One needs to be a risk-taker to *think* beyond habits. How would you rate yourself in the risk-taking area? (Authors' note: risk-taking here is not the bungee-jumping sort; rather, it is being willing to question what one reads and hears, even if it comes from "authority." Questioning expands one's awareness and solidifies new knowledge. One risk of questioning is that it can be interpreted as defiance. Defiance is focused on the power of authority figures rather than on the information being imparted by those sources. Focusing on the issues instead of the source of information decreases the risk of misinterpretation.)

Nurses care for patients who do not fit the textbook recipe as closely as books say they will. When that happens, it is necessary to use other modes of thinking to find alternative explanations and creative interventions. This is called individualization. Imagine yourself as the patient. You would not want a nurse who approaches you only with habits and recipes, and presumes you are exactly like everybody else in the book.

Anxiety

The second-largest obstacle to high-quality thinking is anxiety. Increased anxiety turns down the burner on *thinking* and severely limits the I, N, and K modes. When starting a new field of study as you have, one of the strongest feelings you experience is high-level anxiety. Everything is new—new words, new experiences, new language, new books, new pressures. Nursing as a new experience is probably scarier than other new experiences because nurses deal with life and illness situations. Anxiety decreases one's thinking abilities, even about simple things, like talking. Imagine what it does to higher-order thinking, like learning and problem solving. Learning and problem solving comprise 90% of a nurse's thinking, so it is worthwhile to find ways to decrease anxiety so that you can think more efficiently.

Some techniques that work for students to decrease their anxiety in clinical learning situations are these:

1. Be sure you are well-prepared for clinical assignments. That is, think about what knowledge you might need ahead of time and find resources to increase your knowledge.
2. Request that your instructor ask questions about rationales or procedures either before or after you have done the procedure (e.g., injections). This allows you to focus all your thinking on the new psychomotor task without interruptions.
3. Consciously slow down your breathing.
4. Allow yourself to think aloud. It is sometimes easier to do this unselfconsciously if you start by saying, "I'm thinking out loud here, so, remember, these are not concrete ideas. . . ."
5. Remind yourself that you are a learner and are not expected to have all the answers. In other words, do not fear making mistakes. If you blunder, say to yourself and/or others, "Well, I learned something there."

THINGS THAT MAKE YOUR THINKING UNIQUE

Each of you is unique and special. Each of you brings different types of intelligences, different feelings, different backgrounds, and different ideas to thinking. Below are just a few key factors that make your thinking unique.

Your Gifts of Multiple Intelligences

Intelligence has been studied over the years from many perspectives. Some researchers believe that a person's intellectual abilities are genetically set in stone at conception. Others believe that one's intellect can be modified, enhanced, or inhibited by one's environment. This has been called the great "nature vs. nurture" debate about the intellectual abilities of human beings. A prominent educator from Harvard, Howard Gardner, has taken a much more creative approach to studying human intellect. He not only believes that intelligence is a combination of nature and nurture, he also has proposed that we have "multiple intelligences" (Gardner, 1983). Display 1-3 lists and briefly describes each of Gardner's Multiple Intelligences. His original work included seven intelligences, but he recently added the eighth one: nature/ecological (Checkley, 1997).

   According to Gardner, we all have all of these intelligences in different proportions. He believes we not only have some personal preferences for one or more, but also that different societies and cultures place different values on each one.

DISPLAY **1–3.   Gardner's Multiple Intelligences**

Visual/Spatial: the mind's eye; preference for use of images, pictures, graphical representations

Logical/Mathematical: use of an entire range of reasoning skills, preference for factual data, and both inductive and deductive reasoning

Verbal/Linguistic: embracing speaking and listening, reading, writing, and other forms of communication

Musical/Rhythmic: patterned rhythms of the mind, learning and knowing by sharing, expressing, perceiving, and creating pitch and patterns

Bodily/Kinesthetic: using the body as a conduit for the mind, using action and motion

Interpersonal/Social: using the give and take of communication with intonation and punctuation with a goal of understanding, empathy, and learning from one another

Intrapersonal/Introspective: focusing on knowing self with a goal of internalizing learning through thoughtful connections and transformation of knowledge into meaning

Nature/Ecological: the ability to recognize and differentiate characteristics and phenomena of the plant and animal world as well as inorganic material

⟲**ACTION LEARNING #7: Exploring Multiple Intelligences**

As you refer to Display 1-3, answer the following questions:

1. Which of the eight intelligences do you believe are your strengths?

2. Which of the eight intelligences do you think is most highly valued by Western European cultures? Asian-Pacific cultures? Native American cultures? African-American cultures?

3. Which of the eight intelligences do you think are most important in nursing?

4. Which of your intelligences would you like to enhance? What could you do to achieve this?

Your Other Gifts That Make
Your Thinking Unique

In addition to your multiple intelligences, several other factors are unique to you. Some can be easily modified; others are just part of your personality or the way you approach the world. As you read about these factors, think about how they fit with you and think about other characteristics of yourself and your thinking that are not identified here.

Consistency

In the ideal world, nurses would switch on their *thinking* skills, turn up the power to high, and always (consistently) be great thinkers. In the real world, however, many things interfere with consistent thinking. Food, beverages, room temperature, lighting, clothing, energy levels, sleep deprivation, illness, and many other factors create thinking peaks and valleys. Timing also affects consistency. Sometimes thinkers are "sharp as a tack"; other times they are "dense as a fog." It is important to recognize the inconsistencies in your thinking, be aware of what helps and what hinders you, and maximize your best thinking times.

Organization

Would you describe your thinking as neatly ordered or organized chaos? What one person believes to be organized may seem disorganized to another person. The important thing is to find the organizational patterns that work best for you. Some people need lists; others need sticky notes pasted everywhere; still others just store things mentally. Identify your style and work to improve it for you.

Feelings

Feelings, or emotions, are usually identified in one word: mad, sad, glad, happy, frustrated, confused, angry, elated, scared, anxious, and so forth. Feelings are a part of life; they cannot and should not be ignored. But you can learn to recognize them. You can realize how they affect your thinking and develop ways to modify the circumstances that contribute to the feelings.

Experience

How much experience (a combination of knowledge, understanding, and active participation) do you have? Your experience in nursing may be minimal, but you have had life experiences in which you interacted with individuals, families, and groups. Life experience is a valuable asset in learning nursing. For each life event, coping skills are developed that can be shared with others. Experience in nursing is a key ingredient in moving from a beginner to an expert. The combination of your unique life experience and nursing experience gives you your individual style as you practice the art of nursing.

Self-Perception of Intelligence

Do you think you are smart or of average intelligence? Do you catch on to things quickly or do you mull them over? When you make statements, do they tend to be sure things or do you leave yourself open for other possible answers? Are you a fast or a more meditative thinker? Do you get personal or outside affirmation when you think, or are you put down for not conforming? Answers to these questions indicate how you feel about your cognitive abilities. In general, with the exception of close-minded egotists, the brighter you think you are, the better you use all your *thinking* modes, and the more willing you are to grow in your thinking. It is very important for you to value your abilities, no matter how different they are from those of someone else.

CLOSING COMMENTS

Hopefully, you now have an appreciation for the complexities and challenges of *thinking*. This chapter has addressed some everyday situations and some nursing situations in which the various modes of thinking were used. The purpose of this was to show you how your existing thinking skills can be further developed and used in nursing. Everything nurses do requires one or a combination of the five modes of thinking.

The exercises in this chapter and throughout the book will help you see how you can use all of T.H.I.N.K., not just the "T" and the "H." To nurture your growing awareness of your thinking styles and abilities, you will be talking and writing about your thinking on a regular basis throughout this book (and, we hope, for the rest of your life). At the end of each chapter, you will be writing in your personal "Thinking Log," which is a sort of diary about thinking. It is best to get a notebook that you use just for thinking logs (Fig. 1-2).

FIGURE 1–2   Thinking log.

T.H.I.N.K. Inventory

This inventory provides a brief assessment of existing skills, beliefs, and attitudes in each of the five modes identified in the T.H.I.N.K. model. You might want to re-assess yourself at different times to reinforce growth in your thinking.

TOTAL RECALL (T)

1. On a scale of 1–10, with 10 being the highest, how would you describe your memory?
2. What do you do to move information from your short-term memory to your long-term memory?
3. Do you remember isolated facts easily, or do you search for patterns so you can store information in your brain more easily?
4. What are your five primary sources for finding accurate information?
5. What techniques do you use to remember important information? For exams? For nursing practice? For fun?
6. Is it easier to think about information after you hear it or after you see it, or both?

HABITS (H)

1. How long does it take for you to develop a habit?
2. What are some of your most useful habits?
3. How can you tell when habits are no longer useful?
4. On a scale of 1–10, with 10 being the highest, how important are habits in your daily life? In school? In nursing practice?
5. On a scale of 1–10, with 10 being the highest, how would you rank your intuition skills as they relate to your personal life? To your work life? To your nursing practice?
6. On a scale of 1–10, with 10 being the highest, how do you value your intuition?

INQUIRY (I)

1. Do you tend to accept what you are told by authorities or do you question most things you hear or read?
2. Do you like to examine the reasons behind answers or do you like to be told the "correct" answer?
3. How important is it for you to maintain the "status quo" and not disrupt things that run smoothly?
4. How do you decide when you have enough information to draw a conclusion?
5. How do you decide what information may be missing from a problem you want to solve?
6. How do you deal with ideas that conflict with yours?
7. Are you comfortable with ambiguity or do you prefer situations to have one "right" answer?
8. How good are you at predicting both positive and negative consequences of your decisions/actions? The decisions/actions of others?

9. What are your assumptions (about cultures, health, illness, time, eating, exercise, economic status, education, etc.) and how do they affect the questions you ask? The questions you don't ask? The conclusions you develop?
10. Do you prefer to solve problems in a logical, sequential fashion, in a random, inspirational way, or in some combination of both?
11. Do you like to think about things for a long time before coming to a conclusion or do you like to come to conclusions quickly and save time?
12. Are you comfortable with debate on issues or do you prefer that everyone is in agreement?

NEW IDEAS AND CREATIVITY (N)

1. On a scale of 1–10, with 10 being the highest, how do you rank your creativity?
2. What kinds of things do you do that are creative, but are not traditionally considered to be artistic, musical, etc.?
3. How do you feel about being different?
4. If something doesn't work out as planned, do you give up, see it as an opportunity to be creative, or see yourself as somewhere in between these two extremes?
5. If you had to choose between living with lots of change going on or living with no change, which would you choose?
6. Do you tend to see things pretty much the way most people do or are your interpretations often different from those of the crowd?

KNOWING HOW YOU THINK (K)

By answering the questions under the T.H.I.N. modes, you have already answered many K questions. (Each of those questions asked you to think about your thinking.) Here are a few additional K questions.

1. What happens to your thinking when you are anxious and what makes you anxious?
2. What happens to your thinking when you are experiencing other emotions such as love, hate, loneliness, frustration, sorrow, ecstasy, etc.?
3. Are you comfortable thinking aloud or do you wait to say something when you have your ideas firmly in place?
4. What is unique about your thinking?
5. List as many words or phrases as you can that would describe your thinking skills to a group of high school students who are interested in nursing.
6. How often do you go back and rethink something? Are there certain situations that you rethink more than others?
7. What kinds of things prevent you from reflecting on your thinking? What kinds of things help you reflect on your thinking?
8. How easy is it for you to forgive yourself for "wrong" thinking in the past?
9. When you reflect on your thinking, can you recognize where you have made assumptions as opposed to basing your conclusions on facts?
10. How easy is it for you to see yourself through someone else's eyes?
11. Are you comfortable with enhancing your self-reflection by asking others for constructive criticism?

When you do your first thinking log, you will be examining your thinking. On the preceding two pages is a THINK Inventory. Aside from using the inventory in this thinking log, you will want to return to these questions at many points throughout your career as you examine your thinking.

THINKING LOG #1 ➤

Read each question on the THINK Inventory on the preceding two pages. Write out your responses to each question. At the end of the inventory, create a summary paragraph to describe how *you* think. When you write your paragraph, use as many words as you can from the vocabulary list in Display 1-2.

References

Benner, P. (1984). *From novice to expert: Power and excellence in nursing practice*. Menlo Park, CA: Addison-Wesley.

Benner, P. & Tanner, C. (1987). Clinical judgment: How expert nurses use intuition. *American Journal of Nursing, 87*, 23–31.

Benner, P., Tanner, C.A., & Chesla, C.A. (1996). *Expertise in nursing practice: Caring, clinical judgment, and ethics*. New York: Springer Publishing Company.

Checkley, K. (1997). The first seven . . . and the eighth: A conversation with Howard Gardner. *Educational Leadership, 55* (1), 1–13.

Costa, A.L., Hanson, R., Silver, H.F., & Strong, R.W. (1985). Building a repertoire of strategies. In A.L. Costa (Ed.), *Developing minds: A resource book for teaching thinking* (pp. 141–143). Alexandria, VA: Association for Supervision and Curriculum Development.

Gardner, H. (1983). *Frames of mind: The theory of multiple intelligences* (10th Anniversary Ed.). New York: Basic Books.

Polanyi, M. (1964). The logic of tacit inference. In Grene, M. (Ed.). *Knowing and Being: Essays by Michael Polanyi* (pp. 138–158). Chicago: University of Chicago Press.

2

Doing

�֍ *Learning Outcomes*

After reading and doing the activities in this chapter, you will be able to:

Describe what nurses *do*.

Examine the factors that affect *doing*.

Begin to appreciate how *thinking* and *doing* are intertwined.

DOING IN NURSING

Doing and *thinking* are inseparable in great nursing care, but for now, some concentration on the *doing* alone is helpful. Knowing what one is supposed to *do* as a nurse will help clarify *learning how* to do it. Learning the *how* before developing an appreciation of the broader perspective of what nurses *do* promotes a reliance on TOTAL RECALL and HABIT modes of thinking. A learner might mimic the steps while learning *how* to *do* nursing but would not appreciate how each nursing activity fits into the complex picture of great nursing.

If learners know where they are going (what nurses *do*), they will have a better chance of engaging other *thinking* modes (INQUIRY, NEW IDEAS AND CREATIVITY, and KNOWING HOW YOU THINK) along the way. This will lead to better *doing* in the end.

Doing is the outcome of *thinking* in nursing. The last chapter focused on thinking, something that goes on in one's head that cannot be seen. DOING is the part of nursing one can observe, the part that is more easily recognized; people can put labels on it. For example, nurses can be seen giving medication, making a bed, adjusting the intravenous line, teaching the patient how to change a dressing, and so forth. These *doing* activities are seen in real life, on TV, or in the movies, and are described in books. If the major sources of information were TV, movies, or novels, one might think that all nurses were "attractive" women in high heels and tight, short uniforms flirting with "men of medicine" or gossiping all day. There is no thinking and very little real nursing going on in those depictions of what nurses *do*.

Leaving fantasy behind, it is clear that high-quality DOING in real nursing cannot occur without *thinking*. *Thinking* and *doing* are so interrelated that it is almost impossible to separate them. They will be artificially separated in this chapter, however, so that a strong base of *doing* knowledge can be formed to go along with the *thinking* knowledge. At the end of this chapter, both pieces of the inseparable *thinking–doing* core of professional nursing practice are linked, forming a basis for future chapters on the *how* of *doing* great nursing.

Doing is not as simple as giving a medication or taking a blood pressure. Professional nursing encompasses a gamut of *thinking* and *doing* activities. First, there are many things done that are directly related to patient care. This type of *doing* is called *nursing interventions* or *nursing actions*. Second, there are many other things that provide the background for nursing care; these are called *indirect activities*.

Before studying these basic *doing* categories, it is helpful to consider what you know already. One of the underlying assumptions of this book is that learning occurs best when students can build on what they already know. Triggering one's existing brain patterns gives the learner a place to insert new knowledge. Adding to existing patterns often is more efficient than building entirely new ones for each learning area.

⟳ACTION LEARNING #8: What *Do* Nurses *Do*?

Where have you seen nurses? What have they been *doing*? Write a list of several things you know that nurses DO. Share your list with a classmate and discuss any differences in your perceptions of what nurses do.

THINK ABOUT THIS ■ How many things did you list? Do you see any connections among the things that you listed? Any patterns? How do you feel about your chosen profession's many jobs? How does your list compare with that of your classmate?

During the last decade, nurses in practice, education, and research have taken a long, hard look at what nurses do. One result of these efforts was the development of the Nursing Interventions Classification (NIC) by a group of people at the University of Iowa. The NIC is a taxonomy that is dynamic and continuously evolving as new knowledge about nursing practice is discovered through research. (See Appendix B for NIC Taxonomy—Levels 1 and 2.) The word "intervention" is another way of labeling what nurses do. The Iowa group defined a nursing intervention as "any treatment, based upon clinical judgment and knowledge, that a nurse performs to enhance patient/client outcomes" (McCloskey & Bulechek, 1996, p. xvii).

Let's back up a minute and explain what a taxonomy is before describing the nursing interventions in the taxonomy. A taxonomy is a systematically organized list of things. These things are categorized into groups or patterns based on their similarity to each other. You probably have seen a taxonomy in biology class in which all of the different kinds of animals are classified. For example, all vertebrates whose females have milk-secreting glands to feed their offspring are considered mammals.

The things that nurses do can be grouped into categories as well. For example, putting up the side rails on a patient's bed, preventing a suicidal patient from having access to sharp objects, and removing loose throw rugs from a patient's bedroom all fit into the category of safety interventions. The Taxonomy of Nursing Interventions has many such categories of what nurses do. We discuss this taxonomy in greater detail in later chapters.

The Doing List

Display 2-1 contains a list of the types of things that nurses *do*. This list is a basic one and is not all-inclusive. The list is divided into two categories: "doing direct care" and "doing indirect care." Distinguishing between these categories is like distinguishing between the categories of things students do. "Doing direct patient care" is analogous to going to class, studying, reading books, taking tests, and writing papers—that is, day-to-day student activities. The indirect student activities include registering for classes, getting bookshelves and file drawers organized, and creating a working and living situation compatible with the student role.

This *doing* list of direct and indirect nursing care may seem overwhelming at first glance. It takes time, practice, and a lot of *thinking* to master the multiple nursing actions.

Distinction Between Nursing Interventions and Nursing Activities

A nursing intervention and a nursing activity are not the same thing. A nursing intervention is a term used to label a group of nursing activities. For example, "Bowel Incontinence Care" is an NIC intervention that consists of such activities as washing the perineal area with soap, drying thoroughly after each stool, and monitoring diet and fluid requirements (McCloskey & Bulechek, 1996). Consider nursing activities to be the wheels of a truck that convey a nursing intervention, as shown in Figure 2-1. Nurses do multiple activities to accomplish one or more nursing interventions.

Doing, put together with *thinking*, reveals how these activities fit into nursing situations. Learning skills such as how to use a sphygmomanometer to take blood pressure readings, how to prevent a patient from getting bed sores, and how to

DISPLAY 2–1.   The Basic "Doing" List of Nursing Activity Categories

DOING DIRECT PATIENT CARE

Assisting: Helping patients do for themselves.

Caring: Conveying, through verbal and nonverbal behaviors, nurturing, supportive feelings for patients and significant others.

Care-taking: Doing things for patients and their significant others that they cannot do for themselves.

Counseling: Helping patients and significant others to cope more effectively with situations.

Data collecting: Gathering information about the patient.

Teaching: Providing information so that patients and significant others can understand or carry out activities.

Implementing physician orders: Doing activities ordered by the physician as part of the medical plan of care.

Monitoring: Keeping track of relevant information about the patient and the patient's situation.

Referring: Connecting patients and significant others with helpful resources.

DOING INDIRECT PATIENT CARE

Advocating: Being the patient's "agent," looking out for his or her rights.

Collaborating: Working with other health care professionals and significant others to provide care.

Consulting: Giving professional or expert advice.

Data collection: Gathering information about the environment around the patient and how he or she is interacting with it.

Documenting: Writing down important information about the patient.

Educating self: Being a lifelong learner (even after nursing school).

Managing: Organizing and coordinating the care of several patients at once and supervising other health care workers.

Research, using and doing: Applying new knowledge developed through systematic study, identifying areas of nursing that need further study, and participating in research studies. (This sounds like heavy-duty stuff, but it can be fun and exciting.)

FIGURE 2–1   The things nurses do.

help patients cope with stress, loss, and grief, provides the content for *doing*. *Thinking* allows the nurse to know when such skills should be implemented and how those activities should be tailored to specific patient situations.

To continue your learning about nursing interventions, complete the following Action Learning activity.

⊃ACTION LEARNING #9: Exploring the NIC

Refer to Appendix B at the back of this text. Choose one intervention (Level 3) for each of the classes (Level 2) that you would like to learn more about or are curious about. Find a nursing textbook (or use the NIC book if you have access to it) and look up at least four of those interventions to see what types of activities a nurse would do for each intervention.

THINK ABOUT THIS ■ Did you see any overlap of activities among the four interventions you studied? Why did you choose the interventions you chose? Have you had opportunities to implement such interventions in your nursing career yet? Can you visualize yourself as an expert nurse doing the activities listed in those interventions?

Using the *Doing* List

To discover how this *doing* fits into a real patient situation, read the following situation and the exploration of how nursing care includes all of the *doing* list.

> Mr. Adams cannot dress or bathe himself. He is hospitalized and partially paralyzed after a stroke.

A nurse in this situation might find it helpful to examine the taxonomic structure of the NIC to assist with the identification of applicable interventions. It is premature, in this chapter, to outline the specific parts of the process that are needed to make the decisions for choosing interventions; we will discuss those in greater detail later. For now, consider that the nurse is trying to determine what interventions she will use with Mr. Adams. One method that she may pursue is to review the domains and classes of the NIC taxonomy to identify the categories of nursing interventions that apply. Once the classes of interest have been established, the nurse can examine and select the interventions with the respective activity sets that will be used. For example, a class applicable to Mr. Adams is "Self Care Facilitation," with "Bathing" and "Dressing" being two of the interventions likely to be selected. The nurse will then select the specific activities that will be performed for these interventions, using the activity lists for the interventions.

Now, look at the *doing* list again and think about each item on it as you read a summary of what the nurse did in the situation with Mr. Adams. Obviously, **caring** and **care-taking** apply here. It is likely that a nurse would be **teaching** Mr. Adams adaptive ways to bathe himself. His physician would have ordered treatments and medications that the nurse would **implement**. In a hospital setting, nursing assistants often work with the nurse, so **managing** the part of care performed by assistants also would be part of the nurse's duties.

Although there is no information on Mr. Adams's emotional state, one could assume that he and his significant others might need some **counseling** to help them cope. This *thinking* assumption would be made based on knowledge about situational crises like strokes and how they cause stress. If the patient is to return to a healthy state, he and his significant others must cope with the stress. The nurse would need to find out how much stress this illness has precipitated. This is a good example of what was mentioned earlier; one cannot avoid *thinking* if one wants to *do* great nursing.

There will be many health care providers involved in Mr. Adams's care with whom the nurse will **collaborate** (eg, other nurses; physicians; physical, occupational, and speech therapists; social workers; chaplains; and dietitians). Such people might automatically be part of the treatment team or, if Mr. Adams's needs exceed the nurse's ability to intervene, the nurse might **refer** him to another health care provider, such as a home health nurse or counselor.

Often, nurses have the most consistent and frequent contact with patients and their significant others. Nurses are the key people to **monitor** the patient's status and note any changes in that status. The nurse frequently is the **advocate** for the patient and significant others when their needs and the workings of the health care system are not aligned. Because nurses know the patient and the system, they use **management** skills to get everything to flow as smoothly as possible.

All patient situations require **data collection**; that is how nurses know what is going on and when changes occur with the patient. Nurses need to **document** data, plans of care, and results of care. Proper **documentation** is not only good patient care, it is required by laws and institutional policies.

Every patient situation that involves a nurse is a potential **research** situation. Nurses stay abreast of the literature, reading the latest **research** findings and thinking about how those findings could be applied to care. Practicing nurses also are in the best position to identify gaps in the nursing knowledge base and incite **research** projects.

Related to research is the need to **educate oneself**. Nursing and health care are changing rapidly. The primary ways to keep up on the changes are to read professional literature, go to conferences, and talk to knowledgeable people.

The preceding paragraphs have shown how most of the items on the *doing* list could be put into practice. Obviously, some items are used more than others, depending on the situation. In the example of Mr. Adams, if he had his stroke recently, the nurse might have to provide most of his care for him. If, however, he had his stroke a few days earlier, more time would be spent in teaching than in care-taking because it is important for patients to regain as much independence as possible. The nurse would teach him new ways to bathe himself to compensate for his paralysis, and would collect information to see how well he could help himself. If he were at home, the nurse might teach his significant others how to help him or how to help him help himself.

A lot of factors must be taken into account as nurses put the *doing* list into practice. Mr. Adams's case illustrates the importance of considering the situation itself. A nurse needs to pay close attention to the patient in relation to where he is, how sick he is, what he wants done, when things need to be done, and many other factors. That attention requires thinking.

✔ *Thinking-Learning Check*

Pause here for a thinking-learning check. You should be able to elaborate on these ideas:

✔ What nurses *do*

✔ The differences between Direct Care Activities and Indirect Care Activities

✔ The differences between Nursing Activities and Nursing Interventions

✔ The Nursing Intervention Classification (NIC) work

✔ Tracking what nurses do in a patient situation

FACTORS AFFECTING DOING

What nurses *do* often is dictated by many things other than what nursing books show as "the nursing actions" for "patient problems." Here is where *thinking* makes a big difference. Nurses have to make decisions about how to *do* things by considering all the circumstances of a patient situation. Each patient is an individual with a personal, subjective reality. That reality is shaped by many things, such as cultural norms, values, developmental phase of life, and other influences. There are no recipes for care that apply to all situations.

Display 2-2 lists factors affecting how nurses *do* nursing. These factors, with examples in parentheses, are not all-inclusive. No one could think of all the possible factors and combinations of factors in any given situation. The items listed are meant to stimulate one's thinking about those issues that could affect *doing*.

The details of the environmental factors and patient factors are studied by students in courses such as psychology, sociology, biology, and the like. The "nurse factors," however, need to be addressed immediately because they are vital to beginning-level *thinking* and *doing*. Find a comfortable place to do some serious *thinking* and reading about the nurse factors.

DISPLAY **2–2.   Factors Affecting Doing**

A. Environmental Factors
   1. Setting (hospital, home, clinic, nursing home, school)
   2. Time (Are there 5 minutes available or 2 hours? Will you see the patient again in 20 minutes or in 1 week?)
   3. Resources (supplies, equipment, money, insurance coverage)
B. Patient Factors
   1. Acuity of illness (intensive care, emergency, routine, chronic, health promotion, and so forth)
   2. Values, beliefs, and expectations about health and health care. ("Take care of me totally," "I'd rather do it myself!," "I'm too nervous to do this now," "Leave me alone")
   3. Developmental stage, cultural, ethnic, and socioeconomic factors, and level of education (infant or adult stage; eye contact is inappropriate in some cultures; immunizations are not believed good by some people; level of literacy limits types of teaching tools)
C. Nurse Factors
   1. Values, beliefs, and expectations (the role of nurses; the roles of family and other health care providers; the role of patients)
   2. Standards, laws, policies, and procedures (what a nurse can or cannot, should or should not do to stay within the law and follow the guidelines of the profession and the agency)
   3. Interdependent and independent role functions (collaborative actions or actions taken solely by nurses)
   4. Level of expertise (how much experience a nurse has had with similar situations)

Values, Beliefs, and Expectations

The first factors affecting *doing* are the values, beliefs, and expectations of the nurse. Those values, beliefs, and expectations are formed from a variety of sources—culture, religion, social situations, and so forth—and become the basis for nurses' assumptions and drive nurses' actions.

First, there are the nurse's beliefs—those things that the nurse accepts as true. If, for example, a nurse believes that all things should be sacrificed for the care of the patient, that nurse will be unlikely to take a dinner break if the unit is busy. If a nurse believes that his or her well-being is important to quality care, that nurse will take the time to eat. Second, there are the nurse's values; if a nurse values efficiency more than patient rights, he or she may tell a patient he has to have his bath at 9 AM, for example, with no exceptions. If nurses value themselves and their roles as health care providers, they will do nursing from a position of perceived strength. Those nurses will be comfortable questioning inaccurate physician orders and being strong advocates for patient rights. Expectations often are formed from beliefs and values. I will expect something if I believe it is possible, and I will make sure it occurs if I value it enough. For example, if the nurse values independence and helping patients learn how to help themselves as opposed to having patients stay dependent on nursing care, that nurse will believe that a patient can care for his colostomy safely and will set up expectations for colostomy self care.

One of the factors that strongly influences nurses as a group is their historical heritage—the profession of nursing primarily has been composed of women. Although there are many men in nursing today, nurses continue to be a largely female group. Therefore when looking at the beliefs, values, and expectations of nurses, one must consider the historical and social context of the profession. Women traditionally have had more subservient roles in many societies; their work has not been valued as much as that of men. Theories about human development and ways of thinking and knowing traditionally have been formed from study groups of men. Fortunately some of that history is being counteracted by researchers and writers such as Carol Gilligan and Mary Field Belenkey and her group, who have studied women's development and their ways of thinking and knowing. These recent revelations have helped us to see that, although women may think differently than men, their styles are not necessarily better or worse, just different. Nursing has become more accepting of its female heritage. Intuition, for example, which traditionally was linked to "women's intuition" and not valued in nursing, currently is actively studied as an important factor in patient care from nurses of both genders.

Nurses as a group and as individuals must practice self-reflection (Knowing How You Think) to determine how their values, beliefs, and expectations affect what they do. As an individual, one must question one's assumptions and ask oneself how those assumptions are affecting one's actions. As a group, nurses must question their assumptions about nursing, health, and health care and ask themselves how these affect what they do and the messages they convey to health care consumers.

⊃ ACTION LEARNING #10: Effect of Values, Beliefs, and Expectations on Nursing Care

Study the following two patient assignments and imagine what, if anything, would be different as you plan care for each of them. Record your perceptions and share them with a classmate.

   You are a rehabilitation nurse. Here are two of your assigned patients for the evening.

PATIENT 1

Dolly, a 63-year-old bartender, was in an automobile accident. She suffered a mangled leg that had to be amputated. She has been very quiet and refuses to wear her prosthetic leg to practice walking. The skin on her back is severely broken down. You have concluded that her Impaired Skin Integrity is related to her immobility.

How do you think you will feel as you plan her care?

PATIENT 2

Monty, a 26-year-old nurse, was in an automobile accident while he was stopped on the side of the road to fix a flat tire. A truck swerved as it came around a corner and hit him and his car. His 3-month-old baby, who was in a car seat, also was injured during the accident and currently is in the hospital. Monty also has an amputated leg because his leg was pinned under the car during the accident. He has tried to use his prosthetic leg, but it has been rubbing on his stump. He has refused to get out of bed for the past 2 days and has two areas of skin breakdown on his back. You have concluded that his Impaired Skin Integrity is related to his immobility.

How do you think you will feel as you plan his care?

THINK ABOUT THIS ■ Because these situations are hypothetical, it is possible that what you *think* you would feel would not be exactly what you *would* feel in real life. Hopefully, however, these similar situations have shown you that you might have very different feelings in different patient situations. Notice that the problems of both patients (Impaired Skin Integrity related to immobility) are identical. The surrounding circumstances, however, could make you feel differently. How do your values, beliefs, and expectations influence how you might feel or act with each patient? Would your values, beliefs, and expectations be obvious to the patient because of what you said or did? Or would your values show only in subtle ways—by what you did not do or say, or even by how you said things?

Standards, Laws, Policies, and Procedures

Standards of Practice are set by state and national nursing organizations. These standards are nursing's assurance to society that a basic level of safe care will be maintained. Statements about what nurses can or cannot do are included in state

Nurse Practice Acts. Those are the laws that govern nursing practice. (Make a note to yourself to get a copy of your state Nurse Practice Act if you don't already have one.) Each institution (agency) also has its own set of policies and procedures that govern what nurses can do while employed at that agency. A full description of such laws, standards, policies, and procedures is beyond the scope of this book. They are taught in several nursing courses. For now, remember that they influence what nurses *do*.

Independent and Interdependent Role Functions

Nursing roles overlap with those of other health care professions, and many nursing activities are done collaboratively with other health care providers. These are called *interdependent nursing actions*. An example of interdependent nursing actions is illustrated by this situation: After finding a patient's blood pressure extremely high, the nurse collaborates with the physician so that the patient's medication may be ordered or adjusted. The physician orders the medication; the nurse gives it and monitors its effects. (Except for some nurses with advanced degrees and certification, such as nurse practitioners and nurse anesthetists, nurses cannot prescribe medications.) A nurse who collaborates with a nutritionist to create an acceptable meal plan for a finicky eater on a new diabetic diet also is performing an interdependent nursing action.

Nurses exercise their *independent* roles when they decide what a patient needs and follow through with nursing interventions. For example, a nurse can decide independently to teach a patient how to use relaxation techniques to counteract anxiety. Or, the nurse can give a back rub to help the patient sleep better. The independent role of the nurse is based on nursing knowledge and nursing judgment, not on medical knowledge or that of another health care specialty. The Iowa project makes a similar distinction between a nurse-initiated treatment and a physician-initiated treatment.

> A nurse-initiated treatment is an intervention initiated by the nurse in response to a nursing diagnosis; an autonomous action based on scientific rationale that is executed to benefit the client in a predicted way related to the nursing diagnosis and projected outcomes. Such actions would include treatments initiated by advanced nurse practitioners.
>
> A physician-initiated treatment is an intervention initiated by a physician in response to a medical diagnosis but carried out by a nurse in response to a "doctor's order." Nurses may also carry out treatments initiated by other providers, such as pharmacists, respiratory therapists or physician assistants. (McCloskey & Bulechek, 1996, p. xvii)

Nurses use independent and interdependent actions constantly. In any situation, a nurse may move between the two several times and do the two simultaneously. Nurses engage their *thinking* skills to decide which one is appropriate at any given point.

Here is an example of the interplay between independent (I) and interdependent (ITD) nursing actions:

> A patient with a history of stroke complains of a bad headache. The nurse takes the patient's blood pressure and discovers that it is 160/100 (Independent action). This is a high reading for most people. The nurse might take any or all of the following actions:
>
> > Retake the blood pressure (I)
> > Observe the patient for other physical changes (I)
> > Ask the patient how he is feeling; note any changes (I)
> > Ask the patient what he was doing immediately before the blood pressure was taken (I)
> > Check the patient's record; compare previous readings to the current reading (I)
> > Check the physician's orders for directions related to blood pressure parameters (ITD)
> > Report the blood pressure and other findings to the physician (ITD)
> > Give treatment as ordered by the physician (ITD)
> > Monitor the effects of medication (ITD)
> > Ask the patient what he understands about high blood pressure and how it affects him (I)
> > Teach the patient relaxation techniques that might help lower blood pressure (I)

Think about how using both independent and interdependent roles helps increase the quality of care. What would be different if the nurse just called the doctor and reported the first blood pressure reading? Would that be wrong? No— but it would be the action of a nurse with low-level thinking. (Incidentally, a non-thinking nurse would simply record the data in the chart and not do anything about it, or worse yet, would not even record it!) The *high-level thinking nurse* (you) uses both independent and interdependent actions, providing great nursing care.

Level of Expertise

Level of expertise also influences what nurses *do*. In some situations, nurses are very familiar with patients' problems because they have dealt with similar problems in the past and thus have more expertise. In other situations it is not readily apparent what should be done. Not surprisingly, beginning students of nursing encounter many more of the latter situations than the former. The scale tips in the direction of expertise when experience is gained by nurses who keep their *thinking* caps on.

Much attention has been given in the last few decades to how novices (beginners) and experts differ in their *thinking* and *doing* (Perry, 1970; Benner, 1984; Belenky, Clinchy, Goldberger, & Tarule, 1986; Dreyfus & Dreyfus, 1986). Beginners are less likely to "know" quickly what is occurring in most patient situations. Some beginners look at experienced nurses and are amazed at how "easily" they know what to do. Obviously, they were not born experts; they also started as novices. Table 2-1 outlines some of the differences between beginners and experts. The table does not address the many stages between beginner and expert; one does not just go from one to the other at some point in time. (For more information on the stages of nursing expertise see Benner, 1984.) This simple set of differences between beginners and experts, however, can be helpful. An understanding of the differences can help beginners speed up their transition to the expert level.

Ways of Gaining Knowledge

Beginners sometimes believe that by finding the right books to read, they will find all the answers to nursing questions and will acquire (gain) all necessary knowledge. This is not true. In the first place, there are not enough books in the universe to answer all the possible questions and give solutions to all of the problems that occur in nursing situations. Second, the answers are always changing; what was the best answer yesterday may not be acceptable today.

Clearly, books do have useful information in them; they show what is "typical" or "standard" in many or most situations, or what a procedure ought to be like under controlled circumstances. What books cannot provide are all the possible exceptions to the "rules" (and there are a lot of exceptions). That is where the *thinking* cap and some study skills help. By reading more than one book on a subject, one gets different points of view. Journal articles usually are more current than books; therefore, it is a good idea to read one or two journals on a regular basis and search in journals for specific topics as they come up. Talking to experts and paying attention to one's own experience and common sense also are very helpful. Each of these strategies helps novices move beyond the beginner stage.

Table 2-1 **Some Differences Between Beginners and Experts**		
	BEGINNERS	**EXPERTS**
Ways of:		
Gaining knowledge	Assigned readings and asking authorities	Multiple written and verbal sources, and experience
Thinking	Dualistic	Relativistic
Using rules	Context free	Situation dependent
Looking at situations	Narrow	Broad

⊃**ACTION LEARNING #11: Moving Beyond a Beginner's Way of Gaining Knowledge**

Spend a couple of minutes and think about food intake. (If you need a snack at this point, feel free to partake!)

Probably 90% to 100% of this book's readers have been on a diet or heard about dieting for the purpose of weight reduction. How many different diets can you list?

Pretend you are assigned to a patient who really wants to lose weight, and you do not have access to a dietitian. How are you going to find the "right" diet for the patient? Can you just go to your textbook and hand it to the patient and say, "Read this and see me in a month"? Of course not, but how will you proceed? Briefly describe what you would do and share your ideas with a classmate.

THINK ABOUT THIS ■ Did you find the "right" diet? What makes you think this will work for this patient? How many sources would you use in addition to your textbook? What do you think is the role of the patient in planning this new diet?

Ways of Thinking

Dualistic thinking, common for beginners, involves seeing things as only "right" or "wrong," "good" or "bad," "red" or "blue." It does not take into account the real world, where things are usually poor, good, better, or best, or shades of purple. Relativistic thinkers see the wide range of "purple" hues that make up the real world. Here is how this works. The dualistic-thinking nurse who sees a 5-foot, 140-pound woman eating cookies might assume that the patient is overweight and should not be eating cookies. The relativistic-thinking nurse might consider that the woman could be pregnant and of normal weight, could be an overweight diabetic who, incidentally, needs to eat something sweet to counteract her hypoglycemic reaction (low blood sugar), or would at least get more information before coming to a conclusion about the merit of this person's cookie-eating behaviors.

Ways of Using Rules

Context-free rules are the "steps in the books." Such steps are methods of acting or doing things without considering the unique circumstances of each patient situation. For example, when first learning how to drive a car, the beginner reads the driving manual, which says, "At a four-way stop, the person to your right gets to go through the stop first." This is a context-free rule. Although this is important to know, a driver has to consider each situation before driving through the intersection. The person to the left might be impatient and start into the intersection even though it is Driver A's right to proceed first.

Driver A's action needs to be adjusted to put safety first. Therefore, the rules must be interpreted in context. The same holds true in nursing.

Here is a nursing example. Basic, context-free rules of discharge planning state: "Provide patient with written information on medications and how to take them at home." This is a good idea because written information can be used if a patient forgets what was said verbally. If that patient is illiterate or has a visual impairment, however, the written material is useless. The rule must therefore be adapted to the context of the individual patient situation.

Ways of Looking at Situations

Remember the old expression, "He can't see the forest for the trees"? (See Fig. 2-2.) Beginners often concentrate so hard on the pieces and details of a situation (the trees) that they are unable to see that there is a bigger picture (the forest and maybe even a forest fire coming over the ridge.) Have you ever focused so hard on building a sand castle at the beach that you didn't notice that the tide was coming in and would soon wipe out your hard work? In nursing, missing the big picture is common for beginners because they have to put so much energy into keeping the details straight. Students giving their first injection often concentrate so hard on their technique and hitting the right spot that they may not see other serious situations—for example, that the patient's intravenous fluid has run out, the bed is wet, and the untouched breakfast tray is still sitting at the bedside at 3 PM.

Does all of this mean that all beginners are doomed to think dualistically, be slaves to context-free rules or victims of narrowmindedness? To some degree these attributes of beginners are unavoidable. Beginners can progress beyond this stage, however, if they engage all *thinking* modes right from the start in their nursing careers. Students of nursing advance their *thinking* and *doing* as they progress through school. At the same time, it also is important to realize that no one is an expert by graduation; nurses get there only after several years of experience. Again, nurses move faster along the path to expert *thinking* and *doing* when they pay attention to *how* they think. *Thinking* in all five modes helps compensate for a beginner's lack of experience. This book is designed to help beginners become increasingly aware of their thinking abilities to accelerate their growth toward expertise.

FIGURE 2–2 Missing the big picture (she can't see the forest for the trees).

✔ *Thinking-Learning Check*

Pause here for another thinking-learning check. You should be able to elaborate on these ideas:

✔ Factors affecting *doing* in the categories of Environmental, Patient, and Nurse Factors

✔ Knowledge of environmental and patient factors comes through experience and courses of study

✔ Early attention to the nurse factors that affect doing can help beginners avoid pitfalls associated with those factors

To pull all of the ideas in this section together, another case study is presented. With it, you may test your learning about *doing* and factors affecting *doing*.

⊃ACTION LEARNING #12: What Is the Nurse *Doing* and What Factors Are Affecting the *Doing*?

Read the following case study.

First, list five things that you think the nurse would do in this situation.

Case Study

Julie Wu, RN, has been assigned to Mr. Antler, who is being discharged to his home today. He was hospitalized for 1 week after having a stroke that partially paralyzed his left side. He has had difficulty dressing and bathing himself. He lives with his wife and two teenage sons. Mr. Antler's insurance coverage provides for nursing care at home for 2 weeks. He is having a great deal of difficulty accepting the changes in his body, tries to do things very quickly, and gets easily frustrated. With reminders, he can move more slowly and is able to stand from a sitting position and maintain his balance. His wife also gets impatient and frequently does things for Mr. Antler rather than waiting for him to do things independently.

Second, list five factors that might affect how the nurse does those five things you listed.

Third, explain why you think each of those factors might be affecting Ms. Wu's doing.

THINK ABOUT THIS ■ How easy or difficult was it to think of what the nurse might do? What modes of thinking did you use to come up with your five things? Of the factors you identified that might influence what Ms. Wu did, are those the same factors that would influence you if you were in her shoes? Of the nurse factors listed on page 36, which ones are particularly relevant to you personally?

INTERTWINING DOING AND THINKING

Remember, this chapter started with a focus on *doing*; however, it has been impossible to discuss *doing* without discussing *thinking* at the same time. Although Julie's *doing* was influenced by environmental factors, patient factors, and nurse factors, her actions were strongly influenced by her *thinking*. It is practically impossible to *do* nursing without *thinking*! The next chapter specifically combines *doing* and *thinking* and shows how their intertwining results in quality care.

THINKING LOG #2 ▶

This time you have an interview assignment. Find a registered nurse and ask him or her if you can have 15 minutes of time. Ask the following questions and record the person's response:

1. What are the major things you *do* during a routine day?
2. What are the things you like to *do* best?
3. What are the things you *do* that are most important to good patient care?
4. How much of your day is spent *thinking*?

Make a list of the things the person tells you and compare it with the *doing* list. Share your findings with a classmate. There may be things described by the nurse that are not on the list; be sure to write those things down and discuss them.

References

Belenky, M.F., Clinchy, B.M., Goldberger, N.R., & Tarule, J.M. (1986). *Women's ways of knowing: The development of self, voice, and mind.* New York: Basic Books.

Benner, P. (1984). *From novice to expert: Power and excellence in nursing practice.* Menlo Park, CA: Addison-Wesley.

Dreyfus, H.L., & Dreyfus, S.E. (1986). *Mind over machine: The power of human intuition and expertise in the era of the computer.* New York: The Free Press.

McCloskey, J.C. & Bulechek, G.M. (Eds.)(1996). *Nursing interventions classification (NIC).* St. Louis: Mosby.

Perry, W.G. (1970). *Forms of intellectual and ethical development in the college years.* New York: Holt, Rinehart & Winston.

Thinking and Doing and the Nursing Process: The "How" of Great Nursing

❋ Learning Outcomes

After reading and doing the activities in this chapter you will be able to:

Explain the "how" of great nursing.

Describe the nursing process.

Place the nursing process in its historical context.

Define the components of the nursing process, and the thinking and doing related to each component.

Explore possible nursing process sequences.

The last two chapters have laid a foundation for the examination of great nursing. A basic understanding of the five modes of *thinking* and the many *doing* aspects of nursing provide a beginning for the journey toward great nursing. Keep your thinking caps on as the journey continues.

AN EQUATION FOR GREAT NURSING

A goal of most nurses is to provide high-quality nursing care, or, as some would like to call it, great nursing. Achieving that goal successfully requires high-quality thinking and high-quality doing. For the beginning nurse, it is helpful to examine a simple equation that briefly illustrates *how* to achieve great nursing.

$$\text{Patient} + \text{You} + \frac{\text{Thinking}}{\text{Skills}} + \text{Knowledge} + \frac{\text{Nursing}}{\text{Process}} = \text{Great Nursing}$$

This is a simple linear equation. Obviously, there are many other factors that influence great nursing. Also, what appears to be a simple series of additions of one component to another turns out to be much more complex in real life. In reality, the components are intermingled in a variety of ways. But, for now, look just at the components of the equation. As the chapters continue, the relationships among the components of this equation will be explored and examined in much greater depth.

Who Is the Patient?

The patient may be a person, a family, a group, or a community. The usual description of nursing care for families, groups, and communities is "nursing care for aggregates."

The identical nursing process is used in all cases. The big difference between using the process with individuals and using it with groups is that nurses need different knowledge to determine what is normal and what is not normal to identify problems accurately, formulate plans, and implement and evaluate care. The following is a list of just a few of the different kinds of information and knowledge needed to apply the nursing process to individuals and aggregates:

For *individuals*:
  What is normal oral body temperature?
  What are typical eating patterns of 2-year-olds?
  What are the effects of chronic illness on a person's self-esteem?
For *families*:
  How do members react when one person is ill?
  What happens to family roles after the first child is born?
  What are healthy family developmental stages for single-parent families?
For *groups*:
  What are the norms of behavior for this group?
  How cohesive is the group?
  How do the leaders of the group affect problem solving?
For *communities*:
  What community resources are focused on immunization clinics?
  What is the frequency of drug and alcohol use among the community's 12- to
    18-year-olds?
  What health concerns are resulting from high concentrations of lead in the
    playground soil?

Much more knowledge is needed to provide effective care of families, groups, and communities. Both required and recommended books in nursing school help supply some of that *information*. This text, however, focuses only on the individual.

Understanding the *thinking* and *doing* and the nursing process *with* individual patients is enough for this stage of learning.

Who Are You?

You are a very special, one-of-a-kind person with a desire to be a great nurse. Your personality (feelings, values, and beliefs) as well as your thinking skills will transform the basic skills acquired from textbooks into your own art of great nursing. This will not happen overnight, and it will not even happen by graduation; but it can happen if you accept the challenge to think consistently using all five thinking modes.

What Are Thinking Skills?

The five thinking modes and the nurse's ability to use all of them effectively comprise thinking skills. This text is designed to continue to nurture and expand the reader's existing skills. Patients also have thinking skills. A major part of nursing's role is to help patients engage their thinking skills, or, more generally, to help patients to help themselves.

What Is Knowledge?

Generally speaking, knowledge is what you know. Knowledge has been described as "aggregates of information" derived from many sources and "synthesized information" that results from the interpretation of facts (Saba & McCormick, 1996). Therefore, having knowledge means that one has taken information and organized it meaningfully in one's mind. The many sources of information in nursing include books, journals, interactions with others, and so forth.

All those heavy nursing books provide a great deal of factual information and knowledge. Those texts include many of the facts and concepts required during nursing school **and** during the remainder of one's professional career. The factual information and knowledge from books and articles includes, for example, how illness affects coping skills; what happens to skin if a person is confined to a wheelchair and is incontinent (without bladder control); and all of the multiple nursing needs of a teenager or elderly person with diabetes.

Other major sources of knowledge include clinical experience and nursing research findings. It is impossible to know everything, and it sometimes is barely possible to keep current with the rapidly changing state of knowledge in health care today, but nurses must try to acquire the best knowledge available.

Organization of information as knowledge is most meaningful when nurses can see the relationships between and among what they "know" and what they see in practice. Knowledge in nursing must be usable. Here is an example of using knowledge in practice:

Case Study

Ivan is a 50-year-old farmer who has been having problems with dizziness for the last 6 months. He is 5'5", weighs 210 pounds, and says that he has never been sick in his life. His vital signs are B/P = 180/95; P = 88; R = 18.

KNOWLEDGE USED IN CASE

1. Height and weight are disproportional for a 50-year-old man. This is relevant when the nurse links it with information about norms for height and weight, probably learned in a nutrition class or from reading a book about nutrition.
2. Blood pressure of 180/95 is above the norm for a 50-year-old man and considered hypertensive. This is relevant when the patient data are linked with information about norms for blood pressure learned in a physiology or nursing class or from a textbook.
3. Dizziness is not normal and, combined with data on blood pressure, could indicate a serious cardiovascular problem. This is relevant when several pieces of information are put together as an aggregate. Most nurses originally learn to make such links of information from classes, texts, or articles about circulation norms or cardiovascular disorders. Later in their careers, nurses also add their experience to help link information and knowledge.

What Is the Nursing Process?

Before we answer that, first consider the definition of the word "process." Process is a way of *doing* something. That something could be organic gardening, fly fishing, cutting hair, practicing medicine, repairing cars, or nursing. The word "process" means moving from one point to another and changing things (hopefully, for the better) along the way. Many processes involve problem solving.

The nursing process, which includes problem solving, is how nursing is done. It is presented in its totality in this chapter; subsequent chapters explore the components and the whole process in greater detail.

What Is Great Nursing?

Great nursing is a concept that is hard to capture in a simple definition. It's the point at which the nurse goes beyond good, safe nursing skills. Great nursing practice focuses on patients as human beings with unique strengths and unique health needs. Great nursing is creative and individualized; it is an art as well as a science.

Great nursing is not some elusive ideal that can only be aspired to and achieved in scholarly dissertations. Great nursing is practiced daily by nurses around the world. The key to practicing great nursing is the effective use of all the components of the equation **and** the nurse's belief that every patient is unique.

⤴**ACTION LEARNING #13: _____'s Definition of Great Nursing. _____**

(insert your name and today's date above)

   Think about how you would describe great nursing. Write out a brief description. Share it with a classmate.

THINK ABOUT THIS ▪ Having a description of great nursing is one of the first steps in becoming a great nurse; it provides direction and a personal goal. Save your ideas and look back to them occasionally. You may find that your ideas change as your *thinking* and learning evolve.

With this preliminary understanding of the basic components of great nursing, it is time to focus on some details of the equation's components, specifically the nursing process. Understanding and effectively applying the nursing process requires constant use of thinking caps.

THE NURSING PROCESS

The intertwining of *thinking* and *doing* in nursing is the nursing process. This process is the essence of professional nursing practice. The nursing process is the means by which nurses identify patients' strengths and responses to health and illness situations, design ways to assist patients in dealing with those situations, implement the needed nursing care, and determine the effectiveness of that care by looking for changes in patient behavior. Again, the nursing process is frequently a problem-solving process.

Translated into everyday language, the nursing process would look like this: A nurse meets a patient and *thinks*, "What does this patient need from me, if anything?" To answer that question, the nurse *thinks* about and collects some information. The nurse *thinks* about what the information means and draws conclusions with the patient about what the patient needs. Next, the nurse *thinks* about and works with the patient to identify the best ways to meet the needs. The nurse performs whatever nursing care is required. After the nurse has helped the patient, the nurse and patient determine whether the patient's needs have been met.

The process that the nurse goes through is similar to that used by car mechanics who must find out what is wrong with a car in order to fix it. It also is similar to the process that many others, such as hairdressers, telephone repair people, social workers, and physicians use. Although the processes are similar for these and other groups of workers, the "focus" of each process varies. For mechanics it is car repair; for physicians it is disease care. For nurses it is nursing care.

This process of determining what is needed and taking care of the needs may seem like common sense because it is practiced in everyday problem solving. Nursing, however, like other disciplines, has refined the basic process specifically for itself.

For many years, nurses have used specific terms to identify parts of the nursing process: *assessing*; *planning*; *implementing*; and *evaluating*. Some authors insert *nursing diagnosis* between assessing and planning for the purpose of highlighting the problem identification portion of the process. This appears to lengthen the overall process and is not really necessary, because diagnosing is an integral part of assessing.

Recently the American Nurses Association, in their Standards of Clinical Nursing Practice (1991), moved to a six-step description of the nursing process, comprising assessment, diagnosis, outcome identification, planning, implementation, and evaluation. The original four-part terminology is used throughout this book for these reasons: (1) assessing is a process of both collecting data and forming a variety of conclusions about the data, including, but not limited to, nursing diagnoses; (2) planning includes both outcome identification and choosing nursing interventions; (3) implementing is the care that is based on that plan; and (4) evaluating means determining the effectiveness of that plan.

It is time to talk about how all this works with real patients. Remember, this text concentrates on *thinking* and *doing* and on the nursing process with individuals, but in reality, families, groups, and communities (aggregates) also are recipients of nursing care. Whether it is with aggregates or with individuals, the focus of care is **with** the patient.

The Role of the Patient

In the preceding paragraph, the word "with" was highlighted. Although at times, nurses do things "for" patients who cannot participate in their care, most of the time nurses work with patients collaboratively. Patients' active participation in the nursing process is a key factor in success because it indicates that patients have active roles in care. Active participation in care nurtures the patient's self-esteem and problem-solving skills. When patients are merely the passive recipients of care (when care is provided "for" or "to" them), they become overly dependent on the nurse and cannot achieve their optimum level of functioning.

Working "with" patients implies teamwork. The nurse asks questions and the patient responds. The patient asks questions and the nurse responds. The nurse uses *thinking* skills and professional judgment and, together, they come to conclusions about the patient's strengths and health concerns.

Remember that togetherness is necessary because both the patient and the nurse are using thinking skills and coming to conclusions. The nurse shares conclusions with the patient and must assure the patient that his/her conclusions are an integral part of the nursing process. The nurse does the nurse *doing* activities (teaching, bathing, changing dressings) and the patient does the patient activities (relaxing, exercising, washing, eating). Both evaluate the results—togetherness is the watchword.

Applying the Nursing Process, Thinking, and Doing

What does this nursing process look like when applied to an individual patient? Read the following example, and try to identify the components of the nursing process as well as the *thinking* and *doing* of the student nurse, Ms. Calli Mooradian.

Ms. Calli Mooradian, SN, is assigned to care for Mr. Steinberg. Mr. Steinberg is confined to bed with no weight-bearing on his legs. Both legs were broken when he was hit by a car 1 week ago. While Ms. Mooradian is helping with his bed bath she observes (**assesses**) a pinkish-red area on his lower back. She **thinks**, "This is not normal. The skin over the lower back should be the same color as the rest of the patient's skin." She next **thinks**, "When skin is pink it could mean: (1) sunburn; (2) a normal color for this patient even though it is not normal for most patients; or (3) the beginning of a pressure sore (decubitus ulcer)."

After asking some questions (**assessing**), she comes to the conclusion that this is the beginning of a pressure sore and makes the nursing diagnosis of:

Impaired Skin Integrity, related to decreased circulation to the lower back secondary to immobility

The evidence to support her nursing diagnosis (a conclusion of assessment) is:

The skin on Mr. Steinberg's lower back is pinkish-red.
This is not normal skin color for this patient's lower back.
This patient has been lying on his back without turning for extended periods of time because he is confined to bed (immobility).
Immobility leads to increased pressure and decreased circulation to areas of the body.
Pressure and decreased circulation promote the development of pressure sores (decubitus ulcers).
Decubitus ulcers are not good.

Ms. Mooradian develops a **plan** of nursing care to increase circulation and mobility, which should allow the skin to return to its usual color. She immediately **implements** (*does*) the plan, which includes explaining to the patient the importance of turning off his back at regular intervals. She writes the plan in the patient's chart so that all nurses can follow it.

At the end of her shift, she checks (**evaluates**) to see whether there is any change in the skin color on Mr. Steinberg's back and whether Mr. Steinberg is turning off his back every 2 hours. When asked, Mr. Steinberg says he has been faithfully turning, and there is less pinkish-red color to the skin of his lower back. She **thinks** there is good evidence to validate that she accurately identified a nursing problem and selected an appropriate intervention. She will continue to monitor Mr. Steinberg's skin for several more days.

⊃**ACTION LEARNING #14: Find the Nursing Care with Mr. Steinberg**

Think about what the nurse did that specifically involved the patient as an active participant in his care. Write your ideas down.

THINK ABOUT THIS ■ It is important, as a beginner, to see how the active participation of the patient moves you closer to great patient care. The two episodes that clearly demonstrated patient involvement were explaining to the patient the need to turn, and asking whether he was turning. What else could Ms. Mooradian have done to increase care **with** Mr. Steinberg?

Do you think that all nurses would have applied the nursing process in the same way that Ms. Mooradian did in this situation? Today, the answer is probably "yes" because such use of the nursing process in caring for patients and their skin has become a standard practice. A brief look at nursing's history shows how and why nursing has come to the point at which patients can expect a consistent approach to care from all nurses.

A BIT OF BACKGROUND: TRACKING THE ROOTS OF THE NURSING PROCESS

For many, the idea of looking back at history conjures up unpleasant recollections of memorizing meaningless dates and events. Others appreciate that there are past patterns and events that have significance for the present; such is the case in nursing history (Fig. 3-1).

There were several historical events significant to the development and understanding of the nursing process. Since the time of Florence Nightingale, nurses have attempted to define and describe what nursing is and what nurses do. This text's discussion, however, goes back only to 1967, when a group of nurses in Washington, DC, met and formally described what nurses do and how they do it. They called this the nursing process.

FIGURE 3–1   Tracking the roots of nursing.

The two leaders of this group, Helen Yura and Mary Walsh, compiled the proceedings of the first efforts of the group (Yura & Walsh, 1967) and went on to write four more editions of a book called *The Nursing Process: Assessing, Planning, Implementing, Evaluating* (Yura & Walsh, 1988). Their work on the nursing process has become the standard for nursing for the last 25 years.

Discussion of or references to the nursing process can be found in all current nursing textbooks. The nursing process has become the underlying approach for nursing's Standards of Practice. (Standards of Practice were introduced in the last chapter, under "Factors Affecting *doing*.")

The terms assessing, planning, implementing, and evaluating describe the traditional parts or components of the nursing process. Assessing is the process used by nurses to draw conclusions about patients' strengths and health concerns. Planning is the development of approaches to meet patient needs. Implementing is the actual care. Evaluating is a determination of the patient outcomes and the quality of the care.

Nursing Diagnoses and the Nursing Process

An important addition to the original nursing process work was the development of nursing diagnoses. Until recently, there was no universal set of labels for most of the conclusions reached through assessment. In the early 1970s, work was started by a group of nurses in St. Louis, Missouri, to define more clearly the problems for which nurses provide care (Gebbie & Lavin, 1975). The set of labels identified by the St. Louis group are collectively called "Nursing Diagnoses." In 1976, the St. Louis group expanded into an international nursing organization called The North American Nursing Diagnosis Association (NANDA). Although the nursing process is firmly established, the work of standardizing the terminology for nursing diagnoses is still in progress, and revisions are made every 2 years. The profession currently has a working document called the "NANDA Nursing Diagnoses: Definitions and Classification" (NANDA, 1996; see Appendix A).

The American Nurses Association's Definition of Nursing and the Nursing Process

Another significant development in nursing that affected the nursing process was the publication in 1980 of a "standard" definition of nursing by the American Nurses Association (ANA). The ANA is one of the major professional organizations for nurses. Its definition of nursing is as follows:

> Nursing is the diagnosis and treatment of human responses to actual or potential health problems (ANA, 1980, p. 9).

The term "human responses" was selected to clarify the difference between caring for the actual illness (typically a disease or medical condition—eg, diabetes), which usually is in the domain of medicine, **and** caring for patients as they deal with those health concerns or illnesses (eg, addressing lack of knowledge about giving insulin). Human responses generally include a patient's physical or emotional *reaction* to a disease, change in health status, or potential for reaching a higher level of health (eg, fear of dying, inability to bathe self, or effective coping). Human responses, therefore, are the situations or conditions that nurses diagnose and for which they plan, implement, and evaluate care.

Nursing Interventions and the Nursing Process

In 1992, a group of nurses in Iowa researched and published a standard set of terminology to describe what nurses do, called the "Nursing Interventions Classification" (NIC) (McCloskey & Bulechek, 1992). This work, like that of the NANDA group, is an attempt to define, with standard language, the realm of nursing care. The "Nursing Interventions Classification" does for implementing what the NANDA Classification does for assessing. Classification work is dynamic and involves updating as new information and knowledge become available. The second edition of the NIC was published in 1996 (McCloskey & Bulechek, 1996), and the work continues in preparation for the third edition.

There are other classification schemes that students of nursing may find in their reading and in various practice arenas, such as the Omaha classification scheme for interventions and the Saba Home Healthcare Classification. It is beyond the scope of this text to describe these in detail; therefore, classifications of interventions mentioned in this text generally refer to the NIC.

Nursing Outcomes and the Nursing Process

Similar to the classifications of nursing diagnoses and interventions, there is now a classification of nursing sensitive patient outcomes (Johnson & Maas, 1997). What nurses have available now is a resource for developing plans that provides standardized language for measuring patient outcomes. This work, called "Nursing Outcomes Classification (NOC)," also started by a group of nurses in Iowa, was begun in the early 1990s and continues to be refined. The first edition of the NOC was published in 1997 (Johnson & Maas, 1997).

Nursing Theories and the Nursing Process

One final historical development that is important to align *thinking* and *doing* with the nursing process is the development of nursing theories. The nursing process is just what it says it is—a process; it is the *how* of nursing. But this process cannot stand alone. It needs to be combined with some framework (theory) of *what* nursing is all about. Nursing theories provide direction as to what information needs to be assessed and what to do with that information. The *how* (assessing, planning, implementing, and evaluating) is always the same, no matter what theory (framework) is used, but theories may vary in their conceptualizations of the *what* of nursing.

To appreciate the difference between a theory (framework) and a process, think about gardening.

Gardening theory A says the best way to grow plants is to:

1. Rub the seeds six times before planting them
2. Water the seeds every 10 days
3. Check for insect damage to leaves

Gardening theory B says the best way to grow plants is to:

1. Be careful not to rub the seeds before planting
2. Water the seeds with fertilizer every other day
3. Play music for the plants to get greener leaves

No matter which theory (framework for growing good plants) the gardener uses, the process of planting is the same: you put a seed in the soil, give it water (and maybe fertilizer), and take care of the plant when it comes up. This is basically how nursing theories and the nursing process work together. With all nursing theories, the nursing process of assessing, planning, implementing, and evaluating remains constant, even if different terms are used to describe what nurses do.

Because the nursing process can be used with just about any nursing theory, this book does not try to link the process specifically with one theory or another. Rather, it focuses on the process and shows how **thinking** and **doing** are inseparably intertwined throughout the process. This provides a sound beginning for the practice of great nursing. The preferred nursing theory or theories to support practice can be selected at a later time.

These brief historical highlights provide the basis for a beginning appreciation of the events and time frames of activities that have contributed to the development of the nursing process and the nursing profession. Although the formal terminology "nursing process" is fairly recent, the problem-solving methodology used by nurses is much older. Ongoing nursing research and clinical practice continue to make giant strides in clarifying and refining the use of the nursing process in the achievement of great nursing.

✔ *Thinking-Learning Check*

Pause here for a thinking-learning check. You should be able to elaborate on these ideas:

- ✔ The *how* of great nursing includes the patient, you, thinking skills, knowledge, and the nursing process.
- ✔ The patient, whether an individual or an aggregate (family, group, or community), has unique strengths and health concerns.
- ✔ Knowledge comes from books, clinical practice, and nursing research findings.
- ✔ The nursing process components—assessing, planning, implementing, and evaluating—are constantly intermingling.
- ✔ The roots of the nursing process include:

  Identification of the components of the nursing process and how they work

  Development and refinement of Nursing Diagnoses through NANDA

  Definition of nursing by ANA

  Development and refinement of Nursing Interventions Classification (NIC)

  Development of Nursing Outcomes Classification (NOC)

  Development and refinement of nursing theories

CAUTIONS AND CLARIFICATIONS ABOUT STANDARDIZED LANGUAGES AND STANDARDIZED CARE

Part of the ongoing task of a socially responsible profession is to continue to define and describe clearly what it does for the protection and safety of the public. This movement to continually refine, clarify, label, and develop standards of care, although necessary, is a double-edged sword. Because definitions, descriptions, and standards are professional mandates, they carry with them the danger of making nursing appear to have cookbook-type recipes for care.

Some nurses have criticized the use of standardized classifications (i.e., NANDA, NIC, and NOC), confusing them with standardized care. The major criticisms are based on two beliefs. First, attempts to label and standardize care are too simplistic for the uniqueness of individuals and their needs. Second, the dynamic nature of people, their environment, and nursing care is too complex to infer any direct cause-and-effect relationship between nursing care and the results of care.

It is not the standardized languages that are problematic but rather what is done with the classifications when they are used as cookbook recipes devoid of much thought. The purpose of standardized classifications is to provide a common language for nurses to use in describing their patient care in both written and verbal communication. Unfortunately, the *thinking* and the necessity for focusing attention on the individual can be lost along the road to defining and standardizing terminology and approaches.

A standardized approach, like the nursing process, is similar to a cake recipe. The recipe works fine if the cook has all the correct ingredients in all the right amounts, the right-sized pan, and the correct oven temperature. But what happens if one ingredient is missing? Can some other ingredient be substituted? What happens if the oven doesn't get as hot as the recipe calls for? Can a lower temperature be used, or is it better just to bake the cake longer? Without the ability to think and make adjustments in the recipe, the result will be something much different from the desired cake. The *thinking* cook, however, can modify the recipe and still end up with a great cake.

The same principle applies in nursing. Standards and labels are only guides; the nurse must think and adjust standards and labels to fit each patient's unique needs. Thinking provides the nurse and the patient with multiple avenues to achieve the same goal. It is continually necessary for both beginning nurses and experienced nurses to keep those *thinking caps* on and avoid the rut of cookbook nursing.

Some say that there has always been a focus on thinking in nursing; others say it has been lost. Regardless of the view taken, a brief review of the original work on the nursing process reveals a strong focus on thinking as integral to the components of the process. In their second edition of *The Nursing Process*, Yura and Walsh stated, "The skills the nurse must have to use the nursing process are: intellectual, interpersonal, and technical. Intellectual skills entail problem-solving, critical thinking, and making nursing judgments" (Yura & Walsh, 1973, p. 69).

Nursing has come a long way in 30 years, but there is still much to do. Some may find that prospect overwhelming; others get excited by the challenge. Part of what is exciting is that the nursing leaders, who will guide thinking and doing and the nursing process into the 21st century, are the beginning nurses of today. Keep those thinking caps on and take good care of the profession and the patients.

DEFINITIONS OF THE NURSING PROCESS COMPONENTS

Each of the components of the nursing process serves a special role. To understand those roles better, it is useful to examine the definitions of the components first.

Assessing

Thinking about what information to collect, collecting information, *thinking* about the significance of that information, and drawing conclusions about how the patient is responding to his or her health or illness condition. The conclusions of assessment include two basic categories: strengths and health concerns. Health concerns focus on: (1) issues the nurse can deal with independently (nursing diagnoses); (2) issues that a nurse and another health care provider work on interdependently (interdisciplinary problems); and (3) issues that need to be referred to another health care provider (eg, medical or nutrition problems).

Planning

Thinking about (and usually writing down) how to help with the patient's response to his or her health or illness condition. Working with the patient to decide which problems have priority, developing patient outcomes, and determining what the nurse and the patient need to do to meet those outcomes.

Implementing

Doing specific activities to help the patient meet the goals in the plan, while continuing to *think* about what is being done, how it is being done, and when, where, and why it is being done.

Evaluating

Thinking and collecting information about the patient's responses after some nursing care is provided. Working with the patient to determine whether the patient's outcomes have been met and how well they have been met.

Anyone can memorize these or any other definitions. However, understanding and recognizing the concepts that are defined requires more than TOTAL RECALL. The following learning activity was designed to illustrate how all the components of the nursing process are used with thinking and doing, and to move the reader's thinking beyond the TOTAL RECALL mode.

⟳ACTION LEARNING #15: Identifying Components as the Nursing Process Is Used

Reread the definitions of the components of the nursing process carefully; then read the following case study. Find the components of the nursing process as used by Ms. Louise Lamay, student nurse. Circle the sentence(s) that demonstrate one or more of the components of the nursing process, and write the appropriate label or labels (assessing, planning, implementing, or evaluating) next to your circles.

Case Study

1 Louise Lamay, student nurse, just started her rotation in a pediatric
2 nursing clinic. Preparing for her clinical day, she reviewed information
3 on growth and development, pediatric dosages of medications, immu-
4 nization schedules, and family processes.
5   In the morning before the patients arrived, Louise reviewed 4-year-
6 old Jesse's clinic record and learned the following:

7   Date of birth: 3/4/89
8   Last visit to clinic 1 year ago
9   Normal labor and delivery; successfully breast fed for 9 months
10   Immunizations up to date (needs fourth DPT booster and oral polio
11   vaccination)
12   Ht. = 38 inches (50th percentile for 3-year-old boys)
13   Wt. = 33 lbs. (50th percentile for 3-year-old boys)
14   History of two to three ear infections each winter, effectively treated
15   with amoxicillin
16   Parents' concern about fussy eater after the age of 18 months
17   No known allergies

18   Louise greeted Jesse, who was accompanied by his father, Mr.
19 Frazier. She introduced herself and escorted both to the examining
20 room, where she asked, "How are things?" Jesse smiled and said, "Fine,
21 you want to see my drawing?"
22   While Louise examined the multicolored crayon drawing of teddy
23 bears, Mr. F. stated, "Jesse seems OK, but we are really concerned that
24 he is not eating enough to keep a bird alive. His diet consists solely of
25 American cheese, french fries, peanut butter, white bread, bananas, and
26 milk. He also doesn't want to take naps anymore and gets up three to
27 four times before finally falling asleep at night. He generally sleeps from
28 10 or 11 PM until 8 AM. He hates breakfast! We also see that he gets a
29 rash when he is outside on windy days in the summer."
30   Louise summarized for Mr. F.: "It sounds like you have several con-
31 cerns about Jesse—his eating, his sleeping, and his periodic rashes. We
32 will examine them all, but which one is the biggest problem from your
33 perspective?" Mr. F. replied, "Well, the eating is really our biggest
34 headache."
35   Louise asked Jesse to get on the scale. She found the following:

36   Ht. = 40 inches (25th percentile for 4-year-old boys)
37   Wt. = 35 lbs. (25th percentile for 4-year-old boys)

38   In response to Louise's questions about his eating, Jesse replied, "I
39 don't like other stuff. They feel funny when they crunch and they make

40 my belly hurt. I like fries best, but Mom and Dad won't let me eat them
41 all the time."
42   At this point, Louise looked at the available data and compared
43 them with the norms for 4-year-old boys (height/weight norms, dietary
44 requirement norms, and behavioral norms). She suspected that nutrition
45 was a problem because Jesse's diet was deficient in fruits and vegeta-
46 bles. She also realized that she needed more information—specifically,
47 the amounts of each of the foods he ate during a period of days. She
48 needed a 3-day, 24-hour diet record.
49   After obtaining a diet record through Mr. F.'s recall, she verified her
50 initial hunch that the diet needed more fruits and vegetables. The ques-
51 tion then was, what was causing this eating problem? She considered
52 that he might have food intolerance; he might be trying to control his
53 environment; he might just not like the taste of things; or he might be
54 hesitant to try new things. She asked questions to rule in or rule out
55 these possible causes, and discovered that he was hesitant to try new
56 tastes and textures because they were different. He often interrupted
57 their food discussion with excited remarks about his drawings and new
58 computer painting program.
59   At first Louise thought this was going to be tough. He didn't seem
60 interested in food at all. Then it occurred to her that her mother used to
61 get her to eat new foods by shaping them with cookie cutters. She
62 smiled to herself at the memory of eating stars and hearts.
63   Louise considered what she knew about children's learning styles
64 and, realizing that she must keep things simple, came up with a plan in-
65 volving rewards and short-term goals that would entice Jesse to eat a
66 larger variety of foods. The goal was to get him to eat one new vegetable
67 or fruit each week. The plan included having him create pictures with
68 selected foods, cutting food into bear shapes, and increasing computer
69 time for every new food he tried.
70   Louise told Mr. F. and Jesse that she would call them in a week to
71 see how things were going. She said to Jesse, "When I call, I'd like you
72 to tell me about the food pictures you've eaten and which ones tasted
73 best."
74   After they left, Louise took a minute to review her encounter with
75 Jesse and his dad. She realized she forgot to ask about the rest of the
76 family's eating style. She made a note to ask about this during her
77 follow-up phone call. She also realized that she came up with a very
78 clever plan and hoped it would work. She recorded the plan in Jesse's
79 chart and made a note on the calendar to call next week when she re-
80 turned to the clinic.

> **THINK ABOUT THIS** ■ How easily could you see the components of the nursing process? Could you see the intertwining of the components? Was it sometimes difficult to separate the components?

In Action Learning #15 you focused on what the nurse was *doing*. Now, the focus is on finding the *thinking* in the same case study. Refer back to Chapter 1 to review the five modes of thinking in greater detail, if needed (but the modes are listed below).

⊃**ACTION LEARNING #16: Thinking and the Nursing Process**

Reexamine the case study about Jesse, his father, and Ms. Lamay, this time looking for evidence of the thinking involved. For now, just focus on Louise's *thinking*, not Jesse's and his father's thinking. Use a different colored pen than the one you used in Action Learning #15 and label the thinking according to the *think* mnemonic.

T = Total Recall
H = Habits
I = Inquiry
N = New Ideas and Creativity
K = Knowing How You Think

Remember, the *thinking* may be very evident in the descriptions of *doing* in the case study, or the *thinking* may be implied. Identify the type of thinking that is occurring. Again, a combination of modes may be in operation all at once.

THINK ABOUT THIS ■ What kinds of thinking did you see happening? Do some types of thinking occur more frequently with some components of the nursing process than with others?

Summary of Louise's Thinking and Use of the Nursing Process

Louise's **assessing** involved pre-encounter, encounter, and postencounter **thinking and doing**. **Assessing** started before Louise met Jesse and his dad (pre-encounter). She engaged TOTAL RECALL when she looked up some facts that she thought she should know. She was anticipating her needs and checking things that could help her with **assessing** and **planning** care. As a nurse's expertise grows, more facts are stored in memory for retrieval, but do not ever expect to know it all. Nurses, even very experienced ones, continue to look up facts to help them provide care. Sometimes nurses look up information they anticipate needing; sometimes they find gaps in their knowledge and seek reference material during the patient encounter.

As Louise started **data collection** as part of **assessing**, she reviewed records, which are important sources of pre-encounter data. When she encountered Jesse and his dad, she **collected data** from them. She was **thinking** about the data and **forming conclusions** during the encounter when she verified her hunches about Mr. F.'s concerns.

Louise was also starting to **think** about **planning** care when she asked which problem was a priority. Then she went back to **data collection** to get more information about Jesse's nutritional status. Louise used INQUIRY **thinking** when she **analyzed** the data and considered various **conclusions** about Jesse's problems with eating and the factors that could be contributing to those problems. She didn't jump in with easy solutions as she **planned** what to offer as possible solutions. She used INQUIRY to consider various options, and used her NEW IDEAS AND CREATIVITY when she recruited Jesse's strengths (his interest in art and computers) to improve his eating.

Louise **implemented** the first part of her plan by telling Jesse and his dad her suggestions for how to entice Jesse to eat new foods. She anticipated **evaluation** by letting her patients know she would call to see how things were going. KNOWING HOW YOU THINK was used when Louise reflected on her thinking after Jesse and his dad left; she could see what she needed to do to compensate for her forgetting something.

The review of the thinking and doing in this case study illustrates how the components of the **nursing process** and various kinds of **thinking** are used. All of the *think* modes, except HABITS, were evident. Louise probably used HABITS when she checked Jesse's height and weight. Those measurements are so commonly associated with nutrition that almost anyone would check them automatically.

SEQUENCING THE COMPONENTS OF THE NURSING PROCESS

With the recognition that the nursing process and *thinking* and *doing* are the foundations of successful practice comes the question, "Where does the process start?"

⟲ACTION LEARNING #17: Where to Start

Take a minute now and imagine yourself as the student nurse in the situation described next. Remember that nursing is a process of *thinking* and *doing*. What is the *first thing* you, as a student nurse, are thinking about in the following nursing situation?

You are assigned to care for Mrs. Svensen for the morning. She is 85, very independent, and does not like to bother people. Today she is confined to bed after her hip surgery yesterday. You walk into her room and find her struggling to complete her bed bath even though she can't reach the lower part of her legs.

The first thing I think about is

THINK ABOUT THIS ■ Those of you who wrote, "I need to help the patient finish her bath" are thinking about *implementing* first. Perhaps others wrote, "I need to get some information about the patient first." You are thinking about *assessing*. Still a third group may have written, "I need to sit down and decide what is the best way to help this patient. Should I do it myself, or find another way to help her finish the task so she doesn't have to give up her independence?" Your group is approaching this from the point of *planning*.

Right or Wrong Sequences

Basically, there is no absolute right or wrong place to start. As with most of nursing, it all depends on the situation. Although thinking may focus on any component of the nursing process first, the most logical DOING starts with assessment. Logically, if the nurse has never seen the patient before, some information (assessment) is needed before doing anything if safe nursing care is to be achieved. All encounters begin with some degree of assessment. How much information is needed depends on other circumstances, such as how immediate the patient's need is (eg, is the patient bleeding severely or not breathing?), how much experience the nurse has (is the nurse a beginner or an expert?), and how much time is available to spend with the patient (10 minutes during an office visit or many months in a nursing home?).

Similar circumstances influence how much time and energy nurses put into planning care. Sometimes planning is instantaneous, or on-the-spot. Other times the nurse can sit for an hour or two and write out a lengthy, long-term plan of care. Likewise, implementation may vary depending on the situation.

Evaluation always occurs *after* something is done. It does not make much sense to try to evaluate changes in patient behaviors before any care is provided.

Traditional Assumptions About Sequencing the Components of the Nursing Process

Most traditional nursing books describe the nursing process as a sequence of steps with simple feedback loops. This method provides a basic explanation of the components of the process and the importance of feedback. Unfortunately, this method has several problems. First, it promotes the idea that the nursing process can be effectively used like a "cookbook." The second problem is that the components become a series of concepts to memorize without any appreciation of their dynamic relationship to each other beyond feedback.

Actual Sequencing of the Nursing Process Components

In reading about the nursing process as it was described above, do not be lulled into believing that the nursing process is a simple 1-2-3-4, lock-step procedure. In any given patient encounter, the nurse may assess, plan, implement, and evaluate several times and possibly use all the components at the same time. The nurse also may spend varying amounts of time and energy on each component of the process. Consider this example: the nurse may *assess* for a new problem (eg, diaper rash) while *evaluating* care outcomes for an old problem (eg, how well Mom learned to diaper the baby). Likewise, as the nurse *implements* care for a patient's problem (eg, turning a patient on his side to relieve pain), the nurse may *assess* for other concerns (eg, skin condition, mobility) and even *evaluate* the results of care for another problem (eg, how well the patient has learned to use the trapeze to help with moving in bed), while *planning* care for yet another problem (eg, the best toileting schedule). And, believe it or not, this may be accomplished in several seconds by more experienced nurses. Although it may take a little longer for beginning nurses, the same events in thinking and doing will occur if the nursing process is used effectively.

The "bottom line" here is that there are four key components to the nursing process. All four are critical to high-quality nursing care, and all four are used repeatedly for each nursing concern. Where to start and how much emphasis to place on each component at a certain point in care depends on many factors, including the patient situation, the nurse's expertise, and the amount of time available. Some degree of assessment, even if it takes only microseconds, is usually the starting point.

Examine Figure 3-2 to visualize the sequencing of the nursing process. When the patient and nurse begin the process they join forces. They begin at an entry level assessment in which some information is exchanged and some thinking about that information occurs. Once assessment has started, the nurse and patient make multiple sequencing decisions and can move into any of the following linkages:

Further assessing and planning
Planning and implementing care
Implementing and evaluating care
Assessing and implementing

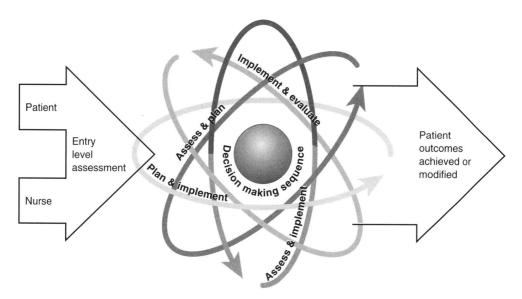

FIGURE 3–2   Sequencing the components of the nursing process.

No matter where they jump in, they will "cross" the lines of the other parts of the nursing process. For example, if the tendency is to start with implementing care, it is highly likely that further assessment will occur almost immediately as the implementation is being tailored to the specific situation. Sometimes, as the nurse is evaluating the effectiveness of actions, it becomes clear that the actions should have been planned more completely, and so forth. Ultimately, the nurse and the patient want the patient to achieve some outcomes that represent a change in health status for the better. The path to that outcome can be extremely varied, however, depending on the thinking processes of the nurse and the patient.

CYCLING AND RECYCLING THE NURSING PROCESS

It is very tempting to view the nursing process as a linear recipe for patient care. When first learning about this process, the pieces are, of necessity, taken apart so that the actions and thinking of each component can be studied. However, in actual practice, the nursing process is a constantly recycled set of thoughts and actions whose components get very "mixed up."

In the next chapter, the details of using the nursing process are addressed. The components are picked apart again. However, it is helpful periodically to *think* back to Louise and Jesse for a full picture of the process in all its complexity. Learning about and using the nursing process along with *thinking* and *doing* is not something that happens with one reading. Rereading, practice, and asking questions will help you continue on your journey toward great nursing.

THINKING LOG #3 ▶

Put yourself in Louise's shoes and identify all the things you would do differently or in addition to what she did. Write out your thoughts below and compare your thoughts with those of a classmate.

References

American Nurses Association (1980). *Nursing: A social policy statement*. Kansas City: Author.

American Nurses Association (1991). *Standards of clinical nursing practice*. Kansas City: Author.

Gebbie, K.M. & Lavin, M.A. (1975). *Classification of nursing diagnoses: Proceedings of the First Conference*. St. Louis: CV Mosby.

Johnson, M. & Maas, M. (Eds.) (1997). *Nursing outcomes classification (NOC)*. St. Louis: Mosby.

McCloskey, J.C. & Bulechek, G.M. (Eds.) (1992). *Nursing interventions classification (NIC)*. St. Louis: Mosby.

McCloskey, J.C. & Bulechek, G.M. (Eds.) (1996). *Nursing interventions classification* (2nd ed.) St. Louis: Mosby.

North American Nursing Diagnosis Association. (1996). *NANDA nursing diagnoses: Definitions and classification 1997–1998*. Philadelphia: Author.

Saba, V.K. & McCormick, K.A. (1996). *Essentials of computers for nurses* (2nd ed.) New York: McGraw Hill.

Yura, H. & Walsh, M.B. (Eds.) (1967). *The nursing process: Assessing, planning, implementing, evaluating*. Washington, DC: The Catholic University of America Press.

Yura, H. & Walsh, M.B. (1973). *The nursing process: Assessing, planning, implementing, evaluating* (2nd ed.) New York: Appleton-Century-Crofts.

Yura, H. & Walsh, M.B. (1988). *The nursing process: Assessing, planning, implementing, evaluating* (5th ed.) Norwalk, CT: Appleton & Lange.

Application of Thinking and Doing in the Nursing Process

❋ *Learning Outcomes*

After reading and doing the activities in this chapter, you will be able to:

Apply your personal thinking approaches to using the nursing process.

Track the thinking path of a student nurse using the nursing process in a patient care situation.

Appreciate the variety of thinking styles used with the nursing process.

The last chapter showed how the components of the nursing process and thinking were used by one student nurse, Louise Lamay. Although many details are needed to understand the nursing process completely, this chapter continues to focus on the whole of the process. Seeing the whole several times helps to make more sense out of the details, which are addressed in later chapters.

This chapter also nurtures beginning students' growing appreciation for their existing thinking skills. Beginning students do not come into nursing with blank slates in their heads, they come with many existing thinking skills. Students bring a whole repertoire of thinking skills that they have developed over the last two to six decades of life. These skills can and should be built on, and not ignored by pretending to start learning at "ground zero." To enhance all thinking modes, especially INQUIRY and NEW IDEAS AND CREATIVITY, students must focus on KNOWING HOW YOU THINK. KNOWING HOW YOU THINK is the key to nurturing all thinking modes.

APPLYING PERSONAL THINKING APPROACHES

To accomplish the task of incorporating personal thinking into the nursing process, the first part of this chapter is one big Action Learning #18. Several questions are posed to stimulate multiple modes of thinking. The second part of this chapter presents another nursing situation accompanied by a report of one style of thinking as the nursing process was applied.

In the following nursing situation you will be asked to *think* through the whole process, even though many questions may remain at this beginning stage. Keep in mind that there are no right or wrong answers here, so be adventurous in your thinking. *Thinking caps on?*

⊃Action Learning #18: The Big Think

Read the following case study and answer the questions. Then find at least two classmates with whom to compare your answers. Remember, the purpose of comparing is not to see whose ideas are better, but to see how differently people approach thinking. Peer collaboration is a great way to learn about a variety of thinking skills.

Case Study

Dan Christopher is a 20-year-old college sophomore in a physical therapy program. He has come to the student health service, where you are a student nurse completing an experience in ambulatory care. Dan is hoping to get a prescription for sleeping pills. He complains of not sleeping well for the last month; midterm exams are coming up soon and he needs some rest. He is 6'1" tall, 170 pounds, neatly dressed, alert, and oriented. He has dark circles under his eyes and yawns several times during the interview. Dan says he is really stressed out this year with his studies, his part-time job, and his roommate who plays hard rock until 3 AM every night. A classmate suggested he get some sleeping pills. He's a little afraid of them because he's never taken anything stronger than aspirin before, but he's willing to try anything.

Questions to Stimulate *Think* Modes

1. How would you feel if you were Dan? Why?

2. What are your first impressions of Dan? Why do you think those were your first impressions?

3. What questions do you have and why do you have them?

4. What do you think Dan wants to see happen in this situation? Why do you think that?

5. What would you do *with* Dan? Why?

6. What do you think is unique about your approach to Dan? Why do you think it is unique?

THINK ABOUT THIS ■ How different or alike were your answers and those of your classmates? Are you beginning to appreciate what is unique about your thinking and theirs? Isn't it interesting how three people can look at the same situation and see some things so differently and some things exactly the same? How did you feel about the differences?

The questions for Action Learning #18 are somewhat broad to allow individual thinking styles to emerge. The questions also are arranged in a typical sequence that many nurses use to begin and follow through on their thinking during patient care. The questions, however, could be arranged differently to fit personal thinking styles. Action Learning #18 also encourages awareness of the feelings associated with thinking, how they might be unique, and how they might be different from other nurses' feelings.

Feelings About Personal Thinking Abilities

Students may have several reactions when they compare their work with that of others. Some feel anxious; others don't. Some feel insecure when they see their work is different from someone else's. Others feel superior when they think they have the best approach or answer. Still others feel all of the above. Although all of these responses are normal, it is important to recognize that they can significantly influence thinking in positive and negative ways.

Think back to how you felt while doing this exercise; on a scale of 1 to 10, with 10 being the highest, what was your anxiety level? Remember, anxiety tends to shut down higher-level thinking skills and shunt thinking energy into survival mode. Therefore, the best thinking occurs when anxiety is not too high. If your anxiety was high while doing Action Learning #18, think about ways to decrease that anxiety. For example, remember that these exercises are for learning, not for grading or even evaluating your ability to do nursing. It is okay to recognize areas for further development—areas you would like to enhance. Acknowledging these areas for development is a great way to learn and to expand thinking, especially in the NEW IDEAS AND CREATIVITY and the KNOWING HOW YOU THINK modes. Recognizing and accepting that there is always room for growth is a true sign of a thinking nurse.

For those who felt insecure after seeing how others responded, consider how this affects your thinking. If feeling insecure hinders thinking, it will hinder nursing care. If feeling insecure is a common response, seriously consider ways to increase your self-esteem. Unfortunately, low self-esteem is a common feeling among college students. The good news is that low self-esteem is a learned behavior; people are not born with low self-esteem. It can, therefore, be unlearned if there is a desire to do so. Many helpful techniques are available besides spending years in psychoanalysis.

Because this text does not allow time for a crash course in improving self-esteem, one simple but effective way is offered. Write a list of 10 of your positive attributes. If you cannot instantly think of 10, list as many as possible. Post the list on your bathroom mirror and read it *aloud* every morning until it is firmly etched in your brain. Add a new item to your list every day and continue to read it aloud. You will be impressed with how much more you can appreciate and respect yourself.

At the other extreme are people who feel they have all the "right answers." This attitude can be a serious threat to patient safety. Students who feel superior are less apt to question their judgments or use INQUIRY in planning nursing care.

No nurse has all the answers, not even those who have worked for many years. Even experts have questions and doubts. If nurses do not ask questions and challenge their own thinking, their patients' health may be in serious jeopardy.

Have all the options for feelings been removed? Don't feel superior; don't feel insecure; don't feel anxious. What's left for those who are human? Well, as with most things in life, balance is needed. Strive for a healthy self-esteem with openness to all five modes of thinking. With that combination, the great nurse in every student can emerge.

TRACKING THINKING THROUGH THE NURSING PROCESS

Now it is time to demonstrate the thinking of a nurse using the nursing process. Thinking is not always easy to track, but it is important to try to visualize this very abstract process. Many textbooks describe what to do and why, but most do not discuss the thinking that occurs. Only recently have educators recognized the importance of describing the thinking process.

Part of the reason that thinking has not been discussed may be that expert nurses and nursing instructors, who have practiced nursing for a long time, find it difficult to explain their thinking, which has become automatic. Think about something you have been doing for years, such as riding a bicycle. How easy is it to describe verbally the balance and coordination that you acquired so many years ago? Most of the process has become second nature for the long-time bike rider. Thinking about how to describe the fine-tuned skills of bike riding is a big challenge.

But challenge or not, describing thinking is one of the best ways to nurture better thinking in beginning students, and examining a case study role model is the next-best thing to real life. The student nurse in this case study is Ken Tanaka. His clinical course focuses on gerontology and rehabilitation care.

Examine Ken's thinking carefully and compare it with yours, keeping an open mind. Draw on the things that make sense and add them to your thinking skills repertoire. Set aside the things that do not make sense, but do not discard them immediately. Read several more chapters on thinking skills, and then decide whether some of these thinking approaches are worth keeping after all.

Case Study

Ken is doing a clinical rotation in a nursing home. This morning, part of his assignment is to care for Mrs. Poski, a newly admitted, 82-year-old patient.

Mrs. Poski came to the skilled nursing home facility after a short hospitalization for malnutrition. She is a retired piano teacher who has been living independently since her husband's death 10 years ago. Three months ago, after her bout with the "flu," her appetite and strength diminished. She lost 20 pounds, which led to her hospitalization.

Mrs. Poski has three sons who visit regularly and are supportive of her returning to her home when her strength improves and her nutritional intake is stable. She is a pleasant woman who is cooperative and agreeable with the current plan for her recovery. Her sons describe her as extremely sociable; she enjoys numerous activities and interactions with others. The nurses, however, have observed her interacting very little with other residents and spending much time in her room alone. When asked about this apparent change in her socialization pattern, Mrs. Poski says she just doesn't want to bother people by asking them to repeat things she can't hear. She is very hard of hearing. She admits that her hearing has gotten worse since the flu and that she should have it checked. However, she assumed she would have to wait until she got home to make an appointment with an ear specialist.

Mrs. Poski is alert and oriented. Her medical diagnoses are osteoarthritis and malnutrition. Her current medications are ibuprofen 200 mg qid and multivitamins, 1 qd. She wears glasses for reading and has her own teeth. Her vital signs this morning were: BP = 106/78; pulse = 76; respiration = 18; temp = 98.6°F. She has no edema or shortness of breath and no history of smoking or alcohol abuse. Her present weight is 95 lbs. With a height of 5'4", her ideal body weight is 120 lbs ± 10%. Before the flu, her weight was 112 lbs. Although she gained 3 lbs. since arriving at the nursing home, her appetite is still poor to fair. She consumes 50% to 75% of meals. She is continent of bowel and bladder and denies problems with constipation. She had a lot of diarrhea during the "flu" and for 1 week thereafter. Mrs. Poski continues to experience decreased strength and stamina since the flu, but is improving with physical therapy five times per week and increased food intake. Her gait is unsteady and her balance is poor during transfers from wheelchair to bed. She is able to bathe and dress herself with moderate assistance. Her skin is intact but fragile.

Assessment

The process of assessment includes data collection and data analysis. Both of these concepts will be explored more fully in Chapters 7 and 8, but for now think about data collection as the gathering of information and data analysis as making sense out of the information. Data analysis includes recognizing important pieces of data, seeing relationships among pieces of data and groups of data, and making conclusions.

Data Collection

Ken began care for Mrs. Poski by listening to the morning report and reading Mrs. Poski's medical and nursing records. This is described as pre-encounter data. He continued his data collection when he talked to (interviewed) Mrs. Poski, observed her during the interview, and took measurements (eg, blood pressure, pulse, respirations, and temperature). The thinking that is required before collecting data is not addressed here, but is dealt with in Chapter 7 ("Health Detectives"). Ken's thinking for analyzing the data will be studied first.

Data Analysis

FIRST IMPRESSIONS

For starters, Ken acknowledged his overall first impression. Mrs. Poski reminded him of his Aunt Millie. He thought: if this were Aunt Millie, I know she'd want really good nursing care and I'd want it for her. Ken thought about what was going through his mind; he knew that when he could positively identify with a patient, he thought more clearly and efficiently. When he didn't like the patient as much, he spent more time making sure he was being nice because he was afraid his feelings about the person would be seen as negative. (Ken was demonstrating the KNOWING HOW YOU THINK mode.)

Overall, he thought, Mrs. Poski is getting better and has good family support. She is likable, but keeps to herself. Her isolation, her nutrition, and her difficulty in transferring are areas of concern that require more thinking. These thoughts all were preliminary hunches that were used to guide his data collection further and refine his conclusions later.

COMPARING DATA WITH NORMS

Next, Ken thought about the information he had. What was normal? He used his recall (TOTAL RECALL) of knowledge from his course work to decide what was standard (normal) for most people, but remembered to check whether these things were normal for Mrs. Poski. He decided that the following data were not normal, or were at least questionable, and therefore considered "relevant data."

20-lb. weight loss during "flu"	Hard of hearing
Ht. 5'4" with Wt. of 95 lbs.	Appetite poor to fair
Consumes 50% to 75% of meals	Decreased strength
Unsteady gait	Decreased stamina
Poor balance	Interacting little
Spending much time alone	Not wanting to bother people
Hearing getting worse	Unable to bathe and dress alone

INITIAL HUNCHES

This list of relevant data helped Ken to sharpen his hunches. His first impressions had been based less on data than on his past experiences. However, once he considered the data, his impressions became more formalized. He began to consider problems with hearing, socialization, nutrition, and mobility. He also suspected that Mrs. Poski had some risk factors for other problems, but he could not be sure just what those were yet. Again, using his recall (TOTAL RECALL) of lectures on aging, he knew that some normal risks accompanied aging. He knew he wouldn't feel sure of his preliminary conclusions until he reviewed some information on aging and on mobility problems for patients with osteoarthritis (again, exhibiting the KNOWING HOW YOU THINK MODE when he was looking for ways to feel more comfortable with his conclusions).

FINDING CLUSTERS

At this point, Ken had lots of ideas in his head, but he had to organize them to come to some final conclusions that could be supported with relevant data. He also thought about what else he needed to know. He decided to jot down the data in clusters (groups) to see what patterns emerged and to see whether there where gaps in information (data gaps). He used INQUIRY to question what else he should consider. He used his RECALL of information about usual patterns of human responses to organize his clusters. Here are five clusters of data he initially developed:

Clusters

Ht. 5'4" Wt. 95 lbs.
Appetite poor to fair
Lost 20 lbs. during "flu"
Gained 3 lbs. in nursing home
Consumes 50% to 75% of meals

Decreased strength and stamina
Gait unsteady
Balance poor
Unable to dress and bathe alone

Interacting little
Spending much time alone
Not wanting to bother people
Hard of hearing
Previous pattern of being very sociable

Assuming she would have to wait for appointment with ear specialist
Hard of hearing

Supportive family
Independent lifestyle
Music interests
Stable vital signs
Communicates effectively
Mentally alert and oriented
Recent weight gain of 3 lbs.

Ken thought about these clusters. The data were so interrelated, he wasn't sure whether these clusters were the best, but he could see that there were definite factors that "painted a picture" of her strengths as well as her health concerns. He also realized that some of the problem areas were primary problems, whereas others seemed to be contributing to the primary problems. For example, Ht. 5'4", Wt. 95 lbs., 20-lb weight loss during "flu," and consuming 50% to 75% of meals showed a picture of nutrition that was less than adequate. Poor appetite was contributing to that problem. The data and the data clusters were interrelated to some extent. He decided he could draw some conclusions that had a good probability of being accurate because he had enough supporting data. More data on the hearing and specific data on the types of food Mrs. Poski liked or did not like would have allowed him to draw conclusions with even higher probabilities of accuracy, so he made a mental note to get more information as soon as possible. This analysis of the relationships among the data exemplified the use of TOTAL RECALL and INQUIRY.

THINKING ABOUT CONCLUSIONS

As Ken prepares to think about his conclusions, part of his thinking involves remembering the basic categories of nursing conclusions. (More detailed discussion of nursing conclusions is included in Chapters 5 and 6.) He recalls that nurses need to identify both the strengths and the health concerns of their patients. He needs to make conclusions about three basic kinds of health concerns: (a) problems for referral (issues that should be addressed by other providers); (b) interdisciplinary problems (issues for which the nurse works collaboratively with other health care providers); and (c) nursing diagnoses (those concerns for which the nurse has primary responsibility for diagnosing and treating).

Ken first concluded that Mrs. Poski had many strengths that could be used in planning her care. He also recognized that there was a definite problem with nutrition, but that it was getting somewhat better. If Mrs. Poski's appetite could be increased, she would eat better, which would increase her strength and speed up her recuperation. He'd have to talk to the dietitian before finalizing plans for nutrition. (This was a possible interdisciplinary problem for his second conclusion.)

His third conclusion concerned the hearing problem; this was a mystery. He decided the doctor should evaluate it, and that perhaps a referral to a specialist would be advisable (possible problem for referral). He knew Mrs. Poski was getting physical therapy (PT), so he would coordinate plans with PT to help with the mobility issues (a fourth conclusion—a possible interdisciplinary problem). He thought that something should be done to help her interact more with people because she seemed socially isolated (a fifth conclusion—a possible nursing diagnosis). He deduced that the hearing problem was a strong contributor to the social isolation. This sixth conclusion about the related factor (the hearing problem) required him to use his knowledge of human behavior and the effects of physical impairment, and then to see a relationship between those two sets of information. Again, TOTAL RECALL and INQUIRY were the major thinking modes used here.

There also were risk factors to consider. The data cluster about decreased mobility led him to think about a potential for falls and injuries (a seventh conclusion—a possible nursing diagnosis). If the nutrition and mobility problems didn't continue to improve, Mrs. Poski's skin would be at risk (eighth conclusion—a possible nursing diagnosis). He recalled from lectures and textbooks that skin, especially that of older people, could break down easily when people didn't move around sufficiently and they were undernourished. This thinking about relationships between pieces of data required the use of TOTAL RECALL and INQUIRY.

Ken then reviewed all the data he collected on Mrs. Poski to be sure he had covered everything. It is always good practice for nurses to go back and forth between the data they collect and the conclusions they make from those data. Ken realized that he had forgotten some very important data that resulted in a missing conclusion.

⟳ACTION LEARNING #19: The Missing Conclusion

Do as Ken did and look back at the data to find the missing conclusion(s). What is missing?

THINK ABOUT THIS ■ How did you approach this task? Where did you start? Did you find more than one missing conclusion?

The conclusion Ken realized he had forgotten to include was Mrs. Poski's problems with bathing and dressing because of her weakness. A ninth conclusion, an additional nursing diagnosis, needed to be made.

CONCLUSIONS

As Ken prepared to write his conclusions in the patient's record, he thought about the best wording to use. He wanted his conclusions to be clear enough that others could understand them. He got out his nursing diagnosis books to look for labels whose definitions fit with his conclusions. When he found similar wording and definitions, he compared his clusters of relevant data with the defining characteristics listed for the textbook diagnostic labels. Because his clusters fit with the clusters in the book, he used the standardized NANDA terminology. (A discussion of NANDA diagnoses is in Chapter 3, and the Taxonomy list is in Appendix A.)

In addition to recording the data clusters that supported his conclusions, he charted the following conclusions:

Ken's Conclusions of Nursing Assessment for Mrs. Poski

I. Strengths (of the patient):

Past history of socialization

Participation in PT

Increased food intake

Supportive family

Vital signs stable

Skin intact

Continent

Artistic interests

Effective communication skills

Mentally alert and oriented

(Ken was aware that many of Mrs. Poski's strengths might be considered for inclusion in a Wellness Diagnosis, but he decided to talk to his instructor before developing one.)

II. Health Concerns:

A. Problems for Referral

Progressive hearing loss (refer to MD)

B. Interdisciplinary Problems

Decreased strength and stamina (PT)

Altered Nutrition: Less than Body Requirements, related to decreased appetite 2° "flu" (dietitian)

C. Nursing Diagnoses (problems and related factors)

Self-Care Deficit for Bathing and Dressing related to generalized weakness secondary to decreased nutrition and prolonged diarrhea after the "flu"

Social Isolation related to increasing hearing loss and not wanting to bother people

Risk for Injury related to generalized weakness, poor balance, and unstable transfers from bed to wheelchair

Risk for Impaired Skin Integrity related to immobility, frail skin, and inadequate nutrition

SHARING CONCLUSIONS WITH PATIENT AND SETTING PRIORITIES

This is the point in the nursing process where assessment and planning start blending together. Sharing conclusions with the patient for validation of those conclusions is part of assessment. Setting priorities is part of planning. For the sake of time, however, both activities usually are done together.

The above conclusions were shared with Mrs. Poski. Ken thought about how important it was for the patient to be actively involved in all aspects of care. He also knew that validating conclusions (making sure the patient agreed with the conclusions) was vital before anything else was done. Mrs. Poski agreed that the conclusions matched her perceptions of her needs. She was most interested in the social isolation diagnosis because she was feeling very alone. She helped to set the priority because no conclusion represented an immediately life-threatening problem or a major safety issue. (See Chapter 9 for more details on setting priorities.) Involving the patient in validating conclusions and setting priorities is another example of using INQUIRY.

✔ *Thinking-Learning Check*

Pause here for a thinking-learning check. You should be able to elaborate on these ideas:

✔ Beginning nursing students have a wealth of life experience and thinking skills to draw on and nurture.

✔ Feelings about personal thinking abilities can help or hinder thinking skills.

✔ Ken's thinking can be tracked in all five modes as he collected data and analyzed data (noting first impressions, comparing data with norms, developing initial hunches, finding clusters, thinking about his conclusions, sharing and validating his conclusions, and setting priorities with Mrs. Poski).

CONTINUED TRACKING OF KEN'S THINKING THROUGH THE NURSING PROCESS

Planning Care

In collaboration with Mrs. Poski, Ken developed a plan of care to address *all* the conclusions and build on her existing strengths. For the sake of time, however, only a portion of the complete care plan is presented here. Refer to Sample Care Plan 4-1 as you read about Ken's thinking and planning.

Patient Goals

Examine the care plan. Study it and then continue to read about Ken's thinking as he prepared his plan. First, consider a "Patient Goal". Patient goals give overall direction to thinking about plans. They may be written or they may be just thoughts. There usually is at least one goal for dealing with each health concern. In this case, we will focus on the social isolation health concern. Here is the goal:

By the end of 1 week, Mrs. Poski will have diminished social isolation

The goal is the first thing Ken thought about after the conclusion (nursing diagnosis) "Social Isolation related to increased hearing loss and not wanting to

▼ **Sample Care Plan 4–1**

Student Ken Tanaka   **Date** 9/3/98   **Patient** Mrs. Poski

Nursing Dx. #2

Social Isolation related to (R/T) increased hearing loss and not wanting to bother people

Defining characteristics: Interacting little, previous pattern of being very social, spending much time alone, not wanting to bother people, hearing loss.

Patient Goal Statement:

By the end of 1 week, Mrs. Poski will have diminished social isolation as evidenced by (A.E.B.):

PATIENT OUTCOMES	NURSING INTERVENTIONS	RATIONALE
1. Sharing her thoughts and feelings about her isolation and hearing loss and their affect on her health (9/3/98).	1. Ask her to share her thoughts and feelings about: Her recent social isolation How the isolation affects her emotional health, physical health, and recovery. How her hearing loss affects her isolation	1.a. Identification of pt's feelings is helpful in planning effective behavior change. Assessing pt's insight into relationship between life situations determines where to start interventions.
2. Discussing ways to obtain information without feeling like a bother (9/3/98).	2.a. Assess her feelings about bothering people. b. Explore with her appropriate ways to get info, without feeling like a bother: Tell people at beginning of a conversation that she needs them to speak slowly, clearly, and in normal tone. Ask if other person would mind if she occasionally reminds them to speak up. Carry pad and pen to offer others as needed. c. Role play an interaction with pt.	2.a. Identification of pt's feelings is helpful in planning effective behavior change. b. Mutual problem solving reinforces pt role as partner in care as well as promoting independence. Providing several suggestions allows pt to expand own thinking of solutions and select ideas best suited to individual needs. c. Role play allows pt opportunity to try new behaviors before using with others.
3. Describing changes in her hearing and things that help and hinder her hearing (9/3/98).	3.a. Assessing hearing loss in depth re: Onset, quality, and quantity of change, chronology of change, aggravating and alleviating factors, associated problems.	3.a. Accurate and complete data collection increases probability of accurate conclusions and effective care plan.

▼ **Sample Care Plan 4–1** *continued*

PATIENT OUTCOMES	NURSING INTERVENTIONS	RATIONALE
	b. Ask her to explain what she understands about hearing and hearing problems.	**b.** Assessing what pt knows saves time in teaching and acknowledges pt as a care partner.
4. Agreeing to participate in hearing exam (9/3/98).	**4.a.** Assess her willingness to have hearing exam. **b.** Obtain M.D. order for exam and schedule exam. **c.** Arrange transportation and be sure results are addressed.	**4.a.** Determining level of pt cooperation avoids waste of time and inappropriate referrals. **b.** M.D. needs to order all exams. Nurse needs to schedule exam. **c.** Facilitating pt attendance at exam and follow-up on recommendations increases chances of behavior change.
5. Participating in two activities/day that require interaction with other residents (9/5/98).	**5.a.** Identify with pt which activities she would be most comfortable with: music group, ceramics, bingo, exercise groups, needle crafts. **b.** Plan daily care to allow adequate time for activities. **c.** Monitor pt participation in activities and talk with her afterward to assess what worked and what didn't, and how to modify plans.	**5.a.** Mutual problem solving reinforces pt's role as a partner in care as well as promoting independence. **b.** Providing opportunity for behavior change increases probability of change. **c.** Evaluating pt behavior and adjusting plan as needed increases chance of successful behavior change and resolution of problem.

EVALUATION:	RELEVANT INFORMATION RE: PARTIALLY MET OR UNMET OUTCOMES	
Outcome # 1 (Met)/Partially Met/Unmet Date: 9/3/98	Actions effective.	
Outcome # 2 Met/(Partially Met)/Unmet Date: 9/3/98	Stated hearing loss hard to cope with. Agreed to all except reminding people.	Was receptive to new ideas. Successful role play.
Outcome # 3 (Met)/Partially Met/Unmet Date: 9/3/98	Helps: Facing patient while speaking, speaking slowly and distinctly in a moderate voice tone. Hinders: High-pitched voice, environmental noise, and lots of people talking in the same room.	

▼ **Sample Care Plan 4–1** *continued*

EVALUATION:	RELEVANT INFORMATION RE: PARTIALLY MET OR UNMET OUTCOMES
Outcome # 4 (Met)/Partially Met/Unmet Date: 9/5/98	Hearing exam scheduled with Dr. Otology for 9/10/98, 10 AM. Son will provide transportation.
Outcome # 5 Met/(Partially Met)/Unmet Date: 9/6/98	Prefers one activity/day for now. Enjoyed the music group. Bingo was too noisy. Will try ceramics and exercise next week.
Outcome # _____ Met/Partially Met/Unmet Date: _____	
Outcome # _____ Met/Partially Met/Unmet Date: _____	

bother people," was validated with the patient and by the data. While developing the goal for socialization, Ken thought about socialization and how personal an issue it was. He knew it was important to have Mrs. Poski develop the plan with him. They agreed that a decrease in social isolation was a reasonable goal to achieve in a week's time.

Patient Outcomes

It wasn't enough just to have the broad goal of decreasing the social isolation problem. The factors contributing to the problem had to be addressed as well.

Looking at those factors, Ken thought about smaller increments of change in Mrs. Poski's behavior that ultimately would reduce her social isolation by eliminating or diminishing the contributing factors. If Mrs. Poski could meet these small increments (patient outcomes), Ken, other nurses, and Mrs. Poski would have tangible evidence that progress toward the goal was being made. For the first outcome, it was important for Mrs. Poski to talk about her feelings. Then, she needed to figure out how to interact without feeling as if she were bothering others. Three other outcomes were developed (see outcomes 3, 4, and 5 on the plan). Ken studied the set of outcomes and, using INQUIRY, asked himself, "Are these outcomes reasonable? Are they measurable? Are they client-centered? Do they address all of the etiologies of the diagnostic statement? If they are achieved, will the goal be met?"

Ken got his ideas for these outcomes from studying the related factors that were contributing to her social isolation and thinking about realistic steps that Mrs. Poski could take to alleviate some of those factors. He also could have found a book, such as the *Nursing Outcomes Classification* (Johnson & Maas, 1997), looked up the nursing diagnosis "Social Isolation.....," read the links between that diagnosis and outcomes, and found suggestions for outcomes that way. You may recall that this resource was discussed in Chapter 3. For example, Ken could have selected the NOC outcomes "Social Support" and "Well Being" to monitor the impact of interventions performed on Mrs. Poski's social isolation status. A baseline measure of these outcomes should be taken at the current visit and each visit thereafter to ascertain changes. The NOC outcomes are five-point scales, not goal statements. This format allows the nurse to assess progress on an outcome over time. If progress is not occurring in the intended direction, interventions can be adjusted and readjusted until the desired changes are achieved.

Nursing Interventions

Once the outcomes were developed, Ken designed the nursing interventions (the middle column in the sample care plan) that would help Mrs. Poski achieve the outcomes to meet the goal. The nursing interventions specifically identify what Ken and other nurses needed to do to increase the probability of Mrs. Poski achieving the outcomes to meet the goal and resolve the problem.

The plan so far may look like a neat package, but not all nurses think or work in this sequence. Sometimes, for some problems, nurses think about the nursing interventions before they think about patient outcomes. This will not seem backward if one remembers that the nursing process is not a linear set of steps. The best way to achieve open thinking with the nursing process is to remember that all the pieces are interrelated, intertwined, and inseparable. The order in which they are written down on paper is rarely an exact replication of the patterns of thinking that produced the plan. In this case, it made more sense to Ken to decide first where Mrs. Poski should be going than to figure out how to get there. Therefore, he developed the goal and outcomes before the nursing interventions. He could have figured out what the nurses needed to do and then related that to what the patient should be achieving. Some books (eg, Smeltzer & Bare, 1992) present care plans with the nursing actions or interventions column preceding the expected outcomes column. Others (eg, McFarland & McFarlane, 1997) put outcomes first, as Ken did. As long as the final plan is consistent in its relationships of goals to outcomes and nursing interventions, the order in which the parts are constructed in the nurse's mind or on paper is unimportant. KNOWING HOW YOU THINK is a mode to use when making decisions about *your* "logical" way to approach planning.

Supporting Rationale for Nursing Interventions

As a student nurse, Ken couldn't just pull the nursing interventions out of a hat (or his head). He used his textbooks to help him find interventions based on sound rationales (reasons). Also, because he was a student who needed to show his thinking to his instructor, he wrote the rationale down next to each nursing intervention (see the right-hand column on the care plan example). *Note:* Many instructors also require students to write down the reference they used for each rationale. For example, for the nursing intervention, "use mild soap," the documented rationale with a reference could read: "these contain no detergents, dyes, or hardening agents" (Smeltzer & Bare, 1992, p. 1456).

There are many sources of information in which students and nurses can find ideas for interventions and rationales. In Ken's case he used his textbooks. There also are books that are focused entirely on care plans. In recent years, as you may recall from discussions in Chapter 3, there has been *Nursing Interventions Classification* (McCloskey & Bulechek, 1996), which categorizes the nursing interventions performed by nurses from all specialties.

Developing the nursing interventions required Ken to use TOTAL RECALL, INQUIRY, and NEW IDEAS AND CREATIVITY modes of thinking. If Ken were an experienced nurse, some interventions would have been HABITS in his mind. Because he was a student, he had not developed nursing intervention HABITS yet. TOTAL RECALL was used when he remembered which books to use, which lectures notes to check, and which nursing care references to locate. He used INQUIRY to make decisions about which nursing interventions were appropriate for Mrs. Poski's care and which were not. He used NEW IDEAS AND CREATIVITY to select the nursing interventions found in a textbook to use as printed and/or appropriately adapt them to Mrs. Poski's unique situation.

Ken repeated the process of planning for the remaining three nursing diagnoses, Self-Care Deficit for Bathing and Dressing related to generalized weakness secondary to decreased nutrition and prolonged diarrhea post flu; Risk for Injury related to generalized weakness, poor balance, and unstable transfers from bed to wheelchair; and Risk for Impaired Skin Integrity related to immobility, frail skin, and inadequate nutrition. These parts of the plan are not included here but, as a review, see what you can do with one of these diagnoses.

⊃Action Learning #20: Developing a Goal and Outcomes

Look at the diagnosis "Self-Care Deficit ... ." What do you think would be an appropriate goal for Ken and Mrs. Poski to be working toward in trying to resolve this problem?

Goal:

What do you think would be one of the outcomes that would show Mrs. Poski was moving toward the goal?

Outcome:

What resources would you use to decide what is appropriate nursing care for this problem?

THINK ABOUT THIS ▪ What was the hardest part about doing this Action Learning exercise? Often, students say it was coming up with concise wording that really said what they wanted it to say. Many students find the wording a challenge at first. Do not despair; you will find that after you have written goals and outcomes for a while, you learn there are patterns to the wording. The goal usually is a restatement of the words in the problem, indicating that the problem is "fixed." (By the end of 1 week Mrs. Poski will have increased her self-care ability.) The outcomes usually are restatements of the words in the related factors, indicating that they are not related factors any more. (Demonstrates ability to bathe and dress self without assistance in 1 hour and not feel worn out.) Note the word "usually" in these sentences. There are no hard and fast rules, only general guidelines. Developing goals and outcomes is addressed more fully in Chapter 9.

More Planning

Planning for Other Conclusions in Addition to Nursing Diagnoses

Back to Ken and Mrs. Poski. In addition to planning the care for all the nursing diagnoses (Social Isolation, Self-Care Deficit, Risk for Injury, and Risk for Impaired Skin Integrity), Ken reviewed his other conclusions. For the hearing problem, he left a note for Mrs. Poski's physician, recommending that her hearing be evaluated. For the nutrition problem, Ken talked to the dietitian, and together they developed an interdisciplinary plan. Likewise, he talked to the physical therapist and learned about realistic mobility goals. The recommendations from the physical therapist were added to the part of the nursing plan that focused on risks for injury and self-care deficits. Some agencies call these collaborative, interdisciplinary, or master treatment plans.

Ken thought about the best way to communicate these parts of the plan to other nurses. He could have developed a specific nursing plan for the mobility and balance problems, but the nursing interventions would have overlapped those on the plan for self-care and preventing injury. To avoid duplication of effort, he picked what he saw as the most logical part of the plan in which to incorporate the recommendations for increasing mobility and balance.

The issues of unstable transfer, poor balance, and weakness were all parts of Mrs. Poski's mobility problems. If Ken had included interventions and outcomes for improved mobility in all parts of the care plan where mobility was a related factor, he would have rewritten the same things several times. To avoid this duplication, he chose to include mobility outcomes and interventions in his plan for the self-care deficit problem. In the other plans, then, he merely said "refer to self care plan for mobility issues." INQUIRY was used to make these decisions about where to write what. Chapter 8 ("Making More Sense Out of the Clues: Cluster Analysis") provides details on the thinking required to consolidate care planning.

Streamlining Care Plans

Decisions about where to write on a plan are sometimes very individual. Nurses do not have time to duplicate efforts, yet they want to make sure that others understand what they and the patient are trying to achieve. Sometimes it is necessary to refer to another part of the plan, for example, "See plan for safety." One thing that will soon become obvious, if it hasn't already, is the interconnectedness of human responses. Few things fit into tidy boxes. The interventions to alleviate one problem usually affect another problem.

Nurses streamline plans to communicate complexities simply (Fig. 4-1). Experienced nurses can shorten plans because they can assume that other experienced nurses have the knowledge necessary to fill in the details. Although it is necessary, streamlining should be approached cautiously. Too little streamlining can cause redundancies and use up too much time; too much streamlining can leave out something important. Students are expected to err on the side of too little streamlining, because they must show what they are learning. As experience is gained, skill in

FIGURE 4-1 Streamlining.

▼ **Sample Care Plan 4–2**

Patient: Mrs. Poski

Nursing Diagnosis #3 Risk for Injury related to generalized weakness, poor balance, and unstable transfers from bed to wheelchair.

GOALS AND OUTCOMES	NURSING INTERVENTIONS
9/3/98 **Goal:** Pt will have no injuries during stay in N.H. **Outcomes** 1. Exhibit enough strength to hold herself up during transfers by 9/9/98 2. Maintain balance during transfers by 9/9/98 3. Demonstrate safe pivot transfers by 9/9/98	1. Reinforce exercises recommended by physical therapist, especially on weekends. 2. Encourage ball squeezing for 10 min tid 3. Remind pt to do body lifting while in chair q 1 hr. 4. Teach pt about keeping feet apart to maintain balance during transfers. Remind pt not to over-lean. 5. Show pt how to transfer by sliding bottom forward on chair, leaning forward, pushing down on arms of chair, and moving hips to new position. 6. Stand-by assist during transfers. Remind pt to call for help before getting up.

streamlining will improve. Below is what a streamlined part of the plan might look like for the problem, "Risk for Injury related to generalized weakness, poor balance, and unstable transfers from bed to wheelchair." Notice that although there is a reference to physical therapy exercises, the specifics are not duplicated. The rationale for each intervention is not written on the plan; it is assumed that experienced nurses know the rationale for their interventions. There are fewer details in the interventions, and the specific interventions are not linked directly to specific outcomes. They are addressed collectively.

Implementing Care

Ken began implementing the plan of care as soon as he and Mrs. Poski agreed it was appropriate. During implementation he continued to assess and also think about how well the plan was working (evaluation). This is another example of how phases of the nursing process overlap. Checking for effectiveness of the plan as the plan is being implemented is a sign of a thinking nurse.

Evaluating Care

The evaluation process actually began when Ken and Mrs. Poski developed outcomes during the planning phase. It is these outcomes that become the criteria for judging changes in patient behaviors after care is provided.

Here is Ken's thinking when he evaluated the implemented plan. First, he thought about the time that was required and compared it with the planned time for the goals and outcomes. When the expected dates for the outcomes on the plan arrived, he reviewed each outcome for that date and asked himself, "Has that outcome been met by Mrs. Poski?" He compared the data he had about Mrs. Poski with what he and Mrs. Poski planned as outcomes. They decided whether each outcome was met, partially met, or not met, and he recorded this information on the patient record.

Look at the evaluation section at the end of the sample plan for Mrs. Poski's social isolation problem. In the left column, notice the circled conclusions about each outcome. In the right column are Ken's comments supporting his conclusions.

Ken's written comments for each outcome serve two functions of evaluation. First, they address the specific patient behaviors that indicate whether or not the outcome was met (this is called outcome evaluation). Second, the comments address how effective the nursing interventions were (this is called process evaluation).

Ken used INQUIRY to do the evaluation. He questioned what he saw, made decisions about the quality of care, and thought about what should and could be done to improve the care. He did this not only for the diagnosis of Social Isolation, but for the whole plan, along with all of the conclusions.

In some ways, evaluation is similar to the initial data collection. Evaluation makes the nursing process a cycle as the nurse moves back to collecting data and, from that data, draws conclusions. These conclusions become the basis for new or changed plans for care. This process continues until all the problems are resolved or the patient is discharged from service.

✔ *Thinking-Learning Check*

Pause here for a thinking-learning check. You should be able to elaborate on these ideas:

✔ Planning includes working with the patient to set priorities and establish goals and outcomes, develop nursing interventions, support nursing interventions with rationales, and write out a care plan.

✔ Streamlined care plans are used by experienced nurses to save time and energy while maintaining high-quality planning.

✔ During implementation of care the nurse continuously assesses and evaluates the results of care.

✔ Evaluation of care involves identifying the impact of nursing interventions on patient outcomes, tracking both the status of desired outcomes over time and the interventions performed with the patient.

REEXAMINING YOUR THINKING ABOUT THE NURSING PROCESS

This chapter, long though it may have seemed, is only the beginning of tracking thinking and using the nursing process. It was designed to show the whole of the nursing process, not *all* the details. However, the missing details may have stimulated many questions for those of you who are developing the finer points of your INQUIRY skills. The thinking log for this chapter was designed to acknowledge your INQUIRY by allowing you to put those questions in writing.

THINKING LOG #4 ➤

Given the large amount of information in this chapter, the complexity of the nursing process, and the thinking that goes into using the nursing process, it is likely that you have identified areas about which you are still fuzzy. List five questions that you now have about *thinking* and the *nursing process*.

References

Johnson, M. & Maas, M. (Eds.) (1997). *Nursing outcomes classification (NOC)*. St Louis: Mosby.

McCloskey, J.C. & Bulechek, G.M. (Eds.) (1996). *Nursing interventions classification (NIC)*. St. Louis: Mosby.

McFarland, G.K., & McFarlane, E.A. (1997). *Nursing diagnosis and intervention* (3rd ed.). St. Louis: Mosby.

Smeltzer, S.C. & Bare, B.G. (1992). *Brunner and Suddarth's textbook of medical-surgical nursing* (7th ed.). Philadelphia: JB Lippincott.

5

Nursing Conclusions

✳ *Learning Outcomes*

After reading and doing the activities in this chapter you will be able to:

Describe the purpose and characteristics of nursing conclusions.

Examine existing conclusion-making skills.

Explain the relationships among hunches, directed data collection, and ruling in and ruling out hunches.

Appreciate the thinking required to develop nursing conclusions with the highest probability of accuracy.

The last four chapters have focused on the big picture of thinking and doing and the nursing process. Now it is time to start looking at the specifics. Nursing conclusions will be discussed first. Conclusions are judgments made after thinking. This chapter examines the purpose of nursing conclusions, the importance of addressing conclusions at the beginning of a study of thinking and the nursing process, several characteristics of nursing conclusions, and the thinking required to develop conclusions.

THE PURPOSE OF NURSING CONCLUSIONS

The overriding purpose of nursing conclusions is to guide effective and efficient nursing care, that is, great nursing. Achieving such nursing care can be challenging because there are so many pieces of information about patients and their situations that the nurse has to address. The nurse needs to make sense of all the information instead of just remembering the individual pieces. The "sense" the nurse makes results in conclusions, which lead to even more conclusions.

Conclusions are part of all phases of the nursing process. Some of those conclusions are major ones; others are smaller steps along the way. With assessment, for example, the major conclusions provide direction for planning great nursing care, but there are many intermediate conclusions leading to the major ones.

WHY LEARN ABOUT CONCLUSIONS AT THE BEGINNING?

It may seem that discussing the details of conclusions before describing the earlier parts of the nursing process, such as data collection, is illogical. By studying conclusions first, however, one can see where one is going. If that destination is known, it is easier to figure out how to get there.

Where one is going is not actually an end point. Most conclusions in nursing are more like rest stops on a journey; they provide guidance for travel along the nursing process path. Consider a driving trip from New York to California. A decision is needed for the first day's end point; otherwise, one might be stuck with no hotel room. If Pittsburgh is selected as the first stop, it allows for some detail planning for the best way to get there at the end of the journey's first day. Likewise, in the nursing process, interim "end points" allow the nurse to move on a well-designed path from data to nursing care.

The conclusions made during the assessment phase of the nursing process are stop-overs that feed into planning. Conclusions made during planning feed into implementation. The conclusions reached during implementation result in evaluation; conclusions from evaluation feed back into planning, and, often, back to assessment. At each of these points, and at other such points in the nursing process, the conclusions represent the nurse's thinking about the information at hand (Fig. 5-1).

PERSONAL CONCLUSION-MAKING STYLE

Because everybody thinks, everybody makes conclusions all the time. Many scholarly dissertations have been written on conclusion making, but what is important here is to get a sense of your personal conclusion-making style. Think about the conclusions you made today—conclusions about what to wear, what to have for breakfast, what to think of the class you are attending, and so forth. And this barely begins to enumerate the numerous conclusions you make on a daily basis. But, have you ever thought about how you come to those conclusions? It is time to use the KNOWING HOW YOU THINK mode.

⊃ACTION LEARNING #21: Tracking Your Thinking Through a Conclusion

Think of an *important* conclusion that you made recently. Write out the process you went through to arrive at the conclusion, paying special attention to what you were thinking *and* how you were thinking. Consider how your conclusion making might have been tailored to the importance of the conclusion. In other words, do you think differently about important conclusions than you do about less important ones? (Reminder: the *how* of thinking can be described with the vocabulary listed in Display 1-2, "Vocabulary for Thinking About Thinking"— assume, infer, interpret, distinguish, perspective, point of view, and so forth.)

THINK ABOUT THIS ■ What did you learn about the process you use for developing conclusions? Does the process vary depending on the situation or the importance of the conclusion? How easy was it to track the *how* of your thinking? As you recall the discussions of nursing in the previous chapters, can you project what parts of your present conclusion-making thinking you will bring to nursing?

FIGURE 5–1 Thinking about nursing conclusions.

NURSING CONCLUSIONS

Nursing conclusions are made the same way conclusions are made in other areas of life. It is important to see these similarities to build on existing skills and not assume that this is a whole new process to learn. After reading about the characteristics of nursing conclusions, the process used to develop nursing conclusions, and the thinking required, compare them with your existing process of making non-nursing conclusions. Some of you may decide that they match very closely; some may discover it is time to enhance and modify your approaches.

Characteristics of Nursing Conclusions

Judgments

Nursing conclusions are judgments formed after thinking about patient data and the relationships among those data. Those judgments form the basis of care. They are part of all phases of the nursing process—assessing, planning, implementing, and evaluating. Nurses make conclusions about patients' needs before they intervene; they make conclusions about patients' strengths and health concerns, how the patient is progressing, and what changes are needed in the care.

Evidence of Thinking

Nursing conclusions, written or verbal, demonstrate evidence of thinking. The necessity of designing care based on conclusions "forces" thinking. The thinking that is required to develop conclusions is discussed in much greater detail later in this chapter. For now, suffice it to say that conclusions reflect the nurse's thinking ability in collecting adequate data, logically analyzing the data, appropriately identifying a label to describe the patient's concerns or state of health, effectively planning, implementing, and evaluating care, and evaluating patient outcomes.

Conclusions are made by analyzing pieces of data and clusters of data. It would be impractical to act on individual bits of information. Think about that for a minute: if a child were crying, one would not act on the crying without getting more information. One would find the source of anguish—whether it was a stubbed toe, a lost toy, or a lost child. Acting on individual pieces of information would be a waste of time and would be potentially harmful because one might be acting prematurely or misinterpreting the problem.

Probability Statements

Nursing conclusions are probability statements. Probability refers to the chances of something occurring. There are many familiar examples of conclusions that are probability statements. The weather forecast is one example. Meteorologists can conclude that an area of the country will get rain by nightfall by using such information as the weather in other parts of the country, temperature patterns, wind velocity and patterns, and past experience with similar weather conditions. Ultimately, they put all of that together and arrive at a conclusion—"70%

chance of rain in the next 24 hours." The percentage is an indication of the probability for accuracy. The higher the percentage, the higher the probability of accuracy.

There are few conclusions, especially those made about human behavior, that have 100% probability of accuracy. However, it is important, sometimes vital, that nurses make conclusions with the highest possible probability. The patient's health and well-being are at stake. High-probability conclusions depend on high-level thinking. Methods to increase the probability of accuracy are discussed later in this chapter.

The Process of Making Conclusions

Some beginning students believe that the process of making nursing conclusions consists of finding the "right" label in a book, writing it down, copying the corresponding care plan, and putting it into action. Unfortunately, the standard conclusions presented in textbooks do not correspond exactly to all patients. Textbooks provide lists of labels for existing nursing diagnoses and lists of the typical signs and symptoms that a patient may demonstrate to qualify for a particular label. But what about all the early- and intermediate-level conclusions that the nurse needs to make to get to the point of selecting one label or another? And what about all the conclusions that need to be made after that label is selected? Don't bother looking; these early- and intermediate-level conclusions are not in the books. There aren't enough resources to address all individual patient situations.

To make conclusions at all levels accurately and efficiently, the nurse must learn an effective conclusion-making process. Again, a nursing conclusion-making process is best learned by enhancing the existing conclusion-making process used in everyday life. A simple example of developing a conclusion follows:

> Mei Song, age 10, has not been feeling well for the last 24 hours.
> Her eyes are red, her nose is running, and she is sneezing.
> Her mother suspects (has 2 hunches) that she may be getting a cold or that her allergies may be acting up.
> To determine which is more likely (more accurate and higher probability), her mother checks things out (collects more data).
> Mei Song doesn't have a temperature, so her mother assumes it probably is not a cold (rules out an infectious process).
> Her mother remembers that it is the time of year that the ragweed is worst, and Mei is allergic to ragweed.
> Her mother gives her the prescribed allergy medicine.
> Mei Song feels much better by dinner time (the accuracy of her mother's conclusion was very high because the intervention worked).

Hunches

In this example, the term "hunch" is used. A hunch is an early-level conclusion or a "possible" conclusion. Hunches are stimulated in many ways. Sometimes a critical piece of information (the allergy history) points to an obvious conclusion because "that's always found with this problem." At other times it is the volume of related pieces of data that points to an "obvious" conclusion. For example, if a patient has pain and difficulty with bowel movements 4 days in a row, when normally he has no problems moving his bowels daily, it is fairly easy to see that "constipation" is a good hunch on the path toward a final conclusion.

Sometimes it is not the significance or the amount of data as much as it is a "gut feeling" or a "sixth sense" that leads to hunches. These gut feelings or sixth senses comprise intuition, and should not be ignored. (You may want to review the discussion of intuition in Chapter 1 [p. 10].) Intuition is being studied with more interest lately. Expert nurses often confide that they do things intuitively. Their thinking skills are so fine-tuned that various levels of thinking occur beyond conscious awareness. It is difficult to explain this thinking by breaking it into steps. Their intuition allows these nurses to make accurate conclusions quickly and seemingly effortlessly; it almost looks like magic. Remember, however, as you admire these "expert" intuitive nurses, that they started at the same point that you did.

Hunches are very important pieces of thinking that lead to accurate final conclusions. Because expert nurses make hunches so automatically, their hunches rarely get discussed, let alone written down anywhere. Thus, hunches rarely get the credit they deserve as significant parts of the thinking process.

Although having and acknowledging hunches is very important, they also must be approached cautiously. "Gut-level" hunches can be triggered by nurse biases or prejudices about certain groups of people. Therefore, a hunch that is not obviously data related should be questioned. If, for example, a nurse has a hunch that a patient would not understand something, that nurse should mentally ask, "Am I thinking that because the patient is young (old), of a certain ethnic group (or not)?" and so forth. Everyone has biases; they become problematic if they are not recognized and challenged.

It is especially important for beginning nurses to acknowledge hunches and nurture their development. Nurturing hunch development can be achieved by writing the hunches as "possible" conclusions. "Possible social isolation," "Possible activity intolerance," "Possible vision problems," and "Possibly delayed development" are examples of how to write hunches (early conclusions).

⊃Action Learning #22: Hunch Development

Read the following situation and write down at least three hunches you have about why this man is not taking his medication.

Mr. Hernandez, a 48-year-old widower and insurance salesperson who travels quite a bit, has been coming to the clinic to have his blood pressure checked every 3 to 4 weeks because he was diagnosed with high blood pressure 6 months ago. At the last visit, Allie Bahe, student nurse, found Mr. Hernandez's blood pressure to be quite a bit higher than usual. She asked Mr. Hernandez if he had been taking his medication as directed, and got this reply, "Well, I know I should, but I didn't take it every day last week; I guess I shouldn't do that." He quickly changed the subject and told Allie about his fiancée, Maria, and about all the social events they had attended lately because of Maria's move to a new modeling agency. He said, with a huge smile, "I feel like a new man these days; I may even be a father again soon."

Hunch #1: Possible ...

Hunch #2: Possible ...

Hunch #3: Possible ...

THINK ABOUT THIS ■ Did some things "jump out" at you, or did you really have to dig to come up with hunches? How strong were your "gut feelings?" If they were strong, why do you think they were? Do you know anyone like Mr. Hernandez?

Consider and compare these hunches about the factors that might be related to Mr. Hernandez's apparent nonadherence to his medication regimen. Think about why a nurse might have these hunches.

Possibly:

- When not feeling bad, he doesn't take the medicine, thinking he would feel bad if his blood pressure were high.
- He thinks high blood pressure is an old man's problem and he feels too young for it.

- He is very busy and forgets to take the medicine.
- When he is traveling, his schedule is unusual and he forgets to take it.
- He is experiencing the side effect of impotence and may be reluctant to talk about it.
- The label on the medicine says not to take it with alcohol and he drinks during social occasions.

Ruling In and Ruling Out

When there are several hunches about one issue, the nurse must differentiate among them to determine which one(s) is (are) the most accurate conclusion(s) about that one situation. This process of differentiation is called "validating hunches" or "ruling in and ruling out" (Fig. 5-2). Collectively, the process of identifying two or more possible conclusions about one situation, distinguishing among them, and arriving at the most accurate conclusion is called "differential diagnosing." This makes sense when one considers that diagnoses are conclusions, and "differential" means "distinguishing among possibilities." A nurse's ability to make differential diagnoses (multiple hunches about one situation) and rule hunches "in" or "out" is directly connected to that nurse's ability to make accurate conclusions. Without accurate conclusions, the rest of the care plan is a waste of time and money for the patient, the nurse, and the health care delivery system.

One of the classic methods for determining which hunches are best to keep and which are best to drop (process of validating hunches) is called *directed data collection*. Gaps in the data picture are identified and the gaps are filled in to give a more complete picture of the patient situation. The additional data collected are "directed" toward supporting or not supporting the hunch(es).

FIGURE 5–2 Ruling in and ruling out.

An example: It is the end of the shift and a new patient is transferred to the unit. The assigned nurse starts to collect data and finds that the patient is breathing very hard after moving from wheelchair to bed. The nurse suspects the patient has Activity Intolerance, but there is not enough information yet to determine that for certain. In this case, the nurse might write on the chart, "possible Activity Intolerance" with a note, "data gap regarding patient's vital signs during exertion."

To know what additional data are needed, beginners usually go to books that have lists of defining characteristics (signs and symptoms or objective and subjective data) for each nursing conclusion (in this case, "Activity Intolerance"). The patient needs to be observed and questioned to determine whether he or she has any of the classic defining characteristics of "activity intolerance" that match those listed in the book. If the patient's data do not fit well, an alternative hunch must be made about an alternative nursing diagnosis. Differential diagnoses in this case could be "Fatigue" or "Impaired Gas Exchange."

Look at the cartoon sequence in Figure 5-3 and explain to a classmate what is being illlustrated.

FIGURE 5–3 Thinking for one of many nursing conclusions.

Which thoughts of the nurse represent analysis as opposed to data?

Where is the nurse demonstrating directed data collection?

How is the nurse seeking validation from the patient?

What can the nurse do to identify data gaps if a nursing diagnosis book is not handy?

What would the nurse do if the patient did not agree with the nurse's conclusion of Sleep Pattern Disturbance?

If you were asked to continue the cartoon, what would be the next logical step in the conclusion-making process once a nursing diagnostic label was validated?

⊃Action Learning #23: Ruling In and Ruling Out Hunches

Look at the hunches you made in Action Learning #22. What additional data (identifying data gaps) would you need to collect from Mr. Hernandez to rule in or rule out those hunches? (Hint: Use your nursing diagnoses texts to look up each of your hunches and compare your data with the defining characteristics listed. Defining characteristics are the pieces of information that support or justify your conclusions.)

Hunch #1 Data Gaps:

Hunch #2 Data Gaps:

Hunch #3 Data Gaps:

> **THINK ABOUT THIS** ■ How did you figure out what additional data were needed? How would you obtain those additional data? How does your experience and knowledge about hypertension, hypertensive medication and its side effects, and middle-aged Hispanic men affect your ability to make hunches and identify data gaps? Could you make any decisions on "ruling in" or "ruling out" at this point? This process of directed data collection to rule in or rule out is discussed further in Chapter 8.

Accuracy and Conclusions

Achieving accuracy in your conclusions *does not mean finding the "one" right answer.* Accuracy means selecting a conclusion that has the highest probability of matching and making sense out of the raw data. It is very important to aim for the highest accuracy because it saves time and allows care planning to focus on the "best" strengths and health concerns. If the focus of care is blurry, the nurse's and patient's time and energy are wasted. Meanwhile, an unidentified problem may be getting worse.

Lunney (1990) developed a scale for degrees of accuracy when examining nursing diagnoses. Her scale ranges from +5 to -1. Nursing diagnoses with a +5 rating have highly relevant data, are precisely worded to reflect the patient's health concern, and have a diagnostic label that is consistent with all the clues. A diagnosis rated -1 may have one clue to support it but has at least two that disconfirm that label.

Although one certainly wants to aim for +5 accuracy, it is important to remember that conclusions are rarely 100% accurate because they are probability statements. There is a certain probability that this or that is the most accurate conclusion to make. In some cases, nurses can be 99.99% sure, but in other cases they have to live with lower odds. The odds of accuracy usually are increased with more data, but not always. Nurses cannot collect data forever; eventually they have to start making conclusions.

Because collecting volumes of data is not always possible or realistic, nurses can increase accuracy by looking for critical data. Critical data (also called critical indicators) are clearly more significant than others. Here is an example: the nurse sees a patient wringing his hands, sweating, and pacing, and has a hunch that the patient is anxious. The probability of that hunch being accurate is perhaps somewhere around 50%. Now, when the patient says, "I'm really anxious," the probability jumps much higher. The statement by the patient is a critical indicator because it is clearly significant for the anxiety conclusion. All the other signs (wringing hands, sweating, and pacing) have some probability of pointing to something other than anxiety. Without that critical indicator, the probability for accuracy is much lower.

High probability for accuracy is directly related to one's skill with the INQUIRY mode of thinking and one's ability to tolerate ambiguity. Remember, from the vocabulary in Chapter 1, "ambiguous" means "having multiple meanings or possible interpretations." INQUIRY skill is necessary to ask the best questions: Do the data support this hunch? What data would make this a stronger hunch? Which data do not support this hunch?

Without adequate use of INQUIRY, diagnoses will be less accurate. Lunney (1990) characterized low-accuracy diagnoses as based on unreliable, invalid, or conflicting cues. They also are less accurate when they are not validated with the patient and when too few differential diagnoses have been considered.

The issue of probability forces one to acknowledge ambiguity in conclusion making. Ambiguity and tolerance for ambiguity can be challenging for many, especially for those who prefer to see the world as having only "right" or "wrong" answers to questions. It is not uncommon for beginning college students, nursing students included, to demonstrate this style of thinking, which is called "dualistic." A "right" or "wrong" perspective for finding answers is, however, extremely unusual for the expert nurse. Expert nurses use more relativistic thinking, which allows for gradations in perspective (awful, poor, good, better, best) and seeing the many shades of green instead of just "yellow" and "blue." The expert not only has learned to deal with ambiguity, but has fine-tuned his or her data collection skills to achieve conclusions with high probabilities of accuracy.

⊃ACTION LEARNING #24: KNOWING HOW YOU THINK About Ambiguity

An awareness of your tolerance for ambiguity will add to your self-understanding. Think about how you feel in situations in which you cannot fit things into neat "boxes." For example, you have a thousand dollars and a week of vacation time. You want to make the most of your time and money; you also know that your car is going to need new brakes in the next six months. What do you do? On a scale of 1 to 10, with 10 being the most relativistic (able to accept the gradations), mark where you think you are comfortable now.

Dualistic	Relativistic
(only "right" or "wrong")	(accepts gradations)

1 - - - - 2 - - - - 3 - - - - 4 - - - - 5 - - - - 6 - - - - 7 - - - - 8 - - - - 9 - - - - 1 0

THINK ABOUT THIS ■ Do you think you are in a good place? Does your dualistic or relativistic perspective vary depending on the situation? Do you think you need to learn to think more relativistically? You will likely find nursing most "comfortable" if you are tolerant of ambiguity and practice relativistic thinking.

Validating Conclusions

When one considers the importance of the patient's verbal report in the earlier anxiety example, it is clear that asking patients about their perceptions is critical to increasing accuracy. In Chapter 1 we discussed the importance of patients' thinking. Their part of the critical thinking situation must never be ignored—not when data are being collected and not when conclusions are being made.

One way to increase the accuracy of conclusions is to validate conclusions with patients (or their significant others, if it cannot be done directly with the patient). Validation also can be achieved by involving the patient directly in formulating the conclusion. The nurse might say something like this to the patient: "It seems to me that these are your strengths and your problems [name the strengths and problems], and these are the things contributing to the problems. What do you think?" It is surprising how different and how similar patients' and nurses' conclusions can be sometimes. As you validate conclusions with patients, you soon see the value of this process.

Another major value of validation is that patients have more control over their care, and nurses do not spin their wheels on problems that patients do not think exist. This seems so logical; however, it is surprising how little validation goes on in health care.

✔ *Thinking-Learning Check*

Pause here for a thinking-learning check. You should be able to elaborate on these ideas:

- ✔ The purpose of conclusions: to guide effective and efficient nursing care (ie, great nursing)
- ✔ The value of studying conclusions at the beginning of a study of the nursing process
- ✔ Transferring conclusion-making skills from everyday life to making nursing conclusions
- ✔ Nursing conclusions as judgments based on thinking, evidence of thinking, and probability statements
- ✔ The process of making conclusions: having hunches, ruling in and ruling out hunches, and validating for accuracy
- ✔ Differential diagnoses: identifying all possible conclusions about one situation
- ✔ Directed data collection: identifying and filling data gaps for all conclusions
- ✔ Ruling in and ruling out: making decisions about which conclusions are the most accurate

TYPES OF THINKING REQUIRED TO DEVELOP NURSING CONCLUSIONS

Many people say "critical thinking" is the key ingredient in making the best nursing conclusions. If critical thinking is defined broadly enough to incorporate all modes of thinking, then that is true. All five thinking modes are necessary to develop accurate conclusions and act on them. Each mode adds an important piece to the process of conclusion making and clinical judgments. Some studies have shown that subjects who demonstrate good critical thinking do not necessarily have good clinical judgment (Kintgen-Andrews, 1991; Miller & Malcolm, 1990). It is a bit like having a lot of "book smarts" but no "common sense." The five modes of thinking must work together to produce skillful clinical judgments.

Total Recall

Think about the *thinking* involved in the conclusion-making process. TOTAL RECALL is used to remember factors that usually go together—cold weather and sweaters, for example, or frail skin, immobility, and incontinence as risk factors for decubitus ulcers. Other information recalled from textbooks may relate to usual clusters of data or critical indicators of certain problems. All of this RECALL knowledge is vital to making accurate conclusions.

Habits

Certain conclusions can easily become HABITS—when nurses see a confused person, they almost always conclude that safety must be addressed. One or two factors just automatically lead to certain conclusions. HABIT-type conclusions can save time and generally reflect conclusions that nurses have made many times with similar sets of information. Although HABITS save time, they also have limitations; they can lead too easily to prejudicial conclusions if the nurse is not careful. Not all old patients are senile, but some people might quickly jump to the conclusion of senility based only on a knowledge of the patient's age.

Inquiry

Although INQUIRY alone is not the whole of critical thinking, it is the "guts" of conclusion making. This kind of thinking is required to make complicated conclusions and important ones. Mentally, nurses put together pieces of information, make early conclusions (hunches), question the validity or completeness of the early conclusions, identify data gaps, use directed data collection to fill those gaps, revise, and make final conclusions. INQUIRY helps nurses keep an open mind to many possible interpretations of data, and keeps them collecting relevant data. But, remember, it is not the amount of data, but the quality of the data that is most important. Thinking about which data provide the best picture helps a nurse to achieve accuracy. Knowing what is needed is not easily figured out. It depends largely on one's knowledge, or TOTAL RECALL (remembering and retrieving that knowledge) about nursing care, biology, psychology, sociology, physiology, and all those other "-ologies" that nurses are required to study.

Knowledge helps nurses avoid a pitfall associated with INQUIRY. INQUIRY, like HABITS, can be a double-edged sword; nurses, especially novices, can get in a rut of endless data collection in the hope of developing the most accurate conclusions, so that they never get to the actual conclusion. At some point, data collection has to be interrupted so that something can be done for the patient. The key is to know when there are enough data. Inquiry, combined with knowledge and experience, provides the ability to zero in on critical data. Recognizing and collecting critical data increase efficiency and accuracy. Efficiency is almost as important as accuracy. The next chapter focuses on how to collect the best data to make the most accurate conclusions efficiently.

New Ideas and Creativity

Some of the best and most innovative conclusions are developed by people with a well developed thinking mode of NEW IDEAS AND CREATIVITY. The NEW IDEAS AND CREATIVITY mode allows a nurse to see different relationships among pieces of data and to consider options not in the books. Thinking in this mode leads to conclusions that are most closely suited to individual patient needs. Individualized care, care that is uniquely suited to the patient rather than copied out of the book, can be provided only when NEW IDEAS AND CREATIVITY are used in developing conclusions. For example, the "standard" approach for colostomy care is to have the patient irrigate and empty the colostomy in the bathroom. If the patient lives in an area with no indoor plumbing, however, it takes NEW IDEAS AND CREATIVITY to modify the plan to suit the patient's environmental constraints.

Knowing How You Think

Because accurate conclusions are a result of high-quality thinking, the better you understand your thinking, the better the conclusions you will develop. Understanding your thinking requires you to KNOW HOW YOU THINK. It's time for some Action Learning to gain more insight into how much you know about your individual thinking while developing conclusions.

⊃ACTION LEARNING #25: **KNOWING HOW YOU THINK and Developing Conclusions**

Think about and write a response to the following questions about your knowledge of your thinking. Share your answers with a classmate.

Identify one of your assumptions about people. For example: "All people are basically good." Do you ever question that assumption? Why or why not?

Identify one of your biases. For example: "Older people don't like to have to
learn new things." Have you ever identified your biases? Why or why not?

Are your conclusions usually supported with data? Why or why not?

Can you usually see more than one "answer" to a problem? Why or why not?

Do you ever make premature conclusions? Why or why not?

How does your point of view generally fit with the views of other nurses, other
student nurses, and patients? Why does it fit or not fit?

What is the best way for you to analyze data and then see relationships among data and data clusters? Why?

THINK ABOUT THIS ■ Did you notice the similarities between this Action Learning and Action Learning #21 ("Tracking Your Thinking Through a Conclusion")? It is important to do many Action Learning exercises focused on the KNOWING HOW YOU THINK mode because self-analysis is a slow, building-up process. Each time you study yourself, you discover aspects of your thinking that you may not have thought about before. Each new discovery then needs to be addressed in relation to other discoveries.

"CONCLUDING" COMMENTS

The first purpose of this chapter was to emphasize the importance of developing conclusions and to begin to examine the process of making conclusions. Without accurate conclusions, the rest of nursing care is on very shaky ground. The second purpose of this chapter was to develop an awareness of existing conclusion-making skills and build on them. If conclusion making in nursing is viewed as a totally new process to be learned "from scratch," learning the nursing process will be significantly delayed. The Thinking Log for this chapter was designed to nurture this growing awareness of your current skills.

As is probably obvious by this point, thinking and conclusion making take time and energy. At first, the pay-off for the time and energy spent may not seem worthwhile. The value is enormous, however. High-level thinking results in accurate conclusions and provides a basis for nursing care that is individualized to each patient, focused on the highest priorities, time saving, money saving, and safe. Beginners will find that the thinking is long and arduous, but, as with any skill, practice makes it easier and quicker. Accepting the challenge in the beginning pays off down the road to great nursing.

THINKING LOG #5 ➤

This log is an extension of what you did in Action Learning #21 but asks for more in-depth thinking. Keep a written journal of your conclusion making for a 3 to 4 hour period of time during your day. This could involve any part of your day, such as deciding what to eat for breakfast, how to drive to work/school when there is road construction in your neighborhood, buying the latest compact disc, or grocery shopping for the day/week/month. When you have finished your journal, find some colored pencils or markers. Identify the following aspects of your conclusion making in your journal, using yellow for hunches, red for directed data collection, green for ruling in and ruling out, and blue for final conclusions. (If you have only other colors, make a color legend for those four things.) Then do one or both of the following:

Write a short paragraph indicating
1. What you see as your strengths in conclusion making
2. What you could do to enhance your conclusion making skills
3. A plan for how to enhance your skills
AND/OR

Draw a diagram that represents how you incorporate hunches, directed data collection, identification of data gaps, and ruling in and ruling out into YOUR conclusion-making process.

References

Kintgen-Andrews, J. (1991). Critical thinking and nursing education: Perplexities and insights. *Journal of Nursing Education, 30*(4), 152–156.

Lunney, M. (1990). Accuracy of nursing diagnoses: Concept development. *Nursing Diagnosis, 1*(1), 12–17.

Miller, M.A. & Malcolm, N.S. (1990). Critical thinking in the nursing curriculum. *Nursing and Health Care, 11*(2), 57–73.

Major Nursing Conclusions of Assessment

After reading and doing the activities in this chapter you will be able to:

Describe the major nursing conclusions of assessment—strengths and health concerns—and the thinking required to develop these conclusions.

Explain the differences among the three categories of health concerns: nursing diagnoses, interdisciplinary problems, and problems for referral.

Explain the differences among diagnosing actual problems, wellness responses, and potential problems.

Diagram the process of making the major nursing conclusions of assessment.

As described earlier, conclusions are made in every phase of the nursing process. Many levels of conclusions, from minor to major, are made throughout the process. This chapter focuses on the major conclusions that are made during assessment. Conclusions made with the other phases of the nursing process are addressed in later chapters.

The major conclusions made during assessment are nursing judgments, based on analysis of data, about patients' strengths and health concerns. Health concerns fall into three categories—nursing diagnoses, interdisciplinary problems, and problems for referral. The nurse's ability to formulate these major conclusions of assessment efficiently and effectively depends on using all five thinking modes. If minimal thinking occurs, inappropriate assessment conclusions may be made, and nursing care ranges from useless to dangerous.

STRENGTHS

Strengths are factors or characteristics of the patient that are positive, are resources, and are important in planning care. It is easy to forget to make conclusions about strengths for at least three reasons. First, because many nurses work with patients who are sick, they often focus on identifying problems they can "fix." (Nurses who work with well populations are less apt to miss strengths.) Second, human nature often seems to direct people toward the negative more than the positive. Third, nurses often see strengths as issues that take care of themselves and therefore do not need to be identified. It takes some extra effort, including a shift in perspective, to *think* about and make conclusions with regard to patients' strengths.

Strengths can be in many areas of one's life. A person with a particularly strong body, who exercises regularly, or one who has a high tolerance for pain, might have physical strengths. Some people have great coping skills; nothing seems to shake them. They have psychological strengths. People with strong family support have social strengths. People who see themselves as an integral part of the universe or those who have faith in a higher being might have spiritual strengths. Those who live in areas where there is easy access to health care, or those who live in certain parts of the country, might have environmental strengths. People who have close relationships with others who come from the same background may have cultural strengths. In the preceding examples, you can see that many categories of strengths—physical, psychological, social, spiritual, environmental, and cultural—have been addressed. You can imagine other examples of strengths in these categories.

Strengths are unique to each patient and must be determined based on the patient's values, not the nurse's values. For example, Demitri, 23 years old, has a very concerned, attentive mother who wants to participate actively in his rehabilitation after his motor vehicle accident. Is his mother's helpfulness a strength in the form of "good family support"? A nurse might come to that conclusion, but if Demitri perceives his mother as domineering, pushy, and always meddling in his affairs, then the mother's actions are not a strength from his perspective.

Nurses need to identify patients' strengths so that they can use those strengths to help overcome the problems. It is not only good practice to help patients recognize all the strengths that can work for them, it is very cost effective to draw on patients' existing resources. Moreover, it is demeaning to patients not to recognize their abilities. For example, Ms. Tohatchi has a medical diagnosis of diabetes mellitus; she needs to learn how to deal with new ways of eating, caring for her skin, and performing routine activities. If Ms. Tohatchi has a college degree in biochemistry, her knowledge about how living organisms function is an educational strength. By building on this strength when designing teaching strategies, the nurse will need less time to teach her self-care.

Strengths usually are identified during the initial assessment but, because assessment continues throughout care, nurses can identify strengths at any point in the care process. Nurses either make a note of patient's strengths mentally or write them down so that they can be incorporated into the nursing care plan.

In this chapter we build an outline of conclusions for you. The first part of the outline is presented here and covers conclusions about strengths:

    I. Conclusions of Nursing Assessment
       A. Strengths
          1. Physical

2. Psychological
3. Social
4. Spiritual
5. Environmental
6. Cultural

⊃Action Learning #26: Finding Patient Strengths

Read this scenario about Priscilla Domphopper. Answer the questions on making conclusions about strengths. Share your responses with a classmate.

Priscilla F. Domphopper is a 46-year-old professor of art history. She describes herself as a basically happy person who enjoys her life and her job. Recently, however, she has "developed sleeping problems." This started about 6 months ago, about the same time that her husband's snoring "escalated to the freight-train-through-the-house decibel level." The sleeping problem is aggravated because Priscilla has become a light sleeper over the last couple of years. She usually gets about 6 hours of sleep each night, waking several times. Because it relaxes her, Priscilla usually drinks a glass of milk or a cup of hot tea right before bedtime.

Priscilla's typical day includes rising at 5:30 AM. She takes a brisk 2-mile walk, showers, and eats a light breakfast of granola cereal, plain yogurt, and 6 oz. of orange juice. Her teaching schedule prevents her from eating lunch most days. After school she picks up her kids, starts dinner, helps the kids with homework, grades papers, and prepares for the next day's work. Because she doesn't have enough time for housework, the house is a bit of a mess. This bothers her husband, but she has gotten used to it. She relaxes by watching one or two of her favorite weekly TV programs.

1. Identify Priscilla's strengths.

2. Describe the process you used to determine Priscilla's strengths.

3. Discuss how you felt about looking for her strengths.

4. Describe the challenges you encountered while identifying her strengths.

THINK ABOUT THIS ■ Think about how identifying Priscilla's strengths might help as you plan care for her sleep problem. If you were not doing this exercise, but were Priscilla's nurse, would you have focused on her strengths as much as you did when you were specifically asked to do so? Do you see that it would make sense to ask her what her strengths are?

It might be helpful to think of reminders for focusing on conclusions about strengths in the future. As you shared your responses with your classmate, did you notice that what some people think is a strength may be seen as a problem by others? The housework issue, for example, can be interpreted several ways. It would be imperative to validate your ideas about her strengths with Priscilla to arrive at the most accurate conclusions about her strengths.

HEALTH CONCERNS

Health concerns are the conclusions many students typically think of as the real nursing issues. These are the illness and wellness issues that usually bring patients to the health care system. There are three categories of health concern conclusions—those that nurses can care for independently (nursing diagnoses), those that nurses work with others to care for (interdisciplinary problems), and those that nurses refer to other health care providers (problems for referral).

Remember the outline that was started at the end of the discussion regarding conclusions about patient strengths. The second part of that outline is presented here:

    B. Health Concerns
        1. Nursing Diagnoses
            a. Problem Responses
                (1) Actual
                (2) Risk for
            b. Wellness Responses

2. Interdisciplinary Problems
3. Problems for Referral

Nursing Diagnosis

The number of books and articles written on the topic of nursing diagnosis is mind-boggling. Refer to those sources for details regarding label definitions, defining characteristics, and related factors (eg, Alfaro, 1994; Carpenito, 1993; McFarland & McFarlane, 1997; North American Nursing Diagnosis Association [NANDA], 1996.) This text, rather than duplicating those other sources, focuses on a few key issues that are critical to the thinking processes involved in making nursing diagnosis conclusions.

To use nursing diagnosis references most effectively, it is important to understand these terms:

Label Definitions: descriptions of the conclusions that are listed as nursing diagnoses

Defining Characteristics: (also called "indicators" or "criteria") the data typically found to support the conclusion as labeled

Related Factors: (also called "contributing factors" or "etiologies") possible patient issues or concerns that are "causing" a problem

Later discussion in this chapter elaborates on these definitions.

Nursing diagnoses are conclusions about those patient phenomena in the domain of independent nursing practice. (Refer to Chapter 2 for the differences between independent and interdependent nursing practice.) These conclusions are health concerns that nurses can and must independently diagnose and treat fully within the legal parameters of their profession. Refer to Appendix A for a review of the current nursing diagnostic labels identified by NANDA.

Nursing diagnoses are labels accepted by the profession to describe patient responses. A response represents the combined signs and symptoms (objective and subjective data) exhibited by the patient that can be grouped together and given a label that means the same thing to most nurses around the world. For example, one of the accepted labels is "Impaired Skin Integrity." This label is defined as "a state in which the individual's skin is adversely altered." The defining characteristics (patient data) are "disruption of skin surface, destruction of skin layers: invasion of body structures" (NANDA, 1996, p. 35). These labels and corresponding criteria (signs and symptoms or defining characteristics) can be found in nursing diagnosis books and most nursing textbooks.

Determining the Nature of Patient Responses

A series of conclusions is required to determine the nature of patient responses and the factors related to the responses. First the nurse must determine whether the response is a problem or a wellness response. If it is a problem, the nurse must determine whether it is an actual problem or one for which the patient is at risk.

The nurse must then make conclusions about the factors that are contributing to the specific problem. Conclusions at each of these points lead eventually to the final conclusion, to which an appropriate diagnostic label can be given.

Conclusions About Problem Responses Versus Conclusions About Wellness Responses

The process of making conclusions is the same whether nurses make diagnoses about problem or wellness responses. In both cases the thinking and the conclusions are based on analysis of groups of data. Whether nurses make more conclusions about problems or more about wellness responses depends largely on the focus of their practice. Nurses whose work involves well populations, such as well baby care, family health promotion, sports health, and so forth, are more likely to make conclusions about wellness responses and intervene to support that healthy behavior. Nurses who work with ill populations are apt to make more conclusions about problem responses and base their practice on restoring healthy responses. Not all responses, however, clearly fit into problem or wellness categories. For example, many problem responses of patients with chronic or terminal illnesses do not lend themselves to restoration of health. Patients with these problem responses need care designed to maintain a current level of functioning or to promote comfort and dignity as the patient approaches death.

If the distinction between wellness and problem responses seems fuzzy, it is because human responses seldom fit into neat boxes (remember the discussion of ambiguity in Chapter 5?). It helps to keep in mind that, ultimately, what the patient validates is the most accurate conclusion. If, for example, a nurse identifies a patient response as a "problem," but the patient says "I'm managing all right with this," then the conclusion could be a wellness diagnosis rather than a problem diagnosis.

Consider the case of Amanda Gayle, the new school nurse. While talking to the parents of Tyler Graham, a kindergarten student, Amanda said, "Mrs. Graham, I think Tyler has a problem with his motor development. His walking is very stiff and he has trouble running." Mrs. Graham smiled and said, "He's doing great. He was born with severely clubbed feet and has had surgery. He wore casts for a long time. A physical therapist and nurse have been working with him and he has made great strides." Amanda then knew that what she thought was a problem was actually a wellness response. She rephrased the conclusion as "Potential for Enhanced Mobility." (NANDA recommends the format of "Potential for Enhanced . . ." as wording for wellness diagnoses [Carroll-Johnson, 1991].) The patient and his family were adapting well, and Tyler would likely improve his mobility. Amanda's care would focus on supporting the family's continued wellness response.

Wellness diagnoses are similar to conclusions about strengths, but they do differ. Wellness diagnoses are focused on transitions in responses, whereas strengths may not be in transition. NANDA has defined a wellness diagnosis as a conclusion about a patient " ... in transition from a specific level of wellness to a higher level of wellness" (Carroll-Johnson, 1991, p. 375). Nurses making wellness diagnoses develop plans to support the patient's move to a higher level of wellness. All nurses, regardless of their practice areas, should make conclusions about patient strengths, but in most cases specific care plans to do something about those strengths are not developed. The strengths are used to help patients overcome problems. Wellness diagnoses, on the other hand, are often the focus of care plans for nurses who work with well populations.

⊃**ACTION LEARNING #27: Identifying Wellness Diagnoses**

Examine the diagnostic labels in Appendix A. Write down all the diagnoses you believe would qualify as wellness diagnoses.

THINK ABOUT THIS ■ How many did you find? What do you think this means? Remember, the NANDA work started only in the 1970s. Early in NANDA's development, there were debates over the necessity of including wellness diagnoses in the taxonomy; it is only in recent years that they have been added. The nursing profession has a long way to go before it has a complete taxonomy of nursing diagnoses. Many more wellness diagnoses need to be developed and added to the taxonomy. Later in this chapter, some suggestions are offered for naming conclusions for which no diagnostic label is developed as yet.

Conclusions About Actual Problems Versus Potential Problems for Patients Who Are at Risk

Conclusions about actual problems and those about problems for which patients are at risk (potential problems) differ in two ways. First, the conclusions for actual problems are based on data that "paint a picture" of an *existing* problem—hence the use of the word "actual." Conclusions about potential problems are based on data that indicate a strong likelihood, or risk, that a problem will occur in the near future if something doesn't change (see Fig. 6-1*A, B* for a graphic illustration of this difference). Nurses make many conclusions about risk factors because a large part of nursing is focused on preventing problems.

There are several differences between diagnoses of actual and potential problems. Table 6-1 summarizes those differences.

Conclusions about risks are conclusions about related factors. If factors are present that usually contribute to a problem, but the problem has not occurred, the nurse would conclude that a patient is at "risk for" that problem.

FIGURE 6–1A   Potential problems.

FIGURE 6–1B   Actual problems.

Table 6–1   Difference Between Actual and Potential Problems

TYPE OF PROBLEM	PROBLEM EXISTS	DEFINING CHARACTERISTICS SUPPORT PROBLEM	RELATED FACTORS EXIST	KNOWLEDGE, EXPERIENCE, THINKING SKILLS	FOCUS OF PLAN'S GOAL
Actual	Yes	Yes	Usually	Good to very good	Usually restore
Potential	No	No	Yes	Very good to excellent	Maintain or promote

A second difference between conclusions about actual and potential problems involves the diagnostic statement. Diagnostic statements for actual problems start with the problem label, for example, "Anxiety," "Ineffective Airway Clearance," or "Constipation." The diagnostic conclusion statement for potential problems begins with "Risk for," for example,"Risk for Impaired Skin Integrity" or "Risk for Infection."

⊃ACTION LEARNING #28: Differentiating Actual From Risk Problems

Read the following three situations and determine whether the patient has an actual problem or is at risk for having the identified problem. Use textbooks with nursing diagnoses to help with this exercise. Explain your reasoning to a classmate.

Situation	**Type of Problem and Reasoning**
#1 Sue, a marathon runner, is confined to a wheelchair for 3 weeks to rest the ligaments damaged in both legs. (Impaired Physical Mobility)	
#2 Bob is 5'10" and weighs 160 lbs. He wants to increase his muscle mass and plans to eat only steak and eggs for the next month. (Altered Nutrition)	
#3 David has attempted suicide three times in the past. His female companion has just left him. (Self-Directed Violence)	

THINK ABOUT THIS ■ How did you come to your conclusions? How did the textbooks help? How did your reasoning compare with that of your classmate's?

Conclusions About Related Factors

The last conclusions made in the larger nursing diagnosis conclusion-making process are those focused on the related factors. Once a nurse concludes that a patient has a problem response, then the factors that are "causing" that problem must be determined. The term "cause" is not used because nurses, dealing with human behavior, know how difficult it is to pin down behaviors in terms of a direct cause-

and-effect relationship. Human beings are so complex, with a multitude of individual coping mechanisms, that the nurse can only say, "there is a high probability" that some factors contribute to problems or influence problems. Therefore, when nurses write nursing diagnostic statements, they link the problem and related factors together with the words, "related to" rather than "due to" or "caused by."

Although related factors are listed along with the label for problem-focused nursing diagnoses, they are used less often with wellness diagnoses. NANDA recommends that wellness diagnoses be written as one-part statements without the related factors, but many nurses add the related factors just as they do with problem diagnoses.

Related factors are also called "contributing factors" or "etiologies." These terms generally mean the same thing in nursing. "Etiology" is used more often in medicine when referring to causes of diseases. Most books that include information on nursing diagnoses also provide lists of related factors that could go along with the nursing diagnosis label. Related factors, however, are unique to each individual, which means that the lists in the books are used only to trigger thinking. For example, one of the related factors listed for the diagnosis "Diversional Activity Deficit" is "problematic time management." That related factor would be individualized to a patient and might be written as, "Diversional Activity Deficit related to excessive amount of time spent with AM care to the point of missing morning craft class."

As demonstrated in the example above, nursing diagnostic statements, as they are used to describe conclusions in the independent nursing realm, are written in terms of actual problems or risks for problems, and are accompanied by related factors (etiologies). The two components of the statement are linked by the words, "related to." Wellness diagnoses, which also are part of independent nursing care, usually are not accompanied by related factors, but some nurses write them in the same format that is used for problem responses. Display 6-1 shows three written examples of diagnostic statements that represent the culminations of the many levels of conclusions that are needed to identify health concerns accurately.

As is shown in Display 6-1, there may be one or many related factors for each problem or response. There is no magic number, but it is important to identify all possible related factors. Otherwise, when care is planned, something important may be left out. Think about this situation. If weight loss occurs because a person has problems preparing meals, a nurse might help that person adapt to alternative methods for meal preparation. But if another related factor exists, for example, the person's income does not allow for adequate food purchase, then dealing only with the meal preparation issue will not solve the problem.

Relationship Between Related Factors and Planning

One of the primary roles of related factors is to start the nurse thinking past assessing to the planning phase of the nursing process. A plan to alleviate or eliminate the problem must be developed. The factors related to the problem must be identified so that something can be done about them. Doing something about the related factors allows for resolution of the problem.

DISPLAY **6-1.**   **Examples of Diagnostic Statements**

ACTUAL PROBLEM	RELATED TO	RELATED FACTORS
Altered Oral Mucous Membrane	related to (R/T)	irritation from dentures that no longer fit properly

POTENTIAL PROBLEM	RELATED TO	RISK FACTORS
Risk for Ineffective Airway Clearance	related to (R/T)	17-year history of smoking two packs of cigarettes a day, impending surgery with 3 hours of general anesthesia

WELLNESS RESPONSE

Family Coping: Potential for Enhanced Growth

To appreciate this close relationship among the problem, its related factors, and planning, read the following description of two different patients with the same problem but different related factors. Patient A has a sleep problem related to worries about school and an inability to relax. Nursing care should focus on helping the patient to relax and deal with the worry to alleviate the sleep problem. Patient B also has a sleep problem. This patient's problem, however, is related to frequent urination at night, secondary to excessive intake of fluids late in the day. Nursing care must focus on helping this patient change the fluid intake to alleviate the sleep problem.

The goal is identical for both patients—improved sleep patterns—yet what needs to be done for each patient is quite different. Examine Figure 6-2 to visualize this situation.

Nursing Diagnosis Taxonomy: How it Helps With Conclusion Making

Chapter 3 introduced readers to the NANDA Taxonomy of Nursing Diagnoses that is included in Appendix A. There have been several references to that taxonomy in the intervening chapters. As a review, remember these points: about 25 years ago nursing began developing a taxonomy of nursing diagnoses so that a common language could be established for those patient responses that nurses encounter. The taxonomic work of revising and adding diagnostic categories and labels continues today through the professional organization, NANDA. The taxonomy is a classification scheme of labels for actual problems, problems for which patients may be at risk (potential problems), and wellness responses.

The list of diagnoses in the taxonomy is most helpful when it is used with a book that cross-references the label with the usual data that "define" the problem, potential problem, or wellness response. (Examples of such books are given in the

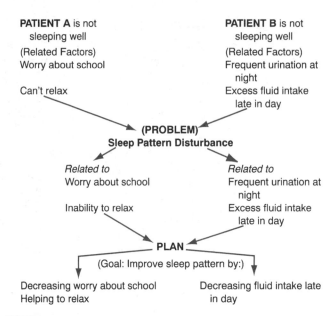

FIGURE 6–2   Relationship between related factors and plan for dealing with a problem.

reference list for this chapter.) The data are the signs and symptoms (defining characteristics) that nurses usually find when that particular diagnostic label is valid. An example, "Impaired Skin Integrity," was discussed earlier in this chapter. Another example of an accepted label for an actual problem is "Impaired Verbal Communication." This label means the patient is experiencing one or all of the following conditions: "unable to speak dominant language; speaks or verbalizes with difficulty; does not or can not speak; stuttering; slurring; difficulty forming words or sentences; difficulty expressing thought verbally; inappropriate verbalization; dyspnea; disorientation" (NANDA, 1996, p. 37).

↻ACTION LEARNING #29: Becoming Familiar With Labels, Definitions, and Defining Characteristics

Find a book that has nursing diagnoses accompanied by lists of defining characteristics and related factors.

Pick two diagnoses that you are interested in.

Study the defining characteristics. Do they "paint a picture" of the diagnostic label?

Study the related factors. Can you think of other factors, not on the list, that might contribute to the health concern identified by the diagnostic label?

Finally, get together with a classmate. Read the lists of defining characteristics for the diagnoses you studied to your classmate and see whether she or he can identify from the list what diagnoses you are describing.

THINK ABOUT THIS ■ Depending on your familiarity with nursing diagnosis books, you may have found this exercise easy or difficult. If you have not used such books yet, you probably gained an appreciation for how helpful such resources can be. How easy was it to find the label for the defining characteristics listed by your classmate?

Arranging labels in the form of a taxonomy helps nurses find diagnoses easily and consider differential diagnoses (other possibilities) with increased accuracy. For example, the response category of elimination has labels for problems with bowel elimination and urinary elimination. When a nurse finds a cluster of data that may indicate "Functional Incontinence," the nurse can look for that label in the elimination group and find other labels (differential diagnoses) to consider as well. The alternative diagnostic labels to consider would be Reflex Incontinence, Stress Incontinence, Total Incontinence, and Urge Incontinence.

Because building the taxonomy is a relatively recent endeavor, it is not yet complete. Nurses may not always find the labels for their independent nursing conclusions in the taxonomy. When no appropriate label is found, nurses develop the best label themselves. As nursing students, the best rule for using the taxonomy is to check it first and use the accepted label if possible; however, if no appropriate label is found, develop one that best summarizes in a word or two the patient response. Developing labels not currently on the taxonomy, which calls on the NEW IDEAS AND CREATIVITY mode of thinking, is particularly useful in the areas of mental health, community health, maternal–child health, and wellness nursing. Most of the current NANDA labels are geared toward the area of medical–surgical nursing.

⊃ACTION LEARNING #30: Finding an Appropriate Diagnostic Label for Priscilla

Look again at the story about Priscilla Domphopper presented in Action Learning #26. Search the list of diagnostic labels in Appendix A and use a nursing diagnosis textbook to find the label that seems to fit best with the data on Priscilla. Write down that diagnosis label along with the data you used to arrive at that conclusion. Remember to identify both the data that "define" the problem, wellness response, or risk response, *and* the data that are related factors. Share your conclusions with a classmate.

Diagnostic label:

Supporting data (defining characteristics):

Related factors:

THINK ABOUT THIS ■ How similar were your conclusions to those of your classmate? If your conclusions were similar, how did your supporting data compare? How sure are you of your final conclusion?

This exercise shows how the taxonomy can help with conclusion making. The taxonomy can be used to stimulate thinking about differential diagnoses, it can remind the nurse of items to include in directed data collection, and it can validate a conclusion by showing how that conclusion usually accompanies that particular set of data.

✔ *Thinking-Learning Check*

The last several pages have addressed some very critical information about strengths and health concerns. Nursing diagnoses, a major category of health concern conclusions, has consumed most of the discussion. Pause here for a thinking-learning check. You should be able to elaborate on these ideas:

   ✔ The major conclusions of the assessment phase of the nursing process: identification of the patient's strengths and health concerns (nursing diagnoses and related factors, interdisciplinary problems, and problems for referral)

✔ Identifying strengths: the need to get the patient's perspective because of the very subjective nature of these responses

✔ Nursing diagnoses: health concerns within the domain of independent nursing practice

✔ Differentiating types of nursing diagnoses: wellness responses, actual problems, and risk responses (potential problems)

✔ Conclusions about related factors: part of the diagnostic statement and importance to planning

✔ Format for writing nursing diagnostic statements

✔ The taxonomy of Nursing Diagnoses: how it is used in developing accurate diagnoses

The rest of this chapter addresses the last two health concerns about which nurses need to make accurate conclusions—interdisciplinary problems and problems for referral. Both of these aspects of nursing require a strong knowledge of the other health professions.

INTERDISCIPLINARY PROBLEMS

Interdisciplinary problems comprise those conclusions about patient problems that are in the interdependent domain of nursing. (For a review of independent and interdependent nursing domains, refer to Chapter 2.) Interdisciplinary problems, as the words imply, require collaboration with other health care professionals (physician, physical therapist, nutritionist, social worker, clergy, and so forth). Depending on the setting and the patient population, there may be more or fewer interdisciplinary problems than there are nursing diagnoses.

The line between a nursing diagnosis and an interdisciplinary problem often is very fuzzy. There are few clean distinctions between what one health care provider does and what another does. Clear differences can be seen only at the extremes; for example, a patient recently diagnosed with renal failure may have the following interdisciplinary problem (Note: the format for an interdisciplinary problem is the same as for a nursing diagnosis):

Risk for hyperproteinemia related to lack of knowledge of renal diet.

This patient needs assistance from a dietitian as well as from a nurse because renal diets are quite complex. In many cases nurses deal with diet issues independently, but as the complexity increases, as in the example above, it is a good idea to collaborate with a diet expert.

In the fuzzier arena, consider a second example, which compares two patients with skin problems diagnosed by the nurse:

Impaired skin integrity related to immobility and incontinence

At first glance this looks like a straightforward nursing diagnosis, not an interdisciplinary problem. However, it is not that simple. With one patient, the nurse may be able to diagnose and care for this problem independently by turning the patient and cleaning the skin frequently. For another patient, this problem may have become so severe that several layers of the skin are involved, and the area has become infected. In that case, the nurse needs to collaborate with the physician because medication and treatments may need to be ordered. In this example, the severity of the problem makes a difference; when the problem gets so severe that medical intervention is needed, the nursing diagnosis moves into the realm of interdisciplinary problems. The written diagnostic statement is the same, but one falls into the independent nursing domain and the other into the interdependent domain.

These two patients with skin breakdown are a good illustration of how all the diagnostic labels have not yet evolved to their most descriptive level. As the taxonomic work continues, there may be labels that will better differentiate, for example, the severity of the patient's response. Whether or not interdisciplinary problems will be added to the NANDA Taxonomy remains to be seen.

A broad knowledge base and sharp thinking skills are necessary for nurses to make accurate conclusions about interdisciplinary problems. Not only do nurses need to know nursing's specific body of knowledge, they need to know quite a bit about the biomedical, social, psychological, and spiritual bodies of knowledge that are the primary foci of other disciplines such as physicians, social workers, psychologists, and clergy. Without that knowledge, conclusions about interdisciplinary problems may be missed or inaccurate.

PROBLEMS FOR REFERRAL

Because nurses assess in a holistic manner ("holistic" means looking at all aspects of the person—biological, psychological, social, cultural, and spiritual), they frequently find problems that fall completely into the domains of other health professionals. Here is an example: a nurse working in an emergency room, while assessing a patient brought in by a spouse, finds that the patient has not been eating for the past week, refuses to come out of her bedroom, won't talk to anyone, and has not been sleeping very well. The nurse recognizes that this patient is very likely depressed, but so severely that the problem requires more intensive therapy than the nurse is qualified to provide. The nurse would refer this patient to a psychiatric clinical nurse specialist, a psychiatric social worker, a psychologist, or a psychiatrist.

The specific person to whom the nurse refers the patient, and the referral process itself, vary from institution to institution. Sometimes there are chains of communication that must be followed, such as the nurse calling the primary physician, who calls a consultant. At other times, the nurse makes the referral directly, such as to a nurse practitioner or to a physician. It is very helpful to know the appropriate ways to refer within an organization; this saves a lot of time for the staff and the patient and improves the quality of care for patients.

✔ *Thinking-Learning Check*

Pause here for another thinking-learning check. You should be able to elaborate on these ideas:

- ✔ Interdisciplinary problems: health concerns within the domain of interdependent nursing practice
- ✔ The importance of basic knowledge about many health care professions in effectively identifying and planning care for interdisciplinary problems and problems for referral
- ✔ Knowing an organization's specific referral system is very time saving and quality-care focused.

CONCLUSION ABOUT CONCLUSIONS

This chapter has examined the major nursing conclusions of the assessing phase of the nursing process. One reading of the chapter may not be enough to integrate all of the ideas and concepts into existing thinking about conclusion making. This chapter's Thinking Log has been designed to foster integration of the chapter's content into your memory.

Examine the outline in Figure 6-3, which provides an overview of the conclusions of nursing assessment. (The conclusions of planning, implementation, and evaluation are discussed in later chapters.) It is important to see all the possible conclusions together so that the range of possibilities becomes clear. Being able to recognize the various categories of these assessment conclusions will be very helpful when you start planning care for the various areas of need.

I. Conclusions of Assessment

    A. Strengths

        1. Physical
        2. Psychological
        3. Social
        4. Spiritual
        5. Environmental
        6. Cultural

    B. Health Concerns

        1. Nursing diagnoses
            a. Problem responses
                (1) Actual
                (2) Risk for
            b. Wellness responses
        2. Interdisciplinary problems
        3. Problems for referral

FIGURE 6-3   Overview of the conclusions of nursing assessment.

THINKING LOG #6 ➤

Take Figure 6-3 with you as you talk to a nurse. Ask the nurse to share with you a brief patient summary. Ask the nurse what he/she has identified as the nursing conclusions of assessment. You may have to explain the difference between interdisciplinary problems and problems for referral. Ask the nurse whether there are any other conclusions that nurses make that are not included in Figure 6-3.

References

Alfaro-LeFevre, R. (1998). *Applying nursing process: A step-by-step guide* (4th ed.). Philadelphia: JB Lippincott.

Carpenito, L.J. (1997). *Nursing diagnosis: Application to clinical practice* (7th ed.). Philadelphia: JB Lippincott.

Carroll-Johnson, R.M. (Ed.) (1991). *Classification of nursing diagnoses: Proceedings of the ninth conference North American Nursing Diagnosis Association.* Philadelphia: JB Lippincott.

McFarland, G.K. & McFarlane, E.A. (1997). *Nursing diagnosis and intervention* (3rd ed.). St. Louis: Mosby.

North American Nursing Diagnosis Association (1996). *NANDA nursing diagnoses: Definitions and classification 1997–1998.* Philadelphia: Author.

Details of Thinking and the Nursing Process

Health Detectives:
Data Collection
and Data Analysis

✳ *Learning Outcomes*

After reading and doing the activities in this chapter you will be able to:

Appreciate the role of the nurse as a health detective.

Demonstrate the ability to find clues (data collection) and make sense out of them (data analysis).

Explain the thinking required to be a great nurse health detective.

NURSES AS HEALTH DETECTIVES: OVERVIEW

Collecting and analyzing data and arriving at conclusions constitute the activities of the assessment phase of the nursing process. The thinking that occurs during assessment allows nurses to make accurate conclusions about a patient's strengths and health concerns. Determining what a patient needs from a nurse and what information the nurse needs from the patient is very much like detective work. The nurse looks for clues to health issues and problems. Once the clues are found, they are validated (checked for accuracy) and put together into meaningful patterns. Like detectives, nurses keep their eyes, ears, noses, and hands open to discover those clues. They also constantly question the validity of the clues; that is, they are careful to not just accept things at face value. Nurses think about what clues they are finding and confirm the accuracy of the clues with other data or other sources of data—just as good detectives validate their information.

  The purpose of this detective work is to arrive at accurate conclusions about the patient's strengths and health concerns. Those major nursing conclusions of assessment were described in Chapter 6. Keeping the purpose of detective work—making conclusions—in mind helps the nurse engage all five modes of thinking to find relevant clues and make sense of them. If this purpose of assessment is not in clear focus, it is easy to fall into an assessment rut; data collection becomes a mindless HABIT, in which the nurse simply asks questions and writes the patient's comments on a form without paying attention to the importance of the data or to the connections among them. If nurses slide into this rut, the information comes in through the ears or eyes and goes straight out the fingers to the paper, without passing through the brain in the process.

To avoid this assessment rut, it is extremely important to recognize that data collection and data analysis **must** occur simultaneously. Data collection is finding clues, and data analysis is making sense of the clues. Both activities must occur in unison, and all five modes of T.H.I.N.K. must be engaged to reach accurate conclusions of assessment.

This chapter focuses on the details of data collection (finding clues) and the initial methods of data analysis (making sense out of the clues). The thinking used to analyze data as they are collected is described. The next level of analysis, clustering data (grouping clues that "fit" together) and making conclusions from these clusters, is described in Chapter 8.

FINDING CLUES (DATA COLLECTION) AND MAKING SENSE OUT OF CLUES (DATA ANALYSIS)

The best detectives use a systematic approach to finding and interpreting clues. Clues in health care are commonly called data. Data are the building blocks of the conclusion-making process. Data are "unstructured raw facts" and "are discrete entities (facts) that have not been interpreted." (Saba & McCormick, 1996, p. 231). Most of this chapter is focused on how nurses gather data. The next chapter gives more details about interpretation, or analysis of those data. However, it is important to realize that data collection and interpretation occur simultaneously. Most importantly, any conclusion made from interpretation must have a firm grounding in the unstructured, raw facts.

The classic approach to collecting data asks six questions, *who, what, where, when, how,* and *why.* A similar approach is useful for nurse health detectives. *Who* are the sources of data? *What* are the types of data? *Where* are the data? *When* are data collected? *How* are data collected? *Why* collect data? Some answers to these questions are listed in Display 7-1 and are discussed in the following pages.

Who

The patient is always the primary source of data and must be listened to and observed carefully, using all five senses. Although that seems like an obvious statement, the issues can be complex. The patient's level of consciousness, cognitive ability (memory and intellectual functioning), mental status, degree of comfort, desire to cooperate, and many other such factors can add to or detract from the amount and quality of data collected. Thinking nurses always keep these factors in mind as they collect data.

DISPLAY **7–1.   The WHO, WHAT, WHERE, WHEN, HOW, and WHY of Finding Clues (Data Collection)**

WHO are sources of data?
  Patient
  Significant others
  Other health care providers
WHAT are the types of data?
  Subjective raw data
  Objective raw data
WHERE are the data or where is the patient?
  Acute and long-term inpatient settings
  Clinics and health care provider offices
  Schools and workplaces
  Homes and communities
WHEN are data collected?
  All the time (during all phases of the nursing process, assessing, planning, implementing, evaluating)
HOW are data collected?
  Observation
  Measurement
  Interaction
WHY collect data?
  To make conclusions (back to the purpose of data collection)

Significant others, an additional source of data, include family members, friends, companions, housemates, neighbors, and so forth. These sources can be valuable for validating information provided by the patient, filling in patient information gaps, or guiding the nurse in exploring additional health concerns not mentioned by the patient. When the patient is unable to communicate because of age, decreased level of consciousness, altered mental state, or other communication deficits, significant others serve as the primary source of verbal data.

Other health care providers also are sources of data and a means to validate data. Although they generally are very objective sources, they, like nurses, have human biases and value systems that can influence their perception and interpretation of information. Nurses need to be alert to the biases and validate these data as well. Other providers also may validate data collected by the nurse.

Except for first-encounter situations, when no one has seen the patient before, data collected by other providers frequently are documented in the patient's record. Most patient records contain past history, laboratory reports, medical orders, consultations by other providers, and progress notes. It is important to read records to avoid frustrating the patient by asking for the same information over and over. A word of caution, however: do not always assume that something in the record is valid. Verify with the patient anything that seems inconsistent with what you observe directly or hear the patient say. For example, a nurse might say to a patient,

"I noticed in your record that you are allergic to strawberries, but you are eating them with your lunch. Can you tell me about this discrepancy in information?"

Making Sense Out of "Who" Clues

The thinking modes required for *who* are primarily H (HABITS) and I (IN-QUIRY). Going directly to the patient and significant others for information can and should become a HABIT. The best nurses combine that HABIT with INQUIRY as they gather data directly from patients and hear reports from other nurses about those patients. Again, nurses should not blindly accept everything they hear about patients, but should validate data with the patients. Most nurses will directly assess patients as soon as possible. In hospital settings, nurses usually get a report from previous shift nurses and, before acting on anything, go on "rounds" to assess their patients directly. This example of INQUIRY thinking does not mean that nurses do not trust the data collected by others. Rather, it is a double-check (validation) that is vital for safe, high-quality care. The same principle of checking and rechecking described here is used with the administration of medications. Validation also reflects the nurse's constant awareness of change.

What

What types of data are available to the nurse health detective? There are different ways of classifying types of data. The first way makes a distinction between raw data and inferences. The second way divides raw data into subjective and objective categories.

Raw Data and Inferences

Raw data (as in "straight facts," not as in "uncooked") are those clues that are subjective (told to the nurse by the patient or significant others) and those clues that are objective (nonverbal data collected with the nurse's five senses). Inferences are judgments made about the data; they are miniconclusions.

Sometimes the distinction between data and inference becomes blurred because in the real world there are many degrees of interpretation. For example, two typical pieces of information about urine include its amount and its color. If 250 mL of urine is measured, there is little doubt that this is a piece of objective raw data (straight fact). But if a nurse says, "The color is amber," is that a fact (a piece of raw data) or is it a judgment (an inference)? A case could be made that "amber urine" is an inference, which depends on the nurse's ability to judge color. However, describing urine as "amber" generally is seen as a piece of raw data because currently there is no more precise way of measuring urine color other than visually examining it. "Amber" becomes a "necessary inference" that is acceptable in clinical practice. Necessary inferences are those inferences for which no better practical method of measurement exists. If, however, the nurse were doing research on urine color, a much more precise measurement would be demanded, requiring the use of expensive color analysis equipment.

Examples of some inferences that are commonly used but really *do need* supporting data include healthy appetite, good activity level, and noncompliance with medication regimen. All of these inferences (judgments) are miniconclusions that nurses make about groups of data. Each inference needs raw data to support the conclusion. For instance, the data to support "healthy appetite" might include: "Patient consumes 100% of all meals within 15 to 20 minutes, and occasionally asks for seconds and evening snacks."

Usually it is best to list the raw data, and not the inference, as a safeguard against making premature judgments. The important thing to remember is that whenever possible, the data should be measured and described as raw data. If too many inferences are showing up in the data base (the total of the information collected on one patient), the nurse may be making premature conclusions that can lead to inappropriate or unsafe care.

Objective and Subjective Data

Objective data, also called "signs," are all those clues (data) that the nurse sees, hears, smells, palpates (feels), or tastes directly. Few data are found through taste, but there are some examples, such as a salty taste when kissing a baby with cystic fibrosis.

Objective data also include descriptive observations and measurements collected by other health care providers and recorded in the patient's record. Objective data generally are acquired through observation and measurement, which are discussed later under "How" data are collected.

Subjective data, also called "symptoms," include direct quotes from patients or significant others. Subjective data are valuable information that provide the patient's personal perspective and interpretation of the concerns. Without subjective data, it is impossible to individualize nursing care. Subjective data are obtained through interaction with the patient and significant others. More details on interaction are given in the "How" section.

Two additional points about distinguishing between subjective and objective data are important. First, the hearing used to collect objective data (heart sounds, breath sounds, and so forth) is the same hearing used to listen to the patient or significant others talk about something. The data, however, are categorized differently. The heart or breath sounds heard by the nurse through a stethoscope are objective data; when the patient says, "My heart is beating too fast," the nurse hears subjective data.

Second, one might ask, "What difference does it make whether one distinguishes signs from symptoms, or objective from subjective data? They are all data." The importance is that if no distinctions are made, the overall database may be lopsided. If only objective data are collected, the patient's perceptions and ideas are being overlooked. If there are only subjective data, important signs (objective data) may be missed. Both objective and subjective data are needed for a complete picture of the patient's health status and concerns.

⊃Action Learning #31: Distinguishing Types of Data and Inferences

PART 1:

Examine the 12 items listed below. Label each according to the following criteria (you can select more than one label for an item if necessary):

"R" for items of raw data
"I" for items that are inferences
"S" for items of subjective data
"O" for items of objective data
"*" for items that are inferences that have no better way of being measured, and are acceptable for clinical practice

    Temp. = 98.6°F
    Height = 68"
    "I feel cold"
    Patient's feet cool to touch
    Overweight
    Had orange juice, toast, and coffee for breakfast
    Patient said he slept from 11 PM to 6 AM
    Patient anxious about surgery
    Normal bowel movement
    Eating well
    Skin over left knee red, warm to touch, and shiny
    "My son has these awful ear infections every fall"

PART 2:

Select two items you labeled as inferences with **no** "*." Write down the data that could be used to validate and support that inference.

Data that Could Support This Inference

Inference #1

Inference #2

PART 3:

Briefly describe to a classmate your thinking as you completed the above tasks.

THINK ABOUT THIS ■ How did you make your determinations? Were some very obvious and others less so? What standards did you use to make your decisions? Where did you find those standards? How did you describe your thinking?

Making Sense Out of "What" Clues

The thinking modes used with *What* clues are primarily TOTAL RECALL, HABIT, and INQUIRY. One valuable HABIT should include making sure that a balance of subjective and objective data is collected. Obtaining accurate raw data and validating any inferences also should become HABITual.

To determine the relevance (importance) of the clues, TOTAL RECALL and INQUIRY are needed. Nurses need a good understanding of people and health and what is normal. For example, when trying to determine whether urine is "normal," the nurse needs to know what is normal for color, specific gravity, and output in a 24-hour period; it also is important to know the frequency with which the patient voids, and whether there is any discomfort or pain during elimination. Determining "normal" requires the use of TOTAL RECALL of this factual information, or at least recalling where to look for the "normals" of urine. It also requires the use of the INQUIRY mode to make comparisons between what is found and what should be found.

Determining whether a piece of data is normal signals the initial thinking required for data analysis. If it is normal, it could be a patient strength or just interesting information. However, if something is not normal, it is considered "relevant" and becomes significant in developing accurate conclusions.

Look at the following three pieces of information. Knowing nothing else about the patient, what do you *think* is relevant?

Eyes = two in front of head
Skin = green color with purple spots and neon stripes
Toes = 10, 5 on each foot

What made you say that the second item was relevant? Because it is not normal. How did you know it was not normal? Because nobody (on our planet, at least) has skin like that. So, in this situation, you compared the available data with a population norm (standard). You used TOTAL RECALL and probably thought about whether or not you had any memory of seeing, hearing, or reading about people with green, purple-spotted, neon-striped skin. More discussion on population norms (standards) is presented in Chapter 8.

This first level of data analysis, which uses TOTAL RECALL and INQUIRY to distinguish relevant data from nonrelevant data, is accomplished by comparing data with population norms. There is another type of norm that must be used for further analysis—the individual's norms. When a nurse looks at separate pieces of information, the only comparison that can be made is with population norms. To find out whether this condition or situation is normal for the individual, however, the nurse must get more data, even if this amounts only to asking the patient, "Is this normal for you?" Here is an example of the distinction between the two types of norms: A patient sleeps 3 to 4 hours each night. Does this meet population norms? No, most textbooks indicate that 6 to 8 hours of sleep every 24 hours is "normal" for adults. To find out whether this is normal for the patient, the nurse has to collect another clue to compare with his individual norm. The patient may say "Yes, this is my usual pattern." In this case, the data, "sleeps 3 to 4 hours each night" *and* "this is my usual pattern," become a set or a cluster of data that is less relevant than the single datum might have been.

In that example, the nurse had to go beyond analyzing one clue to clustering that clue with one additional clue. This clustering process is discussed more fully in Chapter 8, but for now it is important to see that judgments about the relevance of one piece of information constitute only the first step in data analysis.

⟲ ACTION LEARNING #32: Looking for Relevant Data

Examine each item in the following list of data. Using TOTAL RECALL and IN-QUIRY, determine which items may be relevant, based on population norms.

(Hint: As you check books, you will not find the words "population norms." What you will find are descriptions of "typical findings" or what something "should look like." For example, "The usual range for hemoglobin for women is 12 to 15 g/dL," or "When examining the eyes, assess the pupils for roundness and symmetry, size, reaction to light . . .")

Pupils dilated and fixed
Pedal pulses 2+ bilaterally
Hematocrit 39%
Crackles in both lower lung fields
Three bowel movements a day

THINK ABOUT THIS ▪ How easy was it to find the "norms"? How many did you know without having to look them up? Do you see how, after determining the fit with population norms, you would also need to check individual norms to determine whether certain information is relevant?

Where

Where data are obtained depends on the physical location of the patient and the surroundings. Different kinds of data are available depending on whether patients are in acute or long-term settings, clinics or providers' offices, schools, workplaces, or homes. Patients in hospitals, for example, do not have their "things" around them. A patient whose home is filled with books may not be recognized as an avid reader while in the hospital. On the other hand, hospital rooms are not devoid of information that reveal things about a person. Consider a patient who has a rosary on the bedside table; seeing that object in the environment could give the nurse information about the patient's religion. Would an inference (judgment) about the patient's religious preference be wise without collecting more data?

Seeing patients in their homes can provide a wealth of information that frequently goes uncollected in an inpatient setting. Most people surround themselves with things that are extensions of themselves and that reflect their interests. Also, patients on their own "turf" often act differently than they do when they are on nurses' "turf."

It is easy to miss data from the environment, no matter where the location, when the patient is such a strong focus of attention. The nurse's natural tendency is to talk to patients and rely on verbal reports of data instead of looking at the more subtle clues surrounding the patient. These subtle clues, such as plants, clutter, room temperature, lighting, music, and the like, reflect needs, likes, and dislikes.

In addition to asking questions directly about the environment (eg, "Tell me about your sleeping environment, where and how you sleep, and how it helps or hinders your sleep patterns"), the nurse health detective must develop a keen sense of environmental observation. No matter what the setting, the nurse health detective must constantly observe for data about environmental hazards (eg, loose throw rugs in the home, bedrails not locking properly) and environmental impediments (eg, only bathroom is on the second floor of patient's home, patient's call light is not in reach).

Making Sense Out of "Where" Clues

Again, the first three modes of T.H.I.N.K. are required to collect *where* clues. Finding clues in the patient's environment requires a HABIT of constant awareness of the "big picture," or seeing the patient as a unique individual within a larger system. The larger system includes, among other things, the physical space, the family, and the community. How the patient relates or does not relate to the larger system also is important. A broad understanding of people and how they interact with their environments is necessary to recognize clues and make sense out of them. This understanding comes from TOTAL RECALL of information learned in courses such as sociology, psychology, and nursing science. INQUIRY helps nurses question the environmental data and their relevance to the patient's health status.

To see how you measure up, test your current environmental awareness with Action Learning #33. Keep in mind that this skill, like any other, can be nurtured and improved with practice. Environmental awareness should become a useful HABIT.

⊃**ACTION LEARNING #33: Testing Environmental Awareness**

Select a TV show that you do not usually watch. Watch it for 10 minutes with the sound off. Pay attention to the environment and the nonverbal behaviors of the people. Write down what you observed that you might not have noticed had the sound been on. If you write down an inference, also write down the raw objective data you observed to support (validate) your inference.

THINK ABOUT THIS ■ How acute was your awareness? Have you discovered a strength—that you are very aware of environmental clues—or is this an area that needs work? What can you do to enhance your environmental awareness?

✔ *Thinking-Learning Check*

Pause here for a thinking-learning check. You should be able to elaborate on these ideas:

✔ Nurses are health detectives who need to find clues and make sense out of those clues.

✔ Data collection and data analysis *must* occur simultaneously.

✔ Finding clues is focused on questioning *who, what, where, when, how,* and *why,* and using all five modes of thinking to make sense out of the data.

✔ Patients are the primary source of data.

✔ Raw data are subjective or objective, and a balance of both provides the best information.

✔ Some inferences are necessary, but most need to be supported (validated) with raw data.

When

Data collection occurs at every patient encounter from start to finish. In fact, data collection (finding clues) occurs before the nurse encounters the patient, through verbal reports and records, during patient encounters, and after patient encounters through validating data with other data, or with other people. The bottom line on *When* is "always."

Making Sense Out of "When" Clues

The T, H, I, and N are all needed. Observing and listening need to become well-tuned HABITs. But habitually collecting data at all times is ineffective unless the nurse is putting pieces together and making sense out of them using INQUIRY. NEW IDEAS AND CREATIVITY are used when the nurse takes advantage of less obvious opportunities for *when* to collect data. For example, when accompanying a patient to the cafeteria or when facilitating a patient's leisure activity, the creative nurse may find clues that the less creative nurse would miss. These are not "usual" times for collecting data, but patients may be more relaxed and may reveal information that might not be shared in more formal situations.

How

There are whole courses on *how* to collect data; traditionally, these courses are titled "Health Assessment." Although health assessment courses provide the foundation for *how* to collect data, all nursing courses add to the repertoire of data collection techniques. The basic categories of techniques are **interaction**, **observation**, and **measurement**.

Interaction

Interaction is the method for collecting subjective clues. Most beginning students know more about *interaction* than about other techniques because everyone interacts with people every day. Therapeutic interactions, however, require not only everyday experience, but nursing skill in knowing what promotes or blocks communication. Anybody can pick up a form and ask questions from it. Finding the best wording for questioning individual patients, however, takes thought and practice. Also, knowing when and how to ask for more specific information or expand on existing information is important. Most nursing textbooks cover the topic of therapeutic communication very well and should be read carefully. Reading about therapeutic communication before working with patients helps the beginning nurse plan how to ask questions efficiently. Role-playing a patient interaction, with a classmate playing the patient role, is very helpful. An even better learning technique is to videotape the interaction, play it back, and evaluate it for strengths and areas needing further development.

Because of time and space limitations, this text highlights only two specific interaction techniques that demonstrate good thinking skills. Both techniques are similar in that they provide for expansion and elaboration of information. The first is called "branching," and the second is called "DETAIL" (Display 7-2).

Branching is very descriptive of the technique itself. A patient's verbal response stimulates a thinking nurse to ask sequential questions that, when an-

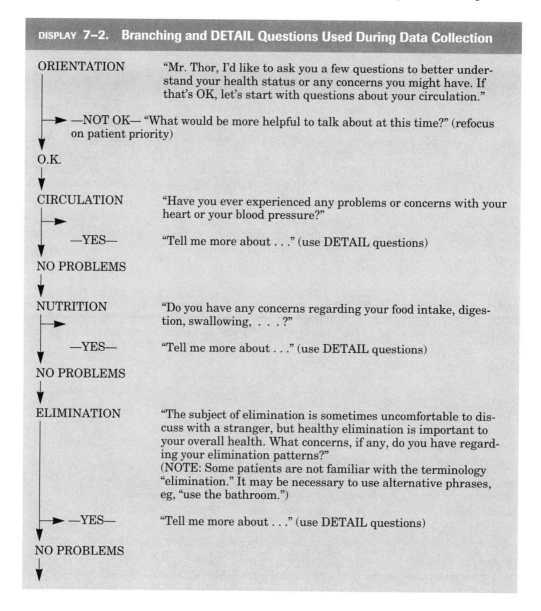

DISPLAY **7–2.   Branching and DETAIL Questions Used During Data Collection**

ORIENTATION   "Mr. Thor, I'd like to ask you a few questions to better understand your health status or any concerns you might have. If that's OK, let's start with questions about your circulation."

—NOT OK— "What would be more helpful to talk about at this time?" (refocus on patient priority)

O.K.

CIRCULATION   "Have you ever experienced any problems or concerns with your heart or your blood pressure?"

—YES—   "Tell me more about . . ." (use DETAIL questions)

NO PROBLEMS

NUTRITION   "Do you have any concerns regarding your food intake, digestion, swallowing, . . . ?"

—YES—   "Tell me more about . . ." (use DETAIL questions)

NO PROBLEMS

ELIMINATION   "The subject of elimination is sometimes uncomfortable to discuss with a stranger, but healthy elimination is important to your overall health. What concerns, if any, do you have regarding your elimination patterns?"
(NOTE: Some patients are not familiar with the terminology "elimination." It may be necessary to use alternative phrases, eg, "use the bathroom.")

—YES—   "Tell me more about . . ." (use DETAIL questions)

NO PROBLEMS

swered, clarify or validate the first piece of information. Branching is extremely helpful for collecting related pieces of data, organizing data, finding patterns, and making sense out of the data (see Display 7-2 for an example of branching questions). Chapter 8 illustrates how important branching is to clustering data in the next level of analysis.

The second useful interaction skill designed for data collection is D.E.T.A.I.L. D.E.T.A.I.L. is a another mnemonic that generates even more branching-type questions when a patient has an identified area of concern. For example, D.E.T.A.I.L.

helps to zero in on key pieces of data regarding a patient's complaint of pain. The categories of data collection in the D.E.T.A.I.L. mnemonic are as follows:

"D," date of onset and course, provides historical data and chronologic data that are useful in determining the chronic or acute nature of the concern. Typical patient responses to questions in this category include: "It started yesterday," "It started three years ago," "It was worse in the beginning," "It is gradually getting worse," or "It is OK in the morning but by noon I have the most trouble."

"E," exact location, provides anatomic data. Typical patient responses include: "The whole top of my head hurts," "Just one very sore spot right here," "It is just sort of all over my body," or "Right behind my knee."

"T," terms (patient's) for description of quality and quantity, provides the patient's perceptions of what the issue or problem is like and its severity. Typical patient responses include: "It's stabbing," "It's a dull ache," " It is like being jabbed with a burning hot poker," or "On a scale of 1 to 10, with 10 being the worst, it's a 12."

"A," aggravating and alleviating factors, help identify what makes the problem worse and what makes it better. Typical patient responses include: "Bright lights really make it worse," "The medicine the doctor prescribed helps some," "A hot bath really helps," or "Small rooms with smoke are the hardest places to be."

"I," intersystem connections, provides information on what else is happening to the person at the same time. Typical patient responses include: "When I have a sinus infection everything else gets messed up too," "I get constipated from the medicine," "I get so tired because I can't sleep at night because I can't breath when I'm lying flat," or "I get a stiff neck because I have to sleep with three pillows to breath and my nose gets so sore from all the blowing."

"L," listening to the patient's interpretation, is always good advice. Patients are the primary source of data, but their perceptions of what causes problems and what might help alleviate problems can be overlooked easily. Patients often will not offer their interpretations, thinking the nurse knows best. When asked directly, however, patients can supply useful insights, such as, "I really think I'm just too stressed out to sleep well," "It feels like I have a sinus infection," or "My baby is coming **now**!"

EXAMPLE OF USING DETAIL

Nora Dakota, SN, is doing a home visit with the Peters family, who have requested help with new baby care and when to add solid foods to the formula feedings. Before getting started with the planned baby bath, Nora asked Mrs. Peters how she was feeling, because this was her fifth day postpartum (after delivery). Mrs. Peters smiled and said she was fine except for a bad stomachache.

Nora thought, "A stomachache is not normal." (She was comparing the data with population norms.) She also thought, "A stomachache for a woman who is 5 days postpartum could be an indication of more serious problems." (She was RECALLing what she knew about postpartum health care issues, uterine bleeding, infections, and constipation.) Nora's first question to Mrs. Peters was, "Do you normally have stomachaches?" (She was asking for an individual norm to compare with the data.) When the patient's response was "No," Nora proceeded to use the DETAIL format to collect more specific information. The following dialogue occurred:

> **Nora:** Tell me when you first noticed the stomachache and if there have been any changes. Is it getting worse or better?
>
> **Mrs. P.:** Well, it started 2 days ago. It does seem worse today.
>
> **Nora:** Show me where you are actually feeling the stomachache.
>
> **Mrs. P.:** It's right here [she rubs the right side of her abdomen below her ribs].
>
> **Nora:** Does it hurt anywhere else?
>
> **Mrs. P.:** Mostly just right here, although sometimes it seems to move a bit over to the left.
>
> **Nora:** Describe for me how it feels, and on a scale from 1 to 10, with 10 being the worst, how bad it is.
>
> **Mrs. P.:** Well, it feels like a block of lead is sitting in me. I can't wear anything tight or it really hurts. I guess I would say it's about a 3 sometimes and a 6 at other times.
>
> **Nora:** Is there anything that makes it worse or makes it better?
>
> **Mrs. P.:** Sitting for a while makes it worse, or if I lie on my right side at night. Sometimes taking a walk helps it feel better. And, this is embarrassing, but passing gas helps too.
>
> **Nora:** Have you noticed this stomachache affecting anything else?
>
> **Mrs. P.:** I don't have much appetite. I'm also much more irritable than I usually am, but I just assumed that was normal for a new mother.
>
> **Nora:** Irritability can be a concern, and we can talk about it too, because it's not necessarily normal. But are you noticing anything else related to your stomachache—for example, have you had much vaginal bleeding? Have you had any diarrhea or constipation? Have you had a fever?
>
> **Mrs. P.:** Let's not forget to discuss the irritability. But, no, no unusual bleeding beyond what the doctor said was normal. I haven't had any diarrhea; in fact I can't remember when I had my last bowel movement. I've been so busy I haven't paid much attention. And, no, no fever.
>
> **Nora:** How often did you have bowel movements before the baby was born?
>
> **Mrs. P.:** Usually about every day or at least every other day.
>
> **Nora:** Have you ever experienced this kind of pain before, and what do you think might be going on here?
>
> **Mrs. P.:** Now that you mention it, I did have something like this several years ago, but a lot worse; I hope this isn't the same thing. I had such bad constipation after a bout with the flu that I almost had an impaction. I'll bet that is what is happening!
>
> **Nora:** The information you are describing does fit that picture. What did you do the last time?
>
> **Mrs. P.:** I had to take this terrible medicine and several enemas. I sure don't want to do that again.

Nora: Let's consult with your obstetrician and try some less drastic measures first, like extra water, prune juice, raisins, exercise, and any other things that normally stimulate your bowels to move.

Nora and Mrs. Peters continued their visit. The baby bath was completed, and they had time to talk about not starting solid foods yet and about irritability. After consulting with her obstetrician, who ordered a mild laxative, they worked out a plan to increase her fluids and exercise. By the next day, Mrs. Peters began to pass small amounts of stool and was beginning to feel better. By Nora's second visit, Mrs. Peter's stomachache was completely gone and her bowel elimination was within her personal norms. She was no longer feeling irritable and was very comfortable with safely bathing her new baby.

⟳Action Learning #34: Collecting the DETAIL Clues on a Headache

Find a person who recently had or currently has a headache. Use the DETAIL format to collect expanded information on the headache. Share your data with a classmate who did this same activity and compare responses.

D = Date of onset and course of the problem
E = Exact location of the problem
T = Terms (patient's) for description of quality and quantity of the problem
A = Aggravating and alleviating factors
I = Intersystem connections of the problem
L = Listen to patient's interpretation of the problem

D.

E.

T.

A.

I.

L.

THINK ABOUT THIS ■ Did you get a full picture of the headache? Do you see how these details give you more direction for planning interventions than you would have had without them? Did you also see how different headaches produce different data?

Observation

Observation is one *How* method used to collect objective data. Like interaction, it is something that all people use daily. Some people are very attentive; others are not. Nurse health detectives must have very attentive, fine-tuned observation skills at all times. When with a patient, a nurse must look at the patient *and* the environment. Sensitive eyes and ears can pick up changes in patients and their environments that the patient may not yet be able or willing to describe verbally.

The things that nurses learn to observe are too numerous to list. A few examples include the patient's nonverbal behaviors (movements, body language, facial expressions, voice tone, gait, and the like), skin color, eating behaviors, sleeping behaviors, condition of teeth, ability to use call lights, and environmental hazards among others.

⊃ACTION LEARNING #35: Using Observation Skills

Find a picture in a magazine or at an art museum that includes people doing something. Describe everything you see that may be related to the health of the people in the picture. Ask your classmate to look at the same picture and do the same activity. Share your findings.

THINK ABOUT THIS ▪ What did both of you find? Were there many differences? What subtle issues did you notice, such as skin tone, unhealthy behaviors, unhealthy environments, and so forth?

Measurement

Measurement, the third *How* technique, is also used to collect objective data. It is generally considered the most precise of the three data collection techniques because it quantifies data (amount, size, and the like) through specific instruments that enhance the nurse's five senses.

It is always best to use a measurement instrument when one is available rather than guessing at measurements. This may seem obvious for things like blood pressure readings, but it is easily forgotten when one measures something like a skin lesion. A specific measurement (4 cm as measured with a ruler) is more descriptive than statements like the "size of a grapefruit." There are too many variations in grapefruit size.

Remember the discussion on inferences and raw data. A good nurse will not substitute an inference for raw data if a specific measurement is possible. For example, instead of documenting the inference, "large lesion on back," measure it and record a clear description such as "2.5-cm, round, flat, red lesion with defined borders on coccyx." The word "large" is too general and open to interpretation, as are the words "lesion" and "back." In the more descriptive example, the word "lesion" was used but clearly modified with descriptive words that narrowed the limits of interpretation. The other parts of the description are so specific that anyone reading it could visualize it.

Although the precision of measurements and numbers is highly respected, the nurse's intuitive "measurements" are equally valuable in the overall picture. Experienced nurses often can make very accurate measurements without tools, but beginners do not have the necessary familiarity with patient situations to rely on their "eyeballing" as experts do.

⊃ACTION LEARNING #36: Practicing Your Measurement Skills

PART 1:

Ask a friend to work with you for this Action Learning exercise. You will need a tape measure calibrated in centimeters. Practice measuring the following items:

A fingernail
A mole

The circumference of the calf of your leg
The great toe
The distance around an ankle
Abdominal girth

PART 2:

Study the back of your hand and your friend's hand and describe them in writing so that anyone would be able to determine which hand was whose by comparing the written descriptions with the actual hands.

THINK ABOUT THIS ■ Can you think of patient circumstances in which such measurements would be critical data? Check a nursing textbook for care of patients with ascites or deep vein thrombosis for examples. As you measured the calf and abdomen, did you think about the importance of specifying precisely where on the leg or abdomen the measurements were taken? What were the key differences in the backs of your hands?

Making Sense Out of "How" Clues

All T.H.I.N.K. modes are needed to determine *how* best to collect and analyze data. TOTAL RECALL is important to organize the data collection and know what to ask, observe, and measure. Establishing therapeutic relationships before collecting data must become a HABIT. Just "jumping right in" and asking questions, observing, and measuring without establishing that relationship could alienate and possibly frighten patients. *How* to use data collection instruments, such as thermometers and blood pressure cuffs, appropriately and safely also may become HABITS. INQUIRY is important for branching and collecting DETAILs because the nurse must constantly mentally ask whether the data need to be expanded. NEW IDEAS AND CREATIVITY are needed to determine *how* to get information in unusual patient situations. Use of the KNOWING HOW YOU THINK mode will help beginning nurse health detectives develop comfort with data collection and analysis. How each nurse thinks influences such things as *how* and *when* data are recorded, how structured the data collection process needs to be, and how easily relevant data are recognized.

Why

The answer to the *Why* question is found in the purpose of data collection. The reason for collecting data is to have raw data from which valid conclusions can be made. Data collection and analysis provide the building blocks for the thinking that leads to valid conclusions. Think about it! How productive and safe is it to pull conclusions out of thin air? Safe, great nursing demands thinking during data collection to develop accurate conclusions. Return to Chapter 5, if necessary, to review the thinking about conclusions.

✔ *Thinking-Learning Check*

Pause here for a thinking-learning check. You should be able to elaborate on these ideas:

✔ Data are always collected during all encounters.

✔ Data are collected through interaction, observation, and measurement.

✔ Branching and D.E.T.A.I.L. are useful skills of interaction.

✔ Data are collected to develop conclusions.

✔ All five modes of thinking are required during data collection and analysis.

CLOSING COMMENTS

This chapter has covered a great deal of basic information that must be incorporated into the skills repertoire of the nurse health detective. These skills will not be developed overnight, but they are essential to great nursing. It takes practice and much repetition for many of these health detective skills to become useful HABITS. It also requires thinking in all five modes to avoid the assessment rut. The next chapter expands this thinking process of data analysis to cluster analysis, from which the major conclusions of assessment can be made.

THINKING LOG #7 ➤

Think about how you learn best. Develop some strategies for remembering and being able to apply all of the things you have just learned from this chapter. If you prefer the written word, you might outline this chapter on a 5 × 8 card. If you prefer a visual format, you might create a diagram or flow chart to illustrate all the concepts in the chapter. Use your creativity to enhance your learning and share your results with a classmate.

References

Saba, V.K. & McCormick, K.A. (1996). *Essentials of computers for nurses* (2nd ed.). New York: McGraw-Hill Health Professions Division.

Making More Sense of Clues: Cluster Analysis

❊ *Learning Outcomes*

After reading and doing the activities in this chapter you will be able to:

Describe what clusters are and how to develop them.

Explain the need for clusters in developing conclusions.

Demonstrate all modes of T.H.I.N.K. in cluster analysis.

Chapter 7 focused on collecting data and the preliminary analysis that occurs as the nurse collects data. Analysis, however, must go much further before major conclusions of assessment can be made by the nurse health detective. This chapter shows how data are arranged and analyzed in groups so that the most accurate conclusions can be made.

To begin to appreciate this additional level of analysis, examine the following case study and the conclusions made by the nurse. Try to determine what the nurse did between point A (collecting the data) and point C (developing the main conclusions of assessment); in other words, what constitutes point B (the additional level of analysis)?

Case Study (Point A)

Juanita Gomez, widow, age 76, has lived in a nursing home for 4 months since she fractured her right hip and had open reduction and internal fixation surgery (ORIF). She is a former teacher. Mrs. Gomez was born in Puerto Rico but has lived in New York since age 5. She has adequate health insurance, with Medicare and supplemental insurance.

Her medical diagnoses are osteoarthritis, non–insulin-dependent diabetes mellitus (NIDDM), and right hip ORIF. The scar on her right hip is pink and dry with no drainage. She is legally blind but can see shapes and light. Owing to neurologic changes, her hearing is slightly diminished.

She wears lipstick each day and gets her hair done every week in the beauty shop. Her hair is shiny and her clothes are neat and clean. She wakes each morning feeling rested. She wouldn't have chosen to live in a nursing home, but says "this one's not so bad." She usually sees her two children, who live out of state, about once a year. She has three grandchildren.

She spends lots of time alone in her room listening to the radio and "talking books" and crocheting potholders for the annual craft show. She says she feels alone and different from others because she is almost blind; she has not made friends.

Her vital signs are: B/P = 110/76; P = 86, Reg; R = 16; T = 97.8°F. She has 2+ ankle edema (swelling). She is 5'2" and weighs 105 lbs. She follows an 1800-calorie diabetic diet. Her skin is dry, very thin, and translucent. She has bowel movements every other day. They are soft and brown, and she drinks prune juice daily to maintain regularity. She wears "Depends" because of some minor urinary dribbling. Her coccyx and elbows are reddened.

Mrs. Gomez sleeps through the night but has lots of trouble getting out of bed because of joint stiffness and limited range of motion of her right hip. She has a bruise on her left shin from hitting against the wheelchair during transfers from bed. She also has a skin tear on her left hand. She complains of discomfort and irritation of her buttocks from sitting in the wheelchair all day.

CONCLUSIONS ABOUT MRS. GOMEZ (POINT C)

1. Strengths:
   Vital signs stable
   Adequate nutrition
   Adequate bowel elimination
   Adequate sleep pattern
   Adequate health insurance
   Well groomed
2. Health Concerns:
   Nursing Diagnoses (actual problems and related factors):
   Impaired Skin Integrity related to mobility deficits, urinary incontinence, fragile skin, and compromised circulation
   Social Isolation related to sensory deficits
   Interdisciplinary Problems:
   Impaired Physical Mobility (physical therapy)
   Problems for Referral:
   None at this time
3. Hunches to be Ruled In or Ruled Out:
   Possible Knowledge Deficit regarding diabetic care
   Possible problem for referral: vision deficits

⟳ ACTION LEARNING #37: **Looking for "Point B"**

Write your responses to the following questions and share them with a class-mate. As you examined the database, what was your first impression?

What could have been done with the database to make it more under-standable?

Did the nurse's conclusions make sense to you? Why or why not?

What other conclusions did you come up with?

Describe what you think the nurse might have done to arrive at the above conclusions.

THINK ABOUT THIS ▪ Did the database provide adequate information from which to develop conclusions? How could the data have been presented differently to allow for some "natural" groupings of related information? Would "natural groupings" have helped your thinking? If so, why? Did you sense the thinking piece between points A and C?

DEFINITIONS AND IMPORTANCE OF CLUSTERS

The above database and conclusions are realistic examples of what nurses process mentally every day. The mental processing required to get from point A (data collection) to point C (conclusions) is rarely discussed, let alone written down. This thinking is so important to great nursing, however, that all of this chapter is devoted to it. The major component of this thinking is the development and analysis of data clusters.

In general, a cluster is two or more similar pieces of anything. A peanut cluster is a tasty example. A data cluster is two or more pieces of information that fit together and have more meaning together than they do when examined separately. The nurse health detective finds clues, analyzes them for significance as described in Chapter 7 (comparing with norms), and then looks for patterns in those clues so that conclusions can be made. The patterns in the clues are clusters, and making sense out of those clusters is cluster analysis.

Importance of Clusters

Making Accurate Conclusions

Clustering and cluster analysis occur simultaneously, as do data collection and data analysis, and are essential in making accurate conclusions. To make sound conclusions, nurses must look beyond individual pieces of data and how they compare with norms, to the relationships among the data and among the clusters. Nurses do not base care on a single datum because accurate conclusions rarely can be made with one piece of information. Think of this for a minute. A nurse finds a patient crying while talking to her husband on the phone. Would the nurse conclude that the patient and her husband are having marital problems? No, of course not. The nurse would certainly note that the crying is relevant, but would collect more data to develop a cluster before concluding anything. Later, the nurse learns that the patient was talking about her mother, who died 2 years ago in this same hospital, and listens as the patient describes her sadness. The nurse then develops an initial hunch that the patient is experiencing grief. (Of course, this conclusion would need to be validated with the patient.)

Taking Necessary Shortcuts

In addition to promoting accuracy of conclusions, appropriate clustering allows nurse health detectives to take necessary shortcuts by consolidating their thinking and communication with other health care providers. Think of the above example. It is much easier to say to another nurse (after validation), "This patient is grieving," as opposed to describing all the raw data that went into that conclusion: "The patient has been crying, talking about her mother who died 2 years ago in this hospital," and so forth. After hearing the diagnosis of "grieving," other nurses can safely assume that the patient is experiencing certain signs and symptoms. They hear the word "grieving" and assume sadness and loss are being experienced. This does not mean the nurse couldn't describe all of the raw data; there simply are not enough hours in the day to do that for all the patient responses that nurses find.

Avoiding Omissions and Finding Critical Data

A third important aspect of clustering is that it prevents nurses from spending unnecessary time on data that "appear" abnormal on the surface, or from missing something important because the individual clues don't signal any concern. With clustering, something that seemed abnormal can be recognized as normal, and something that seems normal may be recognized as abnormal. Consider the following examples. Which of these situations is/are normal?

A person:
    who wets the bed
    whose menstrual cycle hasn't started yet
    who sleeps only 2 or 3 hours at a time
    who has a bowel movement every 3 days
    who needs to have all his teeth pulled
    who is incontinent of urine

At first glance, a nonthinking nurse might say all these are abnormal and jump to premature conclusions. However, these single pieces of information, by themselves, should not be the focus of nursing care. Other data must be collected to round out the picture; there must be a cluster of data before any accurate conclusions can be made.

In the examples above, adding data about the age of the person might provide enough of a cluster to make some conclusions. If the person who wets the bed is 2 years old, it is not unusual; if the person is 11 years old, the same data cluster takes on new importance. In the second example, again, age and gender are important pieces of information to add before any conclusions can be made. In the third example, one more piece of information probably would not be enough. The nurse would want to find out how this person feels with this sleep pattern, what was waking the person, how long this was going on, whether there had been attempts to change this pattern, and other data as well. Then, again, if the person who only sleeps 2 to 3 hours at a time is a newborn baby, it could be very normal.

What these examples show is that data clusters may have two or any number of pieces of information in them. The amount of information depends on the area under study. Generally speaking, the more data in the cluster, the more accurate the conclusion can be, but that is not always the case. It depends on how critical each piece of information is. Look at the following clusters:

Grasping the throat	"I feel really strange."
Unable to talk	"I'm a bit dizzy at times."
	"My husband just left me."
	"I don't know what I'll do."
	"I can't seem to keep food down."
	Abdomen nontender
	B/P 130/88; P 92; R 24

The cluster on the left has two critical indicators of choking. The logical conclusion, which can be made quickly, is that the person is choking and needs a Heimlich maneuver. The cluster on the right, although it has more information, has fewer critical indicators. It is a larger cluster, but a conclusion based on those data would not be as easy to make and would have a lower probability of accuracy.

Taking Advantage of the Brain's Natural Memory System

Finally, clustering is important as a memory aid that is invaluable in health care. The human brain can store a great deal of information, but the way pieces are stored is the key to retrieval. Without effective retrieval systems the information is useless. Brains have a special short-term memory system for storing raw data as separate units of information (Fig. 8-1 characterizes the brain's use of memory and linkages of information). If people try to store too many separate units, however, their brains 'say', "Hold on, there is a better way to do this without using up so much short-term memory space." The brain starts looking for things that fit together into groups or clusters, and uses the cluster labels as triggers to move deeper into its memory levels for storage or retrieval of the details. The brain's memory system seems to work in layers; each layer can hold only so much information. But remembering a label on one level can trigger the memory of the six or seven separate pieces of information (clues) on the level below it that were grouped together and summarized with that trigger label on the higher level (Hart, 1983; Carnevali & Thomas, 1993). This concept about memory and use of patterns was discussed originally in Chapter 1.

Neurophysiology notwithstanding, the important thing is that nurse health detectives can remember things more easily if they group clues (data) together than if they try to remember all the separate pieces. Because there is so much to remember and analyze in health care, it is impossible to practice great nursing without clustering.

WHAT CLUSTERS LOOK LIKE

Clusters are the groups of data that support nursing conclusions. Some conclusions are simple phrases such as "vital signs stable," and other conclusions have more formalized titles, such as "Social Isolation related to sensory deficits," but all conclusions need to be supported (validated) with a cluster of data. Examine the clusters of data that support each of the conclusions for Mrs. Gomez. Note that some of the conclusions have more data supporting them than do others. Some incomplete "conclusions" have so many data gaps that they are still labeled as hunches.

FIGURE 8-1   Memory patterns and linkages.

Conclusions of Assessment and Supporting Data Clusters

STRENGTH CONCLUSIONS	SUPPORTING DATA CLUSTERS
• Vital signs stable	B/P 110/76, P 86, R 16, T 97.8°F
• Adequate nutrition	Ht. 5′2″, wt. 105 lbs. Follows 1800-cal. diet, shiny hair.
• Adequate bowel elimination	BM every other day, soft, brown. Drinks prune juice for regularity.
• Adequate sleep pattern	Sleeps through the night and feels rested in the morning.
• Adequate health insurance	Has Medicare and supplemental insurance.
• Well groomed	Hair shiny, gets hair done every week, clothing clean and neat, wears lipstick daily.

HEALTH CONCERNS	**SUPPORTING DATA CLUSTERS**

A. NURSING DIAGNOSES

- Impaired Skin Integrity R/T mobility deficits, urinary incontinence, fragile skin, and compromised circulation

DIAGNOSTIC LABEL	**DEFINING CHARACTERISTICS**
Impaired Skin Integrity	Coccyx and elbow reddened, bruise on left shin, skin tear left hand, complaints of discomfort and irritation of buttocks.

RELATED FACTORS	**SUPPORTING DATA**
Mobility Deficits	Wheelchair bound, stiff joints, trouble getting out of bed, limited ROM (range of motion) right hip, hitting wheelchair during transfers, osteoarthritis, right hip ORIF 4 months ago.
Urinary Incontinence	Dribbles urine, wears "Depends."
Fragile Skin	Skin dry, very thin, translucent.
Compromised Circulation	Sitting in wheelchair all day, NIDDM, ankle edema.

- Social Isolation R/T sensory deficits

DIAGNOSTIC LABEL	**DEFINING CHARACTERISTICS**
Social Isolation	Spends a lot of time alone in her room listening to the radio, crocheting (noninteractive activities), says she feels alone and different from others because she is almost blind, has made no friends, sees family once a year.

RELATED FACTOR	**SUPPORTING DATA**
Sensory Deficits	Almost blind, hearing slightly diminished.

B. INTERDISCIPLINARY PROBLEM	SUPPORTING DATA CLUSTER
• Impaired physical mobility	Wheelchair bound, stiff joints, trouble getting out of bed, limited ROM right hip, hitting wheelchair during transfers, osteoarthritis, right hip ORIF 4 months ago.

C. PROBLEMS FOR REFERRAL (SEE BELOW)

D. INCOMPLETE CONCLUSIONS: HUNCHES TO BE RULED IN OR RULED OUT	SUPPORTING DATA CLUSTER
• Possible knowledge deficit regarding diabetic care.	Medical Dx: NIDDM Data gaps: Knowledge about NIDDM, knowledge about care needed to maintain health.
• Possible problem for referral: vision deficits.	Medical Dx: NIDDM Legally blind Neurologic changes have already affected hearing Data gaps: Actual visual acuity, use of glasses, last vision exam, patient's description of actual vision limits

Notice how the clusters "paint a picture" that can be summed up with the conclusion label. The type and quality of data in the clusters increase the probability of accuracy of the conclusions. Can you see how the pieces in the cluster logically fit together? Seeing the logic of the fit for some clusters may come from common sense, but, for other clusters it takes practice, experience, and study. Recognizing important data gaps (missing data) takes even more experience. Because this ability is so important, reexamine the clusters for Mrs. Gomez's data and then practice clustering.

⊃Action Learning #38: Examining Clusters

Examine the following clusters and explain why they do or do not fit together.

Cluster A:	Runny nose
	Temperature of 101.2°F
	Watery eyes
	"I feel awful"
Cluster B:	Sedentary job
	Occipital headaches
	Recently married
	Good health insurance
Cluster C:	Bowel movements every 3 days
	Stools hard, dark brown
	Strains with bowel movements
	"I really feel bloated and I can't even button my pants anymore"
	Drinks two cups of liquid a day
	Sedentary job
	Taking calcium and Tylenol #3 for back pain from arthritis
Cluster D:	Wringing hands
	Sweaty palms
	Wide-eyed stare
	Pacing floor
	"I can't think and I don't know what to do"
	"I think I'm going to throw up"
Cluster E:	Sleeps 8 hours a day
	Does not have vegetables in daily intake
	Able to take care of all daily needs
	Has high school education
	"Every time I go to the bathroom it burns so bad, I get tears in my eyes"

What preliminary conclusions (labels) should be considered for the clusters that appear to fit together? Try to make two or three hunches for each cluster.

CONCLUSION HUNCHES

Cluster A:

Cluster B:

Cluster C:

Cluster D:

Cluster E:

THINK ABOUT THIS ■ Do you see how each item in the cluster, taken by itself, takes on a new meaning when it is combined with other items? How did you know which clusters had data that fit together? How easy was it to select preliminary conclusions for the clusters? Why was it easy or difficult to make conclusions for these clusters?

HOW TO CLUSTER

Clustering skill varies greatly, from the beginning nurse health detective to the expert. Examining the thinking and teasing out the details provide some guidance for improving one's existing skills in this area. The primary tasks include determining what data fit together and what data are missing. After these basic tasks are completed, the nurse must choose the best clusters and the best labels for the clusters.

Determining What Fits Together

Sometimes clustering data is fairly easy because one has current knowledge and experience in that area. If a person is 5'2" and 200 lbs., it doesn't take a Ph.D. in nutrition to conclude that this person is overweight. Most people have read or heard something about height and weight being related; if one is a certain height, one is healthiest in a certain weight range. In Western cultures, it is nearly impossible not to have come in contact with such information. To be really sure, one could check a book (probably a nutrition text) for height and weight proportion range norms. Comparing the norms with the actual height and weight would validate the conclusion that this person is overweight. Coming to that conclusion means putting two pieces of data together and comparing them with norms to reach a judgment about what they mean together. Neither piece of information is important on its own, but together they take on new meaning.

For the beginning nurse health detective, however, what fits together often is not so obvious. Luckily, there are tools and aids to assist in this activity. These will be discussed shortly.

Determining Data Gaps

These same tools and aids (to be discussed shortly) also are useful in determining what data are missing from the cluster. Figuring out what is missing is just as important as figuring out what fits together. The missing pieces are called "data gaps." In the case of Mrs. Gomez, the list of conclusions included some "data gaps" when the nurse was ruling in and ruling out the hunches about knowledge deficit and vision problems.

⟩Action Learning #39: Looking for Data Gaps

Look at the example below. For conclusion #1, the data cluster and data gaps are listed. For #2 and #3, the conclusion and the data clusters are given but the data gaps are missing. Write out two or three pieces of data that, if known, would help you develop a better cluster and, therefore, a more accurate conclusion. It might be helpful to use a nursing diagnosis text or nursing theory text to identify data gaps. (Hint: Look at the defining characteristics of the conclusion labels.)

Conclusion	Cluster	Data Gaps
#1 Low self-esteem	Patient very timid Little eye contact Unable to identify any personal strengths	Verbalizes feeling unworthy Believes not worthy of being cared for
#2 Ineffective airway clearance	Abnormal breath sounds Productive cough	
#3 Adequate nutrition	Height = 6′ Weight = 191 lbs.	

THINK ABOUT THIS ■ How did you decide which data were missing? What sources helped? Were there some missing data that were more important than other missing data?

Filling Data Gaps

Filling in data gaps usually is accomplished by using "directed data collection" (discussed in Chapter 5). To set up directed data collection, the nurse's thinking might follow a pattern like this:

The preliminary cluster of data is: straining with stool, complaints of stomachache, states needs laxative every day to have bowel movement.

Hunch #1 is: Constipation

Hunch #2 is: Perceived constipation

(The above two hunches are **differential diagnoses**)

The nurse then thinks," I don't have enough data to be comfortable with either hunch just yet; there are too many **data gaps**."

"I need to use **directed data collection** to fill the gaps with useful data and not waste time collecting irrelevant data."

"**To rule in or rule out Hunch #1**, I know from experience that the additional data might be: hard, formed stools; feeling pressure in the rectum; and decreased frequency in bowel movements."

"**To rule in or rule out Hunch #2**, the textbook indicates that for perceived constipation, the following defining characteristics might be present: patient expects to have bowel movements at the same time every day, patient has been using laxative for extended period of time to maintain proper timing and amount of stool."

With this knowledge, the nurse would go to the patient to collect the necessary data.

Becoming skilled at identifying data gaps and using directed data collection to fill those gaps is a very positive sign that the beginning nurse health detective is moving in the direction of great nursing.

✔ *Thinking-Learning Check*

Pause here for a thinking-learning check. You should be able to elaborate on these ideas:

✔ Clusters of data: two or more pieces of information about patients that fit together and have more meaning together than separately

✔ Cluster analysis: making sense out of the patterns of data

✔ Clusters: increase accuracy of conclusions, allow for necessary shortcuts, help avoid omissions, take advantage of the brain's natural memory system

✔ Clusters are formed by determining what fits together, determining data gaps, and filling gaps.

AIDS TO FORMING CLUSTERS

The challenge of clustering for beginning nursing students lies in figuring out what fits with what. TOTAL RECALL and INQUIRY are the primary thinking modes used. With experience, some clustering of data becomes HABIT—the nurse knows that when one thing is present, another usually accompanies it. For example, if a nurse observes dark circles under a patient's eyes, it becomes automatic to watch for frequent yawning. Until those HABITS develop, INQUIRY must be used to ask "What is usually associated with this?" That ongoing use of INQUIRY is essential to seeing the complete picture of the patient situation. TOTAL RECALL (memory or looking it up) helps answer many INQUIRY questions. What beginners have to work with to develop clusters are knowledge from courses (nursing courses and all those other "-ology" courses), life experience, assessment instruments, and the taxonomy of nursing diagnoses.

Knowledge From Courses

One reason novice students find the thinking process in nursing a challenge is because they have a limited knowledge base. Students are asked to put information together and act on it while they are still learning the importance of the information. Nursing and supporting courses continually provide a wealth of information about patterns of human responses. In physiology courses, nurses learn about the body's biologic processes; in psychology courses they learn about emotional responses; in nursing courses they learn about health and illness responses, and so forth. Each of these courses obviously adds to the nurse's knowledge of what usually fits with what, but it takes time to reach a "critical mass" of information. The challenge is to pull all of that knowledge together and quickly retrieve what is needed in each patient situation. INQUIRY thinking keeps nurses asking what other information is needed, and TOTAL RECALL thinking sends them back to the books or to whatever part of their mind stores the relevant information. For beginners, INQUIRY is more of a challenge because they have less first-hand nursing experience to use as a thinking stimulus. This is where life experience can help.

Life Experience

Remembering that patients are people just as nurses are people may seem like a simplistic notion; however, it merits some thought. As beginners, students may get so caught up in trying to sort through all they have to know that they forget what they do know—all that valuable information not taught in classrooms. Everyone has been sick at some time and can relate to things like lack of sleep and irritability, decreased appetite and anxiety, weight loss diets and frustration, stress and stomachaches, nausea and vomiting, and so forth. To stimulate your thinking about what you have learned from life experience, try the following Action Learning.

⊃Action Learning #40: Tapping Your Life Experience

From the experiences listed below, circle those that you can relate to, either because you experienced them yourself or because you were around someone who did. For each one circled, list what signs and symptoms (objective and subjective data) went along with the item listed.

	Signs	**Symptoms**
Constipation		
Stress reaction		
Anxiety or fear		

Nutrition problem

Sleep disturbance

Parenting issue

Loss or grief

Mobility deficit

Situational crisis

Other (add your own)

THINK ABOUT THIS ■ Do you see how you have identified clusters of data that go along with situations? Some of you probably had experience with many of these; others perhaps have experienced fewer. These and other such life experiences provide valuable information that will help you think. Obviously, you would not base nursing care on just your personal experience, but these experiences can help your INQUIRY by reminding you of questions to ask and leading you to the appropriate resources to help you build from life experience to professional nursing interventions. Life experiences, by the way, also are very valuable in helping nurses relate to patients as human beings.

Assessment Tools

Assessment tools, also called assessment instruments, usually are organized to enhance clustering. Such tools generally are developed from some theoretical model that indicates how human responses are seen as patterns with labels and which patient behaviors are part of which responses. For example, Roy's model (Roy & Andrews, 1991) considers patient responses to be outputs (patient behaviors) in four modes: physiologic, self-concept, role function, and interdependence. Assessment tools based on her theoretical model are arranged according to those four modes. Other models, such as Orem's Self-Care Framework (Orem, 1991), and assessment tools based on her model, categorize patient responses as universal self-care demands. The North American Nursing Diagnosis Association (NANDA) considers response categories with the Unitary Person focus. A nursing assessment tool using the NANDA approach is presented in Chapter 13.

Assessment tools often are used to collect data from patients in a systematic, organized way during first encounters. On repeated encounters with patients, depending on how tools are used in the particular setting, additional data may be added to the tool.

Once data are recorded on a tool, clusters emerge because data from observations, interactions, and measurements of each human response pattern are in one place. Look back to the database on Mrs. Gomez. It would have been easier to see the clusters if the data had been arranged in more appropriate categories. Turn to the assessment tool in Chapter 13 and study how the tool helps with data arrangement.

> ⊃ ACTION LEARNING #41: Discovering
> Assessment Tools
>
> Find at least three different assessment tools. (Clues to help your hunt: If you are
> a student, there is probably one used at your school. Most clinical agencies have
> a specific one geared toward their specialty. There are many books that include
> these tools.) Study the tools and ask yourself how they are similar and how they
> are different. Make a copy of one of them. Refer to the data for Mrs. Gomez on
> the first pages of this chapter. Put all the data into the tool format.
>
> THINK ABOUT THIS ■ How were the tools different? Alike? Could you deter-
> mine why each was arranged in the manner that it was? When you recorded
> the data for Mrs. Gomez on the tool, could you see patterns? Did the data
> form any natural clusters? What conclusions could you see more easily with
> the tool format? How did the tool help you see data gaps?

By using the assessment tool, it should have been easier to recognize how some data fit together. In a sense, some of the preliminary thinking, in the form of sorting, is done for the nurse as data are recorded on the assessment tool. However, not all of the thinking is done. As mentioned before, human responses rarely fit into tidy boxes; any categorization of responses is somewhat artificial. Consider a patient who has a mobility deficit. Data about mobility also are relevant to elimination responses (people who decrease their mobility often get constipated and may have urinary retention), skin responses (decubitus ulcers form when there is prolonged pressure on body parts), and many other responses. Therefore, assessment tools, although they provide a start to clustering, also can provide a false security; a nurse must rely on *thinking* to find the less obvious clusters.

Taxonomy of Nursing Diagnoses

The NANDA taxonomy (Appendix A) can help nurses cluster data that lead to nursing diagnosis conclusions by reminding them of the various diagnostic labels grouped within response patterns. If one piece of information seems to indicate a particular diagnosis, such as urinary incontinence, examining the taxonomy will remind the nurse that there are several types of incontinence. Referring to a book that has the defining characteristics of the diagnoses will trigger the nurse's search for data that can be added to the cluster. Directed data collection can be used, or the nurse can refer back to the database to find the data and form the best cluster. The list of nursing diagnoses, along with defining characteristics and related factors, can help fine-tune the clusters. Guidelines for ruling in and ruling out hunches (differential diagnosis) can be found in Chapter 5. Ruling hunches in or out is really a process of clustering data more and more specifically until the final cluster "paints" the best picture of the conclusion label.

CHOOSING THE BEST CLUSTERS

Clusters have certain characteristics besides being groups of data. There are pure and mixed clusters. In addition, there are different types of clusters for nursing diagnoses, including those that are actual problems and those that are potential ("risk for") problems. It is important to recognize these subtle differences to select the best clusters for the major conclusions of assessment.

Pure and Mixed Clusters

The clusters shown in the Mrs. Gomez example are "pure" clusters; they contain only the specific data for each conclusion. Some nurses used "mixed" clusters, especially when they are forming nursing diagnosis conclusions. They use mixed clusters because they believe it is more logical or easier to include all data supporting the problem statement and all data supporting the related factors in the cluster. For example, nurses who prefer mixed clusters would develop the following cluster for the nursing diagnosis of Impaired Skin Integrity related to mobility deficits, urinary incontinence, fragile skin, and compromised circulation:

Data Cluster

Coccyx and elbow reddened, bruise on left shin, skin tear on hand, complaints of discomfort and irritation of buttocks. Wheelchair bound, stiff joints, trouble getting out of bed, limited ROM right hip, hitting wheelchair during transfers, osteoarthritis, right hip ORIF 4 months ago. Dribbles urine, wears "Depends." Skin dry, very thin, translucent. Sitting in wheelchair all day, NIDDM, ankle edema.

There is nothing "wrong" with forming this type of mixed cluster; indeed, the mixed format may seem more logical at times. One must use this approach with care, however. Remember, there are two conclusions being made—one is the conclusion about the health concern, and the other is the conclusion about the related factors. When a cluster is mixed (supporting two conclusions), it is easy accidentally to have adequate data supporting one conclusion but only limited data supporting the other, and not readily recognize this situation.

The other problem is that this approach can lead to confusion in planning because the pieces haven't been clearly examined. A mixed cluster can decrease the probability of finding all the related factors. The related factors are less evident because there are so many data that the patterns get lost. For example, examine this mixed cluster and its accompanying conclusion:

Data Cluster

- Patient is 76 years old, has fourth-grade education, lives alone
- Recent diagnosis of diabetes mellitus
- Anticipated need for insulin injections

Conclusion: Knowledge Deficit regarding self-care with diabetes.

At first glance this seems logical. A person of that age with limited formal schooling, living alone, and recently diagnosed with diabetes would need to be taught how to give injections and so forth. However, the conclusion of "Knowledge Deficit" has no data to support it. It could be that this patient gave injections to his mother for years. So, what that cluster needs is information about the person's actual knowledge or deficit, if there is one. What the patient does or does not know is critical information to support a diagnosis of Knowledge Deficit.

Clusters for Actual and Potential Problems

There also is a difference between clusters of data supporting actual problems and those clusters supporting potential problems (those problems for which a patient is at risk). Again, consider the Mrs. Gomez case. She had a nursing diagnosis of an actual problem, "Impaired Skin Integrity." One can see why this was an actual problem. The data (defining characteristics for the problem of impaired skin integrity) were there to support the problem. Those data were reddened elbow and coccyx, bruise on shin, skin tear on hand, and complaints of discomfort and irritation of buttocks. These data *actually* existed for the *actual* problem. There also were data that showed the related factors for the skin problem—mobility deficits, urinary incontinence, fragile skin, and compromised circulation.

If the data that supported the problem did not exist (the reddened elbow and coccyx, bruise on shin, tear on hand, discomfort and irritation of buttocks), it seems that one could assume there was no problem. The related factors, however, are still there. Mrs. Gomez still has incontinence; she is still immobile; she still has dry, fragile skin; and she still has poor circulation. Probability indicates that it will be only a matter of time before something happens to her skin. Sooner or later, her skin integrity will break down, and there will be an actual problem to deal with.

Should a nurse wait and see what happens? Of course not; nurses want to prevent health problems before they happen. The way to do this is to draw a conclusion about the risks and design care either to maintain the current status or to promote a higher level of health that puts the patient at less risk. The conclusion in this case would be:

Risk for Impaired Skin Integrity related to incontinence, immobility, fragile skin with poor turgor, and compromised circulation

This can be confusing, so think about it in this way. The "problem" portion of the diagnostic statement, **Risk for Impaired Skin Integrity**, is not an actual problem yet. It is a "potential" problem, one that will become an actual problem if the risk factors are not dealt with soon.

Because it is not an actual problem yet, there obviously are no data (no defining characteristics) and no cluster of data to support a conclusion that a problem exists. In other words, there are no defining characteristics such as "disruption of skin surface; destruction of skin layers; invasion of body structures" (NANDA, 1996).

The "related factors" portion of the diagnostic statement—**incontinence, immobility, fragile skin with poor turgor**, and **compromised circulation**—is the key to this type of diagnosis. These four related factors do exist and do put the patient at "risk for" development of an actual problem if left unattended.

The related factors for a potential problem (or an actual problem) can be single pieces of data (fragile skin) or they can be labels for clusters of data (compromised circulation).

Diagnosing potential problems generally requires a greater amount of content knowledge and experience. Knowing what relationships to anticipate among pieces of data and data clusters is the result of sophisticated, high-level thinking. More discussion of potential problems is presented in Chapter 15.

⊃ACTION LEARNING #42: Another Look at Clusters for Actual and Potential Problems

This Action Learning is similar to the Action Learning #28 in Chapter 6. Consider this as more practice for differentiating data clusters. Using nursing diagnosis books or nursing theory texts, examine each cluster. This time, select a label and write it appropriately. For example, if it is a potential problem, write it as "Risk for . . .", then circle Actual or Potential, whichever is correct.

CLUSTER #1:
Three-day-old infant with hyperirritability; mother addicted to cocaine; infant has great difficulty coordinating sucking, swallowing, and breathing.

Diagnostic Label:
Actual/Potential (circle one)

CLUSTER #2:
Thirty-three-year-old alcoholic in alcohol rehabilitation program; verbalizes feelings of guilt and anger toward husband; admits to diminished interest in sexual activity over the past 5 years; rape victim in early 20s.

Diagnostic Label:
Actual/Potential (circle one)

CLUSTER #3:
Fifty-nine-year-old wife of a 58-year-old man with Alzheimer's disease; caring for
   husband at home for 6 months; currently eating and sleeping well but notes
   that she is gradually getting less sleep because husband wakes and wanders
   through house several times a night; oldest daughter, who is a major support
   system, was recently promoted to company president and had to move out of
   state; wife is hesitant to use local Alzheimer's support organizations.

Diagnostic Label:
Actual/Potential (circle one)

THINK ABOUT THIS ■   How did the nursing diagnosis manuals and nursing
   theory texts help in selecting appropriate labels? What additional data would
   be helpful in validating your selections? Could you identify the data that supported the problem and the data that supported the related factors?

Using the Big Picture to Find the Best Clusters

Clustering data and eventually attaching labels that represent the conclusions
made about the data are not governed by rigid rules. This is especially true with
nursing diagnosis conclusions. There are few "right" or "wrong" ways to go about
these tasks. The ideal for which nurses aim is to have as complete a picture of the
patient's health issues as possible so that nursing care can be planned and implemented in an efficient, yet thorough, manner.

"Efficient" and "thorough" are key words here. As patient data are analyzed,
one can see many, seemingly equally valid, conclusions that could be reached. In
Mrs. Gomez's case, other nursing diagnoses could have been made. For example,
"Sensory Impairment related to decreased hearing and sight," could have been a
nursing diagnosis. There is a clear data cluster "painting a picture" of this actual
problem. The reason why this conclusion was not listed as a nursing diagnosis is
that the nurse cannot really do much about it. The nurse can, however, do something about the social isolation that is the result of the sensory deficit. Putting the
sensory data together with other data led the nurse to a conclusion that, ultimately, will lead to more efficient and thorough care. If the focus were on just the
sensory problems, the social isolation could go unnoticed. By broadening the view a
bit, the nurse can do everything possible for the sensory problem while trying to
decrease the social isolation.

In addition to showing that there are no right or wrong approaches to clustering and conclusion making, this example demonstrates that thinking ahead to the
planning phase of the nursing process helps with finding the best clusters.

The value of looking toward planning as an aid to clustering also is illustrated in the nursing diagnosis, "Impaired Skin Integrity..." The conclusions made from the related factor clusters also could be seen as conclusions about problems. In addition to that one diagnosis, these diagnoses and others could have been made from the same data:

> Urinary Incontinence related to (possibly) neuromuscular changes 2° related to diabetes and decreased circulation
> Impaired Physical Mobility related to osteoarthritis and right hip ORIF
> Altered Peripheral Tissue Perfusion related to immobility and diabetes

Actually, a long list of nursing conclusions could have been generated by clustering the data in various ways.

The decision to cluster in the way it was done for Mrs. Gomez was based on a projection toward planning care. When care is planned for the skin problem, the nurse will automatically deal with the mobility, urinary, fragile skin, and circulation problems because all of these contribute to the skin impairment. Making four or five conclusions by clustering another way would be redundant and inefficient.

Clearly, this is high-level thinking using the INQUIRY mode. The nurse tries out various clusters and thinks about relationships among them. This is a bit like the chicken and egg problem—which comes first? The nurse not only must look at the data and various clusters, but must think toward planning and implementation. The "final" clusters of data will point toward conclusions that are as all-inclusive as possible without overlapping too much. Remember, one "problem" conclusion can be a "related factor" conclusion for another problem. All human responses are interrelated (more on this in Chapter 9).

Differences Between Novices and Experts in Developing Clusters

The thinking described in the preceding section is very sophisticated. Even expert nurses do not make such judgments easily. Beginning students have less knowledge and past experience to tap, so this thinking is particularly challenging. The guidelines given in Display 8-1 are useful in developing this thinking skill.

DISPLAY 8–1.   Guidelines for Choosing the Best Clusters

Write out all clusters and ask the following questions:

- How much overlap is there in my clusters?
- If there is overlap, can another way of clustering combine things and decrease the overlap?
- Of the conclusions reached about the cluster, which ones connect with each other?
- How are they connected?
- As I think about planning, will any of these problems be eliminated if I provide care for other problems?

Novices should not fear redundancy as much as omissions. Trying to move too quickly through the thinking at this stage increases the likelihood of missing important issues.

Take the time to write things out. Do not assume your thinking can process such large volumes of new information without providing time to develop new patterns to add to old patterns of thinking.

PITFALLS TO CLUSTERING

Clustering is seldom easy, and things can go awry when data are not clustered well. The fact that there are no right or wrong approaches to clustering, only acceptable, better, and best ways, should suggest why clustering can be challenging. Low-level thinking and intolerance for ambiguity (a factor hindering thinking that was discussed in Chapter 1) are the major contributors to the pitfalls of clustering.

The first pitfall, and the most serious one, is insufficient clustering so that premature conclusions are made. Data analysis and cluster analysis demand serious INQUIRY work. Constant questioning of the relationships among the data and the clusters will help the nurse avoid premature conclusions.

The flip side of insufficient clustering is forming too many clusters without looking at relationships among the clusters. If this occurs, the nurse will make too many conclusions. As care is planned, there may be much redundancy, and trying to set priorities becomes a nightmare. If there are many repetitive parts of plans, other nurses will have insufficient time to read and implement them.

A balance between these two pitfalls is the best course. Form as many clusters as necessary to address all relevant data; but then analyze the clusters themselves, or cluster the clusters, to see what fits with what.

Not seeing the big picture or not projecting thinking toward planning is a third pitfall. Looking ahead to planning is one of the best ways to test out the usefulness of conclusions about clusters. If there is minimal overlap, and all of the patient's strengths, health concerns, and related factors are addressed, this is a good indication that the best clusters have been identified.

✔ *Thinking-Learning Check*

Pause here for a thinking-learning check. You should be able to elaborate on these ideas:

✔ Aids to forming clusters: knowledge, life experience, assessment tools, and the taxonomy of nursing diagnoses or nursing theory texts

✔ Pure clusters: only the defining characteristics of the problem portion of the diagnostic statement and separate clusters for related factors

✔ Mixed clusters: defining characteristics plus data to support related factors

✔ Actual problems: supported by defining characteristics

✔ Potential problems: supported by related factors; requires higher-level thinking to recognize relationships and patterns that could become actual problems

✔ Seeing the big picture helps clustering

✔ Pitfalls to clustering: low-level thinking, insufficient clustering, too many clusters

SELECTING THE BEST LABELS FOR THE BEST CLUSTERS

Selecting the best labels was originally introduced in Chapter 6 and is briefly expanded on in this chapter. The NANDA taxonomy, which was introduced in Chapter 3 and is in Appendix A, continues to be a primary source of diagnostic labels. The NANDA labels are used internationally to describe the types of patient responses that fall within the domain of independent nursing practice. The current labels in the taxonomy have been "accepted for testing," which means nurses are trying them out. Labels in the taxonomy are constantly being reviewed, researched, and adjusted. The *Proceedings* from each of NANDA's biennial conferences, as well as numerous nursing journal articles, report the ongoing work in refining and adding to the diagnostic labels.

Most (but not all) NANDA labels deal with nursing care in acute medical–surgical settings. For this reason, other professional nursing groups have developed labels more specific to their areas of practice.

For beginners, however, it is most important to be familiar with the NANDA labels. Each label is defined and has both a list of defining characteristics and a list of related factors. Several books, large and small, have been published to serve as references to all the current NANDA labels (see suggested references in Chapter 6). The following guidelines are useful in selecting the best NANDA label:

1. Study the list of NANDA labels to become familiar with all labels by name and with the organization of the taxonomy.
2. Examine the cluster of data that needs labeling and develop a hunch as to which label may be appropriate. (This process may be simplified by using the assessment tool. For example, if relevant data are in the area of elimination, the nurse would focus attention on those labels that describe problems with elimination.)
3. Select one or more labels (differential diagnoses) that might work with the cluster.
4. Read the definitions of the labels to see which fits best with the problem or wellness issue the patient is experiencing.
5. Read the defining characteristics to see which ones currently exist (supporting data) and which ones would be appropriate to search for (data gaps). Note any defining characteristics that are identified as "critical indicators." These are particularly important to have in the data cluster.

6. Read the related factors (contributing factors). These usually are very general descriptions, such as "recent stress." Do any of the patient's data fit with the related factors? For example, a patient who was just fired from her job is experiencing recent stress.

7. If the definition, defining characteristics, and related factors have a good to very close match, there is a very good probability that the label is accurate.

8. If you find that the related factors exist but there are no defining characteristics, consider a "Risk for" label to indicate a potential problem.

9. Keep the label (write it down) for ongoing validation as the nursing process continues.

10. If no label fits well with the patient's situation, consider creating one using the format suggested in Nursing Diagnoses Submission Guidelines from the NANDA *Proceedings* (Rantz & LeMone, 1997).

⊃ACTION LEARNING #43: Selecting the Best Label

Find a nursing diagnostic manual or nursing theory text to use as a reference. Read the following case study and complete the activities listed below.

Case Study

Mr. Richard is 46 years old, has been hospitalized for ulcerative colitis, and recently had a colostomy. It is 3 days after his surgery, and he still refuses to help with the dressing changes or even look at his colostomy. When encouraged to participate in his care, he says, "I don't want anything to do with that 'thing.'"

The nurse considered the following as possible conclusions:

Ineffective Individual Coping
Dysfunctional Grieving
Situational Low Self-Esteem
Body Image Disturbance
Noncompliance with treatment plan for self-care of colostomy

Examine the definitions for each of these, and examine the defining characteristics and related factors. Which conclusion is supported best? What additional data would help to further support the conclusion you selected? Share your thinking with a classmate.

> THINK ABOUT THIS   ■   Were you able immediately to rule out any of the original conclusions based on the case study alone? How confident are you that you have selected the best label at this point? How would you validate this label with Mr. Richard?

CLOSING COMMENTS

If you kept your Thinking Cap on for this whole chapter, it is probably time to take it off, rub your head, and get some nourishment. The content in this chapter required a lot of attention and thinking. Being able to cluster data and analyze the clusters, however, is vital to developing accurate conclusions. Without accurate conclusions, nursing care goes off on minor or major tangents that become a waste of time and energy for both the nurse and the patient. Take time to absorb this material; it probably will require some rereading or referring back to as care plans are developed. Take that time; your patients will appreciate it and you will be more confident in your nursing practice.

THINKING LOG #8 ➤

Chapters 5 through 8 have focused on the thinking needed for the assessment phase of the nursing process. Review those three chapters together and look for the themes of assessment thinking. In your own words, write down those themes. Thinking about how you think, consider what will help you engage all your THINK modes to make high-quality assessments—to collect and analyze data, cluster data, analyze clusters, and develop the best conclusions.

References

Carnevali, D.L. & Thomas, M.D. (1993). *Diagnostic reasoning and treatment decision making in nursing.* Philadelphia: JB Lippincott.

Hart, L.A. (1983). *Human brain and human learning.* New York: Longman.

North American Nursing Diagnosis Association. (1996). *NANDA nursing diagnoses: Definitions and classifications, 1997–1998.* St. Louis: Author.

Orem, D.E. (1991). *Nursing concepts of practice* (4th ed.). St. Louis: CV Mosby.

Rantz, M.J. & LeMone, P. (Eds.). (1997). *Classification of nursing diagnoses: Proceedings of the twelfth conference of the North American Nursing Diagnosis Association.* Glendale, CA: Cinahl Information Systems.

Roy, C. & Andrews, H.A. (1991). *The Roy adaptation model: A definitive statement.* Norwalk, CT: Appleton & Lange.

Designing Care:
A Nurse/Patient
Thinking Partnership

After reading and doing the activities in this chapter, you will be able to:

Describe the connections among planning, implementing, and evaluating.

Examine the conclusions of planning, implementing, and evaluating.

Describe the nurse/patient collaborative thinking partnership with regard to setting priorities and identifying desired outcomes during planning.

Explore the details and complexities of establishing outcomes.

The primary goal of this chapter is to help nursing students see the interconnectedness of the whole nursing process. A strong emphasis is placed on including the patient's thinking and participation in this process. The majority of the chapter focuses on the planning aspects of the nursing process and the end of the chapter brings all of the components of the nursing process together.

The nurse health detective must now expand *thinking* and *doing* from assessment to complete the cycle with planning, implementing, and evaluating care. It is currently necessary to design individualized patient care, follow through on that care, and determine the quality of that care. This chapter provides an overview of these processes, and Chapter 10 addresses more details to complete the nursing process.

THE CONCLUSIONS OF PLANNING, IMPLEMENTING, AND EVALUATING

As mentioned in the beginning chapters of this book, it usually is easier to understand how to do something if one knows what is suppose to be achieved at the end. Therefore it will help to briefly examine the conclusions of planning, implementation, and evaluation before looking at how these components of the nursing process work together.

Chapter 5 described how many conclusions in the nursing process (judgments made after thinking) were made in relationship to assessment. The discussion of assessment focused on the conclusions the nurse made with patients about their strengths and health concerns. There are two more major areas of conclusion making in the nursing process; these include conclusions about the best approaches to care for health concerns, and conclusions about how well those concerns are addressed. In short, the three major conclusions in nursing answer these questions:

- What is the concern (**conclusions of assessment**)?
- What should be done about the concern (**conclusions of planning and implementation**)?
- Is the concern resolved (**conclusions of evaluation**)?

As was the case with assessment, many interim conclusions are necessary along the way to these major conclusions. Before deciding on the best course of action, nurses work with patients to make conclusions about the best resources to use, the most creative solutions, the ideal time frames, and the highest priorities, among others. Likewise, as nurses implement care, they work with patients to make decisions about what to do first, what to record in the patient's record, which things require additional attention, and so forth. Each judgment and decision is a conclusion within the nursing process.

Unlike many books on the nursing process that describe the phases of planning, implementing, and evaluating in relatively isolated segments, this text addresses the principles behind these phases of the nursing process to emphasize their interconnectedness. This interconnectedness is accomplished as the nurse and the patient think ahead during planning to how the plan will be carried out, whether the plan can achieve its purpose, and how the outcomes will be evaluated. Likewise, as a plan is implemented, it must be continually adapted to the patient's changing circumstances through an ongoing evaluation of its effectiveness. Doing all of this at once can be a monumental juggling act if careful thought is not a key ingredient. Continual assessment, which occurs simultaneously, compounds the task. Showing how to keep all these balls in the air at the same time to achieve great nursing is the overarching purpose of this chapter (Fig. 9-1).

Although all the components of the nursing process are intertwined in reality, to learn them one must artificially separate the components. This artificial separation allows for a clearer understanding of each component as well as a beginning understanding of how each relates to the others. Thus, the overview, the definitions, the purposes, and the interrelationships of the three components of the nursing process—planning, implementing, and evaluating—are part of the beginning of this chapter.

FIGURE 9–1 Nurse and patient juggling all of the nursing process.

COMPLETING THE CYCLE
OF THE NURSING PROCESS

Great nursing is impossible without completing the cycle of the nursing process. Being skilled in one or some of the phases but not in the whole process is useless. It is like having the skill to survey a plot of ground *or* design a floor plan *or* construct walls *or* judge the soundness of a building, but not being able to do all four phases of home construction. A house will never be built.

Completing the cycle of the nursing process requires the use of all T.H.I.N.K. modes. Probably the best advice for planning, implementing, and evaluating care is to keep Thinking Caps on and well secured. TOTAL RECALL of resources gives the nurse a sound knowledge base to use for planning, but individualized plans that are unique to each patient cannot be copied out of books because they don't exist. To design individualized plans, the nurse must use INQUIRY and NEW IDEAS AND CREATIVITY. Implementing plans requires TOTAL RECALL of safe practice standards and HABITS for efficiency and effectiveness. Evaluating outcomes demands INQUIRY to determine quality and quantity of results and

KNOWING HOW YOU THINK to analyze and make conclusions about planning, implementing, and evaluating.

The nurse, however, is not the only person doing the thinking. The patient's thinking also is essential. Consider, for a moment, what would happen if you were a patient. Would you stop thinking? Would you use a radically different style of thinking than you do for other aspects of your life? Of course not; the idea is preposterous. Nevertheless, nurses and other health care providers often forget that simple fact. Nurses are quick to make statements about patients' rights—to self-determination, to be part of decision-making, and so forth—yet frequently forget how the patient's thinking enters the picture.

It may be that patients cannot articulate how they think. Articulation often is difficult, even for people studying critical thinking. However, patients will know something about how they think. Nurses must not make the mistake of assuming that patients are not thinking just because they cannot verbalize their thinking processes. Patients *are* thinking, and they use all of the modes of T.H.I.N.K.

Earlier, in reviewing the data collection part of assessment, it was easy to see that patients use TOTAL RECALL. They recall facts about their health. However, they also make conclusions about their needs; this conclusion-making process requires at least some level of INQUIRY. They often demonstrate NEW IDEAS AND CREATIVITY thinking as well. Some patients literally say, "This is what I think is going on"; others do not say this for a variety of reasons. They may feel it would be insulting to a health care provider, who is the "expert" in knowing what is going on; they may feel too intimidated to make such comments. What the nurse must keep in mind is this: whether patients verbalize their conclusions or not, they make them in their minds.

Inviting patients to verbalize their thinking promotes the combined nurse and patient thinking that leads to better quality care designs. If patients do not or cannot verbalize their thinking processes and their conclusions automatically, asking them to validate our nursing conclusions signals to patients that their thinking is valuable to their care.

It also is valuable for the nurse to know the patient's usual HABIT mode of thinking. What are the patient's usual approaches to problems? What type of thinking is "second nature"? Answers to these questions and a consideration of the patient's use of all five modes help in planning the best care and certainly are relevant to the implementation of care.

When the nurse is focusing on the patient's thinking about care planning, it is the perfect time to consider the adage, "Two heads are better than one." Why are they better, you might ask? Well, put yourself in the patient's shoes again. If a nurse asked you about your thinking relative to your health care situation, would you feel valued as a person? Would you know that you are expected to be an active participant in your care? Would you feel a sense of ownership in the plan that you and the nurse developed? Would you be more likely to follow that plan?

Advocating patients' rights has always been an important part of nursing. Patients have a right to be active, educated consumers of health care. If a patient does not seem to be exercising that right—that is, if the patient seems passive and does not show how he or she is thinking—the nurse has an obligation to discover what it is about the patient's thinking that is leading to this behavior. What are the reasons behind the patient's passivity? Some patients may desire a passive role and like being dependent. Other patients may have cognitive deficits limiting their thinking contributions. In those cases, family members and/or significant others may take on participatory roles in decision-making. However, in all other cases, the thinking of the patient is as important as that of the nurse. What the nurse brings to the situation is more knowledge about health and health care. The nurse is the knowledge "expert" but not the individuality "expert." Patients are the experts on their individual perceptions of their health care needs and on how a particular kind of care best fits them.

In 1983, Schon wrote about collaboration in thinking under the title *The Reflective Practitioner*. Although Schon did not mention nursing per se, he did use other health care providers as examples to make his points. Schon wrote that in the real world, problems do not present themselves as givens; they are part of puzzling, uncertain situations. Clarifying and organizing those situations requires what he called "reflection-in-action" (p. 49). This reflection is done in the context of the professional/client contract through reflective conversation. This interaction style results in a deeper understanding for both the nurse and the patient. Schon's ideas, although not couched in the same critical thinking terms and modes that are used in this book, certainly provide similar perspectives. If nurses want to organize and understand the patient situation, they must interact reflectively with their patients. This reflection is the thinking process shared through language, and it is essential to designing, doing, and determining quality nursing care with a patient (Fig. 9-2).

FIGURE 9–2   Nurse and patient "reflecting" together.

DESIGNING CARE (PLANNING)

The next several pages are devoted to examining the second component of the nursing process—planning. This discussion is only an overview that will allow you to start (or perhaps add to) your repertoire of planning skills—skills that you will be building on for the rest of your professional career.

Defined broadly, planning is time and resource management—a basic skill for any profession. In nursing, planning includes such things as organizing time to complete five patient home visits during the day, making sure that *all* the equipment needed to properly change the catheter is in the room, or having adequate, well organized information to support one's proposed suicide precautions policy change at the departmental meeting. Planning with the patient affects how one collects information, how one uses the information, how one delivers care, and whether or not one makes the time to evaluate the results of care. This broader view of planning as it relates to time and resource management is discussed in greater detail in the section on implementation of care (doing), because the two are so closely related.

The planning phase of the nursing process refers to working with patients to design care for all the conclusions of assessment, including nursing diagnoses, interdisciplinary problems, and problems requiring referral. Although the resulting written plan of care is often equated with the "planning phase of the nursing process," it is essential to recognize that there is more to planning than a written care plan. The thinking behind the designing of care is much more indicative of the true definition of "planning."

Definition of Designed (Planned) Care

Designed (planned) care is the most effective, efficient approach to handling all of a patient's health concerns and promoting the patient's strengths. The best plans reflect thinking by the nurse and the patient about setting priorities, establishing clear goals and outcomes for the patient to achieve, and choosing nursing interventions to meet those outcomes. These planned courses of action are based on sound rationales. Plans usually are documented (written) as part of a patient's record.

Purposes of Designed Care

This section describes four major purposes of designing care for and with patients. When nurses and student nurses understand and appreciate the value of designing care they are more likely to do a thorough job, resulting in a quality plan that meets the patient's needs.

One of the primary purposes of designed care is to have an organized, systematic, safe, and well thought-out plan before actually doing anything for or with the patient. This takes more time for beginning nurses than it does for experienced nurses. As beginners gain experience, however, their thinking and planning skills can be applied more quickly.

The second major purpose of planning is to design criteria that will serve as guides for evaluation. It is not enough to design and provide care for patients;

nurses and patients need and want results. Nurses and patients must have a way to determine whether changes actually occur in the patients' health conditions. The outcomes of the plan are "preset" parameters (criteria) for evaluation. They are "preset" because they are determined before the care is implemented. For example, an outcome might be, "By the end of 1 week the patient will use relaxation techniques to fall asleep within 30 minutes." The planned nursing interventions would center on helping the patient learn the relaxation techniques. When the week ends, the nurse and the patient determine whether or not the change (using relaxation techniques to fall asleep within 30 minutes) has occurred as planned. If it hasn't, different approaches can be tried.

A third purpose of planning—that of having written plans of care—provides for continuity of patient care and for communication among health care providers. Think about that. In most health care settings—whether inpatient, outpatient, or home care—patients are cared for by several nurses. Without a written plan to serve as a guide to care, each nurse could be doing something different with each patient during each encounter. Patients would not get very good care, and the amount of time and money that would be wasted is unthinkable.

The fourth purpose of planning is to meet professional and legal expectations for accountability. The Professional Standards of Practice established by the American Nurses Association (ANA) require that nurses plan care, and not just haphazardly do things. Nurses who plan well are less likely to encounter litigation issues in their practice.

Nursing's accountability has improved during the last few decades. This is largely because of the standardization of language for nursing diagnoses, nursing interventions, and nursing outcomes. In Chapter 3, the Classifications for Nursing Diagnoses (NANDA), Nursing Interventions (NIC), and Nursing Sensitive Patient Outcomes (NOC) were discussed. The European Nursing Community currently is working to develop a unified international classification system of standardized nursing terms for diagnoses, interventions, and outcomes. That project, which started in 1992, is called the Association for Common European Nursing Diagnoses, Interventions, and Outcomes (ASCENDIO).

Although the North American classifications (or taxonomies, as they are called in the literature) are in their infancy, they have, for the first time in nursing's history, provided standardized terms for use in documenting and communicating consistently three elements of nursing care: diagnoses, interventions, and outcomes. These classifications have been mentioned at various points in this and other chapters. Chapter 11 addresses other issues related to standardized language, such as the move toward computer programs and reimbursement for nursing care. For now, you need to know that standardized nursing languages are evolving and will have a significant influence on your professional career as you design care for your patients.

Design Components

Care must be designed for all conclusions of assessment. In some cases, such as with interdisciplinary problems, nursing engages in planning with other health care providers. The care designed for nursing diagnosis conclusions is primarily under the direction of the nurse (and, of course, the patient).

Completion of the following tasks is necessary to effectively design care:

- Set priorities about health concerns as they relate to the whole patient situation.
- Identify desired patient outcomes for each health concern.
- Determine nursing interventions for all outcomes.
- Identify sound rationales for all interventions.

The first two of these components, setting priorities and identifying desired outcomes, are addressed in this chapter, and the last two, determining nursing interventions and identifying rationales, will be addressed in Chapter 10. This division requires the collaborative thinking of both the nurse and the patient to set priorities and identify established outcomes. Determining nursing interventions and identifying rationales requires primarily the thinking skills of the nurse. Remember, however, that these artificial separations of the different aspects of the nursing process are only for the purpose of conveying information in a textbook. In real life, the distinctions among assessing, planning, implementing, and evaluating are very fuzzy. What can be separated on paper must be blended in reality.

SETTING PRIORITIES

Setting priorities enables nurses and patients to make the best use of their time, energy, and health care dollars. Nurses set priorities during many aspects of care, but this task is particularly important in planning. Because nurses design plans *with* patients and their significant others, and not *for* them, setting priorities can and should be done *with* patients. All conclusions of assessment must be discussed with the patient so that the conclusions can be validated and the patient can say which concerns are most important. For example, a nurse working with Ms. Romero, who recently had an amputation, has identified the following conclusions of assessment for this patient:

> **Nursing Dx:**
> Body image disturbance R/T feelings about recent below-the-knee amputation (BKA)
> **Interdisciplinary Problem:**
> Altered nutrition: less than body requirements. Need to consult nutritionist because of complexity of diet needs.
> **Problem for Referral:**
> Patient currently is homeless after mudslides and floods and will be discharged tomorrow.

The patient must be consulted for confirmation of all of these conclusions of assessment and to determine priorities. At first glance, the problem for referral may be the highest priority, but the nurse will never know unless the patient is consulted. Ms. Romero could have a large network of friends and extended family who are willing to have her live with them.

Setting priorities is no simple task because there are so many things that are unique to each patient and each situation. There are, however, general guidelines that are helpful. Obviously, an immediately life-threatening problem such as bleeding is a high priority and needs to be dealt with ASAP (As Soon As Possible, if not sooner!!). The next priorities are safety issues. If the patient is at risk for injury, a plan must be made to decrease that risk. The remaining issues, however, do not fall into place so automatically. What the nurse thinks is a priority may not be what the patient thinks is a priority. If patients can communicate in any way, they should make the final decisions about priorities. The general guidelines for setting priorities, therefore, are:

1. Immediately life-threatening issues
2. Safety issues
3. Patient-identified priorities
4. Nurse-identified priorities (based on the overall picture of each health concern in relation to other concerns, the patient as a whole person, and availability of time and resources)

These four guidelines seem straightforward, but they do not always work neatly. This is where INQUIRY thinking is needed. Within these guidelines, nurses must make finer distinctions. They rely on their TOTAL RECALL of ethical and moral reasoning, accepted models of human needs, and other knowledge of human behavior.

Sometimes the patient does not value an issue that the nurse thinks is important and should be addressed. For example, suppose a nurse in a community health nursing setting finds parents who have not had their 2-year-old child immunized. The parents think the child's sleeping habits (waking twice a night) are more important. Should the nurse set the lack of immunizations aside and focus on sleep first? Suppose the reason the parents have not immunized their child is that they have religious beliefs against immunizations? Should the nurse try to change their beliefs?

In this situation, most nurses would try to deal with both issues (the sleep and the immunizations). Using principles of ethical and moral reasoning, the nurse would avoid criticizing the parents' beliefs, but would make sure that they were completely informed about the pros and cons of immunizations. The nurse also might decide to focus initially on the sleeping issue for a week or two with the hope of achieving the following: (1) resolving the sleep problem; (2) demonstrating willingness to focus on the parents' concern first; and (3) developing trust and rapport that might increase the parents' receptiveness to working with the immunization issue.

Further INQUIRY and TOTAL RECALL are needed when nurse-identified priorities must be ranked, or when the patient is unable to participate in setting priorities. Suppose a patient is learning about wound care after a mastectomy and the nurse also identifies Body Image Disturbance and Diversional Activity Deficit as problems. Which should be dealt with first? Maslow's hierarchy of needs often is used in nursing as a method of determining priorities. Maslow (1970) promoted the idea that certain needs must be met before others—in this order: first, physiologic needs; second, safety and security; third, love and belonging; fourth, self-esteem; and, finally, self-actualization. Using Maslow's scheme, the nurse would plan and implement care to teach the patient how to perform safe wound care first, deal with the body image disturbance second, and attend to the diversional activities deficit third. Suppose, however, that the body image problem was interfering with the patient's ability to learn wound care? Wouldn't it make more sense to deal with the body image disturbance first? This kind of judgment requires TOTAL RECALL of the nurse's experience with other patients and INQUIRY thinking to focus on the patient's highest priority, even if it doesn't fit in the Maslow hierarchy or other models.

To complicate matters further, consider the impact of decisions about actual and potential problems. Remember that potential problems are ones that do not yet exist.

Logically it would seem that the actual problem should be dealt with before the potential problem, the reason being that an actual problem exists and a potential problem does not exist. However, this is another one of those times when the nurse has to T.H.I.N.K. beyond the obvious. For example, Mary has the following two nursing diagnoses:

(Actual Problem)

Altered nutrition: more than body requirements R/T consumption of 3000+ calories a day and a sedentary life style.

(Potential Problem)

Risk for violence: self-directed R/T history of suicide attempts, active thoughts of suicide, and plan to drive car into a tree (high lethality).

Which of these two nursing diagnoses for Mary should have the highest priority? Obviously the "Potential Problem" should take priority because it has life-threatening and safety-related consequences, even though it is not an "Actual Problem." This example may be extreme, but it is used to emphasize the necessity of thinking when using any type of guidelines.

To do the best job of setting priorities, the nurse must blend a standard system of establishing priorities with an overview of the individual patient's situation. It is important to remember that knowledge about human needs and priority setting is useful, but setting priorities also must take into account the patient as a whole person, with strengths and health concerns, and not just as a list of problems. INQUIRY must be used.

Viewing the individual patient as a whole person means looking at the relationship among the conclusions. Sometimes, if care is planned and implemented for one health concern, other concerns, because of their interrelatedness, are taken care of. For example, if a patient has a Fluid Volume Deficit related to insufficient intake and excessive diuresis, and that same patient has Constipation related to insufficient fluid intake, caring for the first problem could automatically take care of the second (or vice versa). Looking at these types of interrelationships can save planning time, energy, and health care dollars as well as decrease repetition of care planning.

All priorities set during planning are significantly influenced by the length of time that the nurse has contact with the patient, the resources available, and the setting. In an acute care setting, it is typical to plan care for two or three high-priority nursing diagnoses that will quickly restore the patient to an acceptable health status for discharge. In long-term care settings, such as nursing homes or the community, the list of planned priorities usually expands. The expanded time frame allows for planning in more areas.

In case anyone has started to think that priority setting is linear, one final reminder is worthwhile. Setting priorities, as described on paper, may seem to imply that nurses work on one thing first, finish it, and then work on the second priority. This is neither true nor realistic. If there are no immediate life-threatening or safety concerns, the nurse may, for example, work on two patient-identified concerns and one nurse-identified concern during a single shift or encounter with the patient. Thinking and expertise allow the nurse to address several concerns simultaneously.

Taking into account the complexity of each patient situation, then, a visual framework might help the nurse to remember the guidelines for setting priorities (Fig. 9-3).

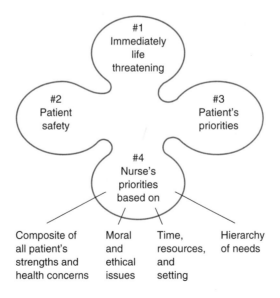

FIGURE 9-3   Guidelines for determining priorities.

Setting Priorities for All Conclusions of Assessment That Are Health Concerns

Keep in mind that the guidelines for setting priorities work with all the conclusions of assessment that are health concerns (including Nursing Diagnoses, Interdisciplinary Problems, and Problems for Referral). The nurse and the patient (and/or significant other) are the thinkers and doers of planning derived from nursing diagnoses.

With interdisciplinary problems, it may be the nurse, the other health care professional, or both people together who design the plan. How this interdisciplinary collaboration is achieved often depends on the setting and the usual types of problems addressed. Generally speaking, however, most disciplines take the same approach to planning that nurses take in designing plans for nursing diagnoses. Typically there are goals, outcomes, and interventions to be taken by health care providers. In some settings, such as mental health, these are called Interdisciplinary Treatment Plans or Master Treatment Plans.

Planning for problems for referral also requires thinking. The nurse usually refers the patient to another health care provider for the identified problem. The other provider either plans the care or comes back to the nurse to design an interdisciplinary plan. Documentation indicating that the nurse made the referral and explaining the reason for the referral is important. Where this information is documented depends on the agency or institution; generally, it is recorded in a progress note. The key is to remember to *do it somewhere.*

As priorities are established, nurses must look at all conclusions collectively. It may be that an interdisciplinary problem or a problem for referral has a higher priority than a nursing diagnosis, as in the example involving Ms. Romero, who was homeless after the mudslides and flooding.

Figure 9-4 highlights whose thinking is essential when designing care and setting priorities.

Type of Health Concern	Participates in thinking and doing of designing care and setting priorities	Example
Nursing Diagnosis	Nurse and patient (or significant other)	Risk for aspiration R/T dysphagia secondary to CVA **Nursing Intervention: raise head of bed 30 degrees and monitor all food and fluid intake**
Interdisciplinary Problem	Nurse, patient, and other health care professional	Social isolation R/T fears of persecution secondary to delusional thinking **Interdisciplinary team of nurses, psychiatrist, mental health techs, and patient**
Problems for Referral	(Nurse-initiated), patient, other health care professional	Patient complains of severe toothache. Lower left jaw swollen, warm, and very sensitive to touch **Referral needed to dentist**

FIGURE 9–4 Whose thinking is needed?

⊃Action Learning #44: Setting Priorities

Read the following situation and the initial nursing conclusions. See if you can find other conclusions that would be appropriate. For other nursing diagnosis conclusions, use the NANDA taxonomy in a nursing diagnosis book or Appendix A of this text. Record the data clusters to support the existing conclusions and any new ones you add. Add your new conclusions to the list below and describe in writing how you would determine the order of priority for your conclusions. Share your work with a classmate.

> Mrs. Partridge is the mother of a 2-week-old baby girl. She had excessive bleeding because of a vaginal tear during the delivery, so she is anemic. She was told by her obstetrician to eat foods high in iron and to take iron supplements, but she says the pills are making her constipated. She says, "I know I should drink more fluids because of the breastfeeding, but it is a real struggle to remember everything I should be doing." The baby is not sleeping well, waking several times each night. Mrs. Partridge is having difficulty breastfeeding. She states, "I don't have much milk yet and the baby seems to cry a lot. I'm so tired all the time, I barely have the energy to feed the baby, much less myself. I feel like my body is telling me not to breastfeed, but I know it's best for the baby. Everyone says I should just keep at it, feed the baby more often, and try to pump my breasts to increase the supply. All I do is lie around all day feeling tired, napping and feeding the baby. I haven't been out of the house or done anything physical for two weeks. I don't know how or when I'll ever return to my jogging and reading novels." Connie Ticket, RN, made the following conclusions of assessment during a home visit to Mrs. Partridge:

Strengths
Confers with obstetrician for follow-up care
Has a house to live in
Has visits from RN at home

Nursing Diagnoses
Fatigue related to insufficient sleep, new mothering role demands, breastfeeding energy expenditure, and anemia
Decisional Conflict about breastfeeding related to conflicts between self-care and care of baby
Diversional Activity Deficit related to fatigue and time demands of new mother role

Interdisciplinary Problems
None identified

Problems for Referral
None identified

Additional Conclusions   Data Cluster

Order of Priorities of Nursing Conclusions

1.

2.

3.

4.

5.
    or more

THINK ABOUT THIS ■ What additional nursing conclusions did you make? Did you consider the nursing diagnosis of constipation? Did you consider additional strengths, such as Mrs. Partridge's enjoyment of jogging and reading novels? Did you consider a referral to LaLeche for professional help with breastfeeding? How did your conclusions compare with your classmate's? Was it possible to establish priorities in this situation? Did you find that some conclusions overlapped others? How did the overlapping affect priority setting?

What you very likely discovered was that this process of priority-setting is not linear at all. There is no "right" or "wrong" approach. One must consider the whole context of the situation. Consider your "K" thinking mode; how does this ambiguity make you feel? Consider your "I" thinking mode; how did this system of setting priorities work? How would you change it to make it more helpful to your thinking as a nurse?

✔ *Thinking-Learning Check*
_____

Pause here for a thinking-learning check. You should be able to elaborate on these ideas:

✔ Incorporating the thinking of both the nurse and the patient into planning, implementing, and evaluating care is essential.

✔ Completing the cycle of the nursing process requires that planning, implementing, and evaluating be added to the thinking begun during assessment.

✔ Guidelines for setting priorities involve looking at the whole patient in relation to immediate life-threatening concerns, safety concerns, the patient's priorities, and the nurse's priorities.

IDENTIFYING DESIRED PATIENT OUTCOMES

We will start with the assumption that you have at least a beginning level of comfort with assessment. You and your patients can agree on the conclusions of assessment and set priorities. If so, you are now at the point where you need to establish patient outcomes. One of the conclusions of planning asks the question, "What should be done about the patient's health concerns?" Or, how do we get the patient from his current status (trouble with walking, for example) to a point where he is able to walk without problems?

If a patient has had a stroke and can no longer walk well on his own, do we simply say, "We want the patient to walk better!"? Sure, we can say it, but what does it do for us? How do we determine "better"? Does the patient have to be "ALL better" or can he be "somewhat better" or a "little bit better"? What does "better" really look like?

For the last several years, nursing has been looking for ways to specify and clarify the results that patients and nurses are looking for—to zero in on what is "better" for many different situations. A big part of this process has to do with the language we use to describe behaviors that are expected of patients. These specific behaviors lead to a status that is "better" than the patient's current status.

The nurse and patient think and work together to identify or develop statements that are written down in the patient's plan of care. These outcome statements describe what will be different about the patient toward the end of care. The next section of this chapter describes the process of establishing outcomes, which become the guideposts with which both the patient and the nurse can judge the patient's progress. These outcomes give direction to the patient's overall care. Outcomes are patient behaviors, not nurse behaviors. They always are written in a format that reflects a patient state, that is, "The patient will . . ."

Traditionally, patient outcomes have been divided into two types: goals and objectives. Goals are broad statements of intent or what the patient should achieve to show that the health concern is resolved. Objectives are the specific, measurable outcomes that are used as standards by which evaluation is determined. There are two schools of thought about goals. One is that goals should be written down to remind everyone of the general end-point that is being sought in a particular situation. The other is that the goal is so obvious that it does not need to be written down—that it is the specific, measurable, objective that counts.

Sometimes the terminology becomes very confusing because "goals," "objectives," and "outcomes" are used interchangeably in textbooks to mean "a measurable, specific criterion for evaluation." When the label "goal" is used alone, it generally is interpreted as a measurable outcome. When "goal" is used along with the term "objective" or "outcome," the former is a general direction and the latter is the measurable outcome. Goals are broad statements of intent, but outcomes are desired measurable patient states (see Figs. 9-5 and 9-6 for examples). This confusion may be lessened as nursing continues to develop the classification of patient outcomes (NOC). As you can see, the term "outcomes" is used with NOC. NOC outcomes are patient states that are measured on a 5-point scale. The American Nurses Association (ANA) also has endorsed the use of the phrase "outcome identification" as a component of the nursing process. As the NOC classifications and the ANA terminology are used more often and become commonplace, it seems likely that nurses will use the term "outcomes" to mean measurable patient states or specific objectives.

In the meantime, whether goals are written in the nursing plan or not, it is helpful to the nurse's thinking to consider the overall goal of care for a specific health concern. The goal sets the stage and keeps the "end point" (patient state) in mind while the other planning is done. In this text, we advocate the identification of goals as well as specific outcomes.

Establishing Goals

To develop goals, the nurse and the patient first determine a direction for care based on the nursing diagnosis (or interdisciplinary problem). For example, if the diagnosis is a problem, the goal would be to reverse the problem, or at least get it under control. For example, if the nursing diagnosis is "Ineffective Individual Coping," the goal would be for the patient to attain or regain effective coping or to increase coping skills. If the diagnosis is a wellness issue, the goal would be to maintain or promote that healthy behavior. For example, if the nursing diagnosis is "Effective Breastfeeding," the goal would be for the patient to maintain effective breastfeeding. If the nursing diagnosis is a potential problem, the goal would be to reduce the risk of the problem occurring. For example, if the nursing diagnosis is "Risk for Injury," the goal would be for the patient to decrease the risk for injury or to have no injury.

In the preceding examples, the words "attain," "regain," "increase," "maintain," "promote," "continue," and "decrease" are used. These verbs sum up the "directions" for care goals. If something about a patient's health response is altered, the patient would want the usual response *restored* or would want to *regain* the usual response. Sometimes the patient needs to *attain* some new type of response or *improve* the present response. If a response is healthy, the patient would want to *maintain, continue,* or *promote* that response. Sometimes, when there is an excess of something (usually of risk), the patient needs to *decrease* the potential for the problem. When there is a lack of something, the patient needs to *increase* what is lacking. These are useful verbs for the nurse to use habitually because they cover the ideal goals for most health issues or concerns for which nurses plan, implement, and evaluate care.

Most goals need a time frame. Exceptions include goals of maintaining, continuing, or promoting responses, which imply that something should stay the same, making a time frame unnecessary. However, when goals are to attain, restore, regain, improve, decrease, or increase a response, a time frame should accompany the goal. The time frames for goals may be long- or short-term, but these terms mean different things in different settings. Long-term goals in an acute care setting may be projected for a week or so, or until discharge. In a long-term care setting, long-term goals might be achieved over months or years; likewise, short-term goals may be defined in terms of hours or months. One value of short-term goals is that they divide up a long-term goal into more manageable increments for the patient.

FIGURE 9-5   Relationship between nursing diagnostic statement and goal statement.

⊃**ACTION LEARNING #45: Establishing Goals**

What might the goals be for these nursing diagnoses? You will not be able to set time frames because you do not have the contexts for these diagnoses, but focus on the wording for each goal. Also, remember that goals are patient goals, not nursing goals. Share your goals with a classmate.

Diversional Activity Deficit related to immobility secondary to fractured leg
GOAL:
Constipation related to low-fiber diet and immobility
GOAL:
Activity Intolerance related to extreme fatigue
GOAL:
High Risk for Aspiration related to neurologic deficits and impulsiveness during
  eating
GOAL:
Functional Incontinence related to difficulties transferring from chair to toilet
GOAL:
Family Coping: Potential for Growth related to effective communication
GOAL:

THINK ABOUT THIS ■ Congratulations! You have mastered an important part of planning care. Hopefully, you have seen the link between the nursing diagnosis and the goal. How closely worded were your goals and those of your classmate?

Before preceding to Action Learning #45, study the example of the relationship between the nursing diagnostic statement and the goal statement given in Figure 9-5.

Establishing Outcome Indicators

Although goals provide general directions for a plan of care, specific nursing-sensitive patient outcomes must be predetermined to serve as a basis for evaluation. NOC outcomes are patient states that are expected to be influenced by nursing interventions. The outcomes are measurable and can be tracked over time to determine if change has occurred in the desired direction.

Remember, there are a variety of terms in the literature that describe patient outcomes. "Objectives," "goals," "outcome criteria," and "expected outcomes" are just a few of the synonyms that can be found. As mentioned earlier, with NOC, it is expected that "outcome" will become the standard term.

The Iowa Outcomes Project (Johnson & Maas, 1997) is a classification system for patient outcomes that can be used for patient care planning. This project is very helpful, especially to beginning-level students, because determining measurable patient outcomes was a very difficult task to learn in the past. The Nursing Outcomes Classification (NOC), which will be further developed during the next few years, provides a "dictionary" of outcomes that can be used to choose and evaluate outcomes. Choosing is a complex thinking process that is discussed later in this chapter.

(Authors' note: We suppose that many of our readers are beginning-level students of nursing. If so, they may already be exposed to the NOC. With the growing use of computers in health care, we believe the nursing classifications, which are computer compatible, will become commonplace in the very near future.)

The NOC system provides nursing-sensitive patient outcomes, outcome indicators, and outcome measures. This is like having a multi-level system of outcomes that can be tailored to individual patient situations. To translate the thinking about outcomes into an everyday situation, consider an analogy to shopping.

Your wardrobe is deficient (unhealthy) because you do not have an appropriate pair of just the right shade of navy blue slacks. A pair of the right shade of navy blue slacks would definitely enhance the "health" of your wardrobe. To increase the probability of finding what you need (achieving the outcome), you go directly to the slacks area in the store. You do not go to the shoe department (although if you are a "true" shopper, a pair of matching shoes would surely add to the health of your wardrobe and the outfit!).

On the racks of slacks you search for blue slacks. Blue is your outcome indicator. Not any blue will do, however; you need a specific shade of navy blue (outcome measure) to match your special sweater (and, maybe, now the new shoes, in case you did stop in the shoe department—just to look!). You find a pair of navy blue slacks (in your size) in just the right shade (they fit your criteria), and your task is achieved. In summary, you pre-planned a desired outcome, with a specific indicator and measure; you met that outcome by implementing action directed toward that outcome.

Now let's see how an example from the NOC works. Think back to the patient described at the beginning of this chapter. He was having trouble walking after a stroke. As you plan his care, you find the outcome "Ambulation: Walking" (Johnson & Maas, 1997, p. 80) (see Display 9-1, an excerpt from the NOC book).

As you look down the list of indicators, you find descriptions such as "bears weight, walks with effective gait, walks at slow pace," and so forth. You stop and think, what do I want to focus on here as outcomes for this patient? What are his expectations? What is realistic in a given period of time? You might select "walks with effective gait" because that will not only ensure safety for the patient but will meet the patient's desire to avoid looking "helpless" when he walks.

With this outcome in mind, you would then look at the measures listed as indicators. In this case, the measures are a scale from 1 to 5, corresponding to these descriptions:

1 = Dependent, does not participate
2 = Requires assistive person and device
3 = Requires assistive person

DISPLAY **9–1.** **Ambulation: Walking**

DEFINITION: Ability to walk from place to place

AMBULATION: WALKING

	Dependent, does not participate	Requires assistive person and device	Requires assistive person	Independent with assistive device	Completely independent
	1	2	3	4	5
Indicators:					
Bears weight	1	2	3	4	5
Walks with effective gait	1	2	3	4	5
Walks at slow pace	1	2	3	4	5
Walks at moderate pace	1	2	3	4	5
Walks at fast pace	1	2	3	4	5
Walks up steps	1	2	3	4	5
Walks down steps	1	2	3	4	5
Walks up inclines	1	2	3	4	5
Walks down inclines	1	2	3	4	5
Walks short distance (< 1 block)	1	2	3	4	5
Walks moderate distance (> 1 block < 5 blocks)	1	2	3	4	5
Walks long distance (5 blocks or >)	1	2	3	4	5
Other _____ Specify	1	2	3	4	5

Background Readings:

Dittmar, S. (1989). *Rehabilitation nursing: Process and application.* St. Louis: Mosby.

Jirovec, M.M. (1991). The impact of daily exercise on the mobility, balance, and urine control of cognitively impaired nursing home residents. *International Journal of Nursing Studies, 28*(2), 145–151.

Mikulic, M.A., Griffith, E.R., & Jebsen, R.H. (1976). Clinical application of a standardized mobility test. *Archives of Physical Medicine and Rehabilitation, 57*(3), 143–146.

Pomeroy, V. (1990). Development of an ADL-oriented assessment-of-mobility scale suitable for use for elderly people with dementia. *Physiotherapy, 76*(8), 446–448.

Tinetti, M.E. (1986). Performance-oriented assessment of mobility problems in elderly patients. *Journal of the American Geriatric Society, 34,* 119–126.

(Johnson, M., & Maas, M. [1997]. *Nursing outcomes classification* [NOC]. St. Louis: Mosby. Reprinted with permission.)

4 = Independent with assistive device
5 = Completely independent

Your thinking should focus on: What is the patient's current status on the outcome and indicators? Let's assume your patient with the stroke is getting some return of motor innervation in his affected side. He currently is functioning at approximately a #2 level on a scale because he still needs a person walking with him and he uses a cane. This point is called a "base line" or the current status of the patient—in this case, on the indicator of "Ambulation: walking."

The next phase in your thinking is to work with the patient to identify a realistic level that he would like to attain by the time he is discharged. Let's say the two of you come up with #4 for your outcome measure. He will still need the cane, but should be able to walk safely by himself and not look "helpless." You have used your expertise, along with the NOC book and the patient's input, to identify the outcome "Ambulation: Walking"; the outcome indicator "Walks with effective gait"; and an outcome measure #4, "Independent with Assistive Device." You would then identify the specific nursing interventions that you and the other nursing personnel would use to help this patient achieve the outcome. Nursing intervention details are discussed in Chapter 10. However, we must first consider other available ways to determine outcomes.

It may seem obvious that you could have come up with something close to the outcomes mentioned without having to look things up in the NOC book. You might use different words and measurement scales, but you would likely come up with a very similar end point. You might use one of the many nursing care plan books that are currently available. Such books have sample plans that include outcomes and interventions. No matter what resource one uses to help with planning, what is crucial is to recognize that somewhere in a patient's plan of care, **outcomes that can be measured must be chosen or developed**. Without measurable outcomes, we have no standard for evaluating nursing care and have only anecdotal, subjective feelings that our patients are making progress. This is not enough; we must be more precise.

Measurable does not mean that the patient's behavior literally can be measured with a ruler. However, with the development of NOC, nurses have the beginnings of scales that can be used for more precise measurement. With or without NOC, the words and scales used to assess outcomes must be sufficiently descriptive to capture changes in patient states over time. The outcome measures should also be reliable, which means that if several people are measuring the same outcome and indicators on the same patient, their measurements should be very similar.

⊃Action Learning #46: Finding Outcome Measures

Listed below are some outcome states, some of which are precisely measurable, some of which are somewhat measurable, and some of which cannot be measured. Mark the most precisely measurable with a "B" for best; the somewhat measurable with a "G" for good; and the unmeasurable with an "NM" for not measurable.

1. The patient will eat at least three quarters of all meals.
2. Mrs. Jones will feel better.
3. The decubitus ulcer will decrease to 1 cm in diameter, with no signs of infection.

4. The patient will have a better appetite.
5. The patient will be able to perform self-care.
6. The decubitus ulcer will improve.
7. The patient will wash her hair independently
8. Mr. Frank will describe his mobility needs.
9. The patient will use an alphabet board to communicate his needs.
10. Mr. Smith will understand diabetic foot care.

THINK ABOUT THIS ■ If you were a nurse using a plan developed by another nurse, which outcome states do you think would be easier to aim for? What makes some easier to measure? How could the others be changed to make them measurable?

In addition to focusing on patient behaviors and being measurable and clear, outcomes should be accompanied by a time frame. The time frame defines the point at which one would expect the patient to achieve an outcome, that is, the time when that part of the plan should be evaluated. Time frames are highly individual. Nurses must know their patients well to adapt standard time frames to them and their specific situations. This is where knowing a patient's strengths helps. Viewing the total picture of the patient's problems and available resources allows the nurse to determine a realistic time frame for outcomes to be reached.

⊃ACTION LEARNING #47: Adding Time Frames

Go back to Action Learning #46 and identify two or three pieces of data you would need to make some reasonable conclusions about time frames for the outcomes you selected as most precisely measurable ("B").

THINK ABOUT THIS ■ What was the most helpful kind of information for determining time frames? How are time frames influenced by a patient's situation, setting, and resources?

The Relationship of Outcomes to Nursing Diagnoses

Generally speaking, to start planning for a patient's particular nursing diagnosis, the nurse looks at the problem part of the diagnostic statement to get ideas for goal setting. The related factors then help with the selection of patient outcomes. Think about that for a minute with a humorous example. Suppose I am your patient and I come to you complaining that I'm lonely and have no friends. You, the nurse, quickly see why, because I have a very strong odor of old perspiration. You conclude: "Social isolation related to deficient hygiene practices." Now, consider a plan of care. The goal would be to find me some friends. However, that goal would not be met unless some preliminary outcomes were met—namely, that I exhibited a more pleasant smell. In this example, the overall goal came from the "problem" (my lack of friends), and the specific outcome indicator came from the related factor (my deficient hygiene).

Each related factor is considered an obstacle to the goal of getting rid of or controlling the problem. When outcomes addressing all the related factors are met, the problem logically should be resolved. See Figure 9-6 for a patient with the nursing diagnosis "Sleep Pattern Disturbance related to worries about work and excessive intake of caffeine." The goal is to restore usual sleep patterns and the outcomes are focused on reversing the worries and the caffeine intake. One outcome could be "The patient will devise a plan to deal with the worries about the work situation," and another could be "The patient will decrease caffeine intake to one cup of coffee after 6 PM." In short, if the patient can do something to alter or eliminate the related factors, the goal can be met and the problem can be resolved.

When Related Factors Do Not Provide Guidance

Most of the time, related factors provide guidance for selecting outcomes, as in the examples described. But sometimes they do not. Consider the following situation and nursing diagnosis.

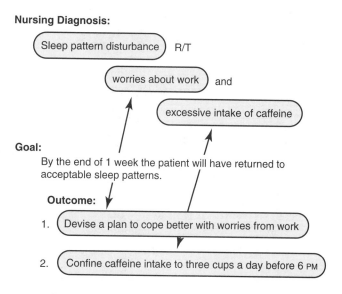

Nursing Diagnosis:

(Sleep pattern disturbance) R/T

(worries about work) and

(excessive intake of caffeine)

Goal:
By the end of 1 week the patient will have returned to acceptable sleep patterns.

Outcome:

1. (Devise a plan to cope better with worries from work)

2. (Confine caffeine intake to three cups a day before 6 PM)

FIGURE 9–6 Relationship of outcomes to related factors.

Jennifer is 18 years old. She is confined to bed for 4 to 6 weeks in a body cast. She fractured both femurs and her pelvis in a skiing accident.

Nursing Diagnosis: Impaired Physical Mobility related to fractured pelvis, fractures in both femurs, body cast, and bed confinement.

Now examine the thinking that the nurse used in moving from assessment to identifying desired outcomes. Highlights of the nurse's thinking are shown in Display 9-2, the Thinking Flow Sheet. *If this kind of thinking does not occur*, the care plan that eventually gets written on paper ends up being useless or, at best, of only minimum benefit to Jennifer.

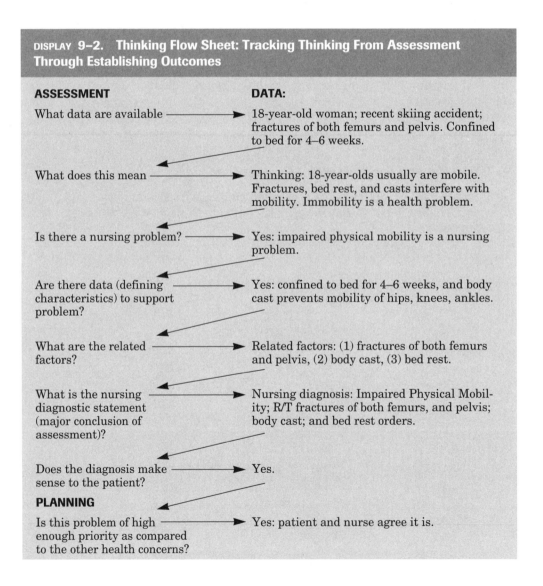

DISPLAY **9–2.   Thinking Flow Sheet: Tracking Thinking From Assessment Through Establishing Outcomes**

ASSESSMENT

DATA:

What data are available ⟶ 18-year-old woman; recent skiing accident; fractures of both femurs and pelvis. Confined to bed for 4–6 weeks.

What does this mean ⟶ Thinking: 18-year-olds usually are mobile. Fractures, bed rest, and casts interfere with mobility. Immobility is a health problem.

Is there a nursing problem? ⟶ Yes: impaired physical mobility is a nursing problem.

Are there data (defining characteristics) to support problem? ⟶ Yes: confined to bed for 4–6 weeks, and body cast prevents mobility of hips, knees, ankles.

What are the related factors? ⟶ Related factors: (1) fractures of both femurs and pelvis, (2) body cast, (3) bed rest.

What is the nursing diagnostic statement (major conclusion of assessment)? ⟶ Nursing diagnosis: Impaired Physical Mobility; R/T fractures of both femurs, and pelvis; body cast; and bed rest orders.

Does the diagnosis make sense to the patient? ⟶ Yes.

PLANNING

Is this problem of high enough priority as compared to the other health concerns? ⟶ Yes: patient and nurse agree it is.

What is a proper goal for ————▶ Goal: "Patient will have improved mobility
this problem?   by the end of 2 weeks."
(Patient-focused, broad
statement of direction to
change the problem in a
given time frame.)

Does the goal statement meet ——▶ Yes.
the criteria of a proper goal?

Does the goal make sense? ————▶ Thinking: decreased mobility has many prob-
                                lems related to it (ie, skin breakdown, consti-
                                pation, muscle atrophy). So it isn't good to be
                                immobile and it's important to strive for im-
                                proved mobility. Yes, this part makes sense,
                                but does the time frame make sense? Maybe,
                                maybe not; it may have to be changed later if
                                necessary.

What are appropriate out- ◀—
comes for this goal? (Outcomes should be patient-
focused, measurable, clear,
have a time frame, and **reflect
how the patient can fix or
eliminate the related factors.)** ——▶

                                SCREECHING HALT IN PLANNING!
                                The patient cannot eliminate or modify the
                                fractures, the cast, or the bed rest orders. Now
                                what do I do?

MORE INQUIRY THINKING ◀—

Does this mean that these are the wrong related factors?

Does this mean that the nurse should ignore this problem?

Does this mean that immobility really isn't a nursing problem?

What happens if the patient is left to be immobile?

Maybe it is time to go back to assessment and reexamine the data and the conclusions.

Data are unchanged, and nursing does need to address the issues of immobility.

Alternative conclusions (differential diagnoses) are considered:
1. High risk for complications of immobility
   secondary to fractures, cast, and bed rest.
2. High risk for disuse syndrome secondary to fractures,
   cast, and bed rest.

⊃**ACTION LEARNING #48: Thinking Through to Establishing Outcomes to Select the Best Nursing Diagnosis**

After reading the Thinking Flow Sheet (Display 9-2), answer the following questions and share your answers with a classmate.

1. At what point do you think the nurse began to suspect that something might not be on track?

2. Did the nurse's thinking follow a logical sequence? What, if anything, would you have done differently?

3. How does this situation illustrate the interconnectedness among the assessment, planning, implementation, and evaluation phases of the nursing process?

4. What are the next questions the nurse would ask to rule in or rule out the two differential diagnoses?

> **THINK ABOUT THIS** ■ How easy or difficult was it to answer these questions? What happens to patient care if you don't ask these kinds of questions? What parts of T.H.I.N.K. are required for this task? Give some examples of your thinking, including especially your use of "I." A word of encouragement: the answers come more easily and more quickly with experience. Your thinking becomes HABITUAL and you suspect problems as soon as you develop the first hunch about the original diagnostic label.

Multiple Related Factors, Not All Providing Guidance

Another situation that affects the "content" of outcomes occurs when there are multiple related factors, only some of which lend themselves to outcomes. In those cases, unlike in the impaired mobility example earlier, the nursing diagnosis (problem label) still may be the best one, but only some of the related factors lend themselves to outcomes and interventions. In such cases, the outcomes focus on those factors for which the patient can achieve change; other related factors are not addressed. A logical question might be: should those "unfixable" related factors even be listed in the nursing diagnostic statement? Yes, they should, because they help to clarify the dimensions of the problem and indirectly help with the design of outcomes. If a related factor to a patient's self-care deficit is his inability to grip because of a stroke, even though nothing can undo the stroke, outcomes will be different than they would be if the inability to grip was because of arthritis. The patient with a stroke might be able to increase his grip with exercises, but the patient with arthritis might have to augment his grip with an assistive device.

Multiple Outcomes for One Related Factor

There also could be more than one outcome for each related factor, especially in long-term settings. A nurse and a patient dealing with a work-related stress problem may have as an outcome for the first week that the patient will list the work problems; an outcome for the second week may be to consider options for dealing with the work problems; and, for the third week, an outcome may be to devise a plan to change the work situation. The time frames in this example could be appropriate when the patient is coming into a clinic weekly. If the patient were in an inpatient setting, the time frames would most likely be much shorter.

In addition to time frames necessitating multiple outcomes for each related factor, outcomes also can focus on different types of patient behaviors for one related factor. There are three general categories of patient behavior: affective (eg, sharing feelings), cognitive (eg, describing, explaining, listing, and stating), and psychomotor (eg, doing an activity, demonstrating, and participating). In reality, there is a lot of overlap among these three, but it is helpful to consider patient behaviors in all three categories. The following is an example of what these type of outcomes look like:

Nursing Diagnosis: Risk for Injury related to knowledge deficit regarding daily insulin administration.

Goal: Patient will decrease risk for injury from insulin injections by the end of this visit as evident by:

1. Sharing feelings about self-administered injections (affective)
2. Explaining safe procedure after being taught (cognitive)
3. Demonstrating safe insulin injection (psychomotor)

Outcomes That Address Changes in Patient Conditions

To make life even more complicated, there is one additional area of content for outcomes that reflect patient behavior but are not generally within the patient's conscious control. This area deals with "pure" physiologic changes in patient conditions that are monitored by such things as vital signs, laboratory values, and urine output. Some nursing diagnoses are very specific with respect to the patient's physiologic status; for example, "Fluid Volume Excess related to fluid retention secondary to congestive heart failure." The goal is to decrease the fluid volume, and changes are measured with outcomes that break the goal into smaller increments. Outcomes for the previous nursing diagnosis could be stated as follows:

1. The patient's body weight will return to its usual range within 3 to 5 days.
2. The electrolytes will return to a normal range in 3 to 5 days.
3. Dependent edema will decrease to no more than 1+ within 3 days.

In this case, the outcomes are clear, measurable, and include a time frame. They differ from the earlier examples of behavioral outcomes, however, because they focus on the patient's physiologic responses rather than on behaviors in the conscious control of the patient.

In summary, outcomes are patient-focused and measurable; they have expected time frames for completion; and they usually focus on controlling the related factors of the nursing diagnosis. Collectively, they should help the patient meet the goal of resolving a problem. Outcomes also are the basis for evaluating patient status. They are preset in the nursing plan as standards or criteria toward which the patient and nurse work. At a preselected time, the nurse and patient determine whether the outcomes have been met.

⊃Action Learning #49: Establishing Outcomes

Review Mrs. Partridge's situation in Action Learning #44. For the nursing diagnosis (that you hopefully found), "Constipation related to iron intake, insufficient fluid intake, and decreased mobility," develop outcomes with time frames for Mrs. Partridge to achieve this goal: By 1 week, Mrs. Partridge will restore her usual pattern of bowel movements, as evidenced by:

Outcomes:

THINK ABOUT THIS ■ Are your outcomes patient oriented, clear, measurable, and accompanied by a time frame? Did you address all related factors? How did you address the iron intake? If you are using an NOC book, how did you figure out where to look?

✔ *Thinking-Learning Check*

Pause here for a thinking-learning check. You should be able to elaborate on these ideas:

✔ Goals set the direction for care and outcomes establish criteria for evaluating changes in a patient's behavior, situation, or status.

✔ Goal statements are patient focused, flow from the problem part of the diagnostic statement, and include a time frame.

✔ Expected outcomes are patient focused, measurable, include a time frame, and should address the issues of the related factors identified in the diagnostic statement.

✔ Clear, organized thinking about the structure and content of goals and outcomes is necessary for great nursing care.

CLOSING COMMENTS

This chapter focused your attention on the portion of planning care that requires the nurse and patient to think together. Setting priorities is done more effectively when the patient is an equal partner in the process. Establishing appropriate and useful outcomes also requires patient input because the patient is the one who has to achieve the outcomes. The more collaboration that occurs at these two phases of planning, the more likely the plan of care will be successful.

The next phase of planning involves primarily the thinking of the nurse—it involves determining nursing interventions with sound rationales. Chapter 10 addresses this next phase of planning as well as the role of evaluation of care and care outcomes, which again includes nurse and patient thinking.

THINKING LOG #9

Ask two or three people who recently were patients what part they took in their care. What specifically did they do? What would they have liked to do, given the opportunity? What were they expected to do but did not want to do? How much do they think a patient should participate in designing care?

Record their responses and read what you have written. Think about the following questions as you read, and then summarize your answers.

1. What themes or patterns did you hear from patients about their perceptions of their care, their participation in their care, and their feelings about their care?

2. What did they say that surprised you?

3. How can you use what you heard to develop your professional nursing practice?

Share your findings with classmates to see whether the feedback from patients shares some common features.

References

Johnson, M. & Maas, M. (1997). *Nursing outcomes classification (NOC)*. St. Louis: Mosby.

Maslow, A. (1970). *Motivation in personality*. New York: Harper & Row.

McCloskey, J.C. & Bulechek, G.M. (1996). *Nursing interventions classification (NIC)*. St. Louis: Mosby.

Schon, D.A. (1983). *The reflective practitioner*. New York: Basic Books.

10

Designing, Doing, and Determining Quality of Care: a.k.a. Planning, Implementing, and Evaluating

❋ Learning Outcomes

After reading and doing the activities in this chapter you will be able to:

Describe the DOING aspect of nursing care.

Develop appropriate nursing interventions with supporting rationales.

Demonstrate beginning skill with outcome evaluation.

Explain the thinking partnership of nurse and patient during the evaluation component of the nursing process.

This chapter begins with a brief discussion of DOING and the principles of implementation. Understanding the principles of implementation helps to set the stage for the nurse's thinking about the last two phases of planning, determining nursing interventions and identifying sound rationales. For these last two phases of planning the nurse does the majority of the thinking with all five thinking modes, but with a special emphasis on New Ideas and Creativity. This mode promotes the most individualized approaches to meeting the patient's unique needs.

The chapter concludes with an exploration of the final component of the nursing process—evaluation and determining the quality of care. Here again the nurse and patient become thinking partners as they determine whether and how well the plan worked and whether or not outcomes were achieved based on the outcome criteria established during the early phases of planning.

DOING (IMPLEMENTING) CARE

Now is a good time to return to Chapter 2 for a review of the *DOING* part of nursing. Reconsider *all* the types of *DOING* and the factors that affect those actions. Also, review the section on independent and interdependent nursing actions. With an expanded understanding of the nursing process gained through the several intervening chapters, do you see things in Chapter 2 that you did not see previously? How has your appreciation of the complexity of nursing changed?

The focus of this portion of the chapter is to briefly examine two key aspects of *DOING*: first, DOING as it relates to the implementation component of the nursing process, and, second, doing as it is inseparably interwoven with the time management part of planning all areas of nursing—from patient care to delegation of care. Although the administration, supervision, and leadership aspects of DOING also are essential to the nurse, this text does not have the space to do justice to those aspects of DOING.

Doing (Implementing) as the Third Component of the Nursing Process

Definition and Purpose of Doing

Doing (implementing) as it relates to the nursing process means carrying out the nursing interventions in nursing care plans, and the nursing parts of the physician's plan and the interdisciplinary plans, while also assessing for new problems, evaluating previous care, and keeping an open mind for subtle or major changes that need to be made in the current plan. Doing also includes documenting all parts of care so that others on the health care team know what is happening. More on documenting is addressed in Chapter 11.

The basic purpose of implementing is to provide the interventions that patients need to attain, maintain, and regain health or—in cases in which the patient is terminally ill—maintain comfort and dignity in dying.

Guiding Principles for Implementation

The three guiding principles for implementing care are (1) maintain patient safety, (2) provide effective care, and (3) provide care as efficiently as possible. Safe, effective, and efficient care are professional standards.

SAFETY

No matter what actions are implemented, they must focus first and foremost on patient safety. Actions that jeopardize patient safety are not only ethically in violation of professional nursing standards but also are subject to litigation, depending on patient outcomes.

Although maintaining patient safety sounds fairly straightforward, it is not always that simple. The simple version requires a good understanding of patient behaviors (eg, confused patients tend to wander off), implementation of nonharmful interventions (eg, soft restraints must not cause skin damage or decrease circulation), awareness of environmental hazards (eg, hot liquids cause burns), and thinking about all these factors as they work together. A more complex version arises, however, in the attempt to decide individual safety priorities and quality-of-life issues. This is where T.H.I.N.K. comes into play.

In some situations, a balance is needed to maintain as safe an environment as possible without violating a patient's other needs, such as growth and development, rights to freedom of movement, or quality of life. For example, Steven, age 11 months, is starting to walk and climb on everything in sight. He is being kept in a playpen all his waking hours to avoid falls and injuries. Or Adam, age 92 years, is confined to a chair several hours a day with a vest restraint because staff are worried about his falling owing to his poor balance and his forgetting to use his walker.

Both of these interventions (confinement to playpen and confinement to chair) will maintain patient safety, but to the exclusion of other, equally important patient needs, including growth and development and quality of life. This is where thinking becomes the critical ingredient in planning and implementing care. Thinking is required to achieve safe care within the context of the total needs of the patient. Discussing overall care needs with patients and family members can provide guidance for implementing safe care.

EFFECTIVENESS

Effective care means the kind of care that does what it is supposed to do. For example, the nurse who is trying to help the patient sleep better must include interventions focused on improving sleep, not on teaching how to inject insulin, or some other problem not related to sleep.

The better the nurse's knowledge base, the more likely it is that the nursing interventions will be effective. One of the best ways to develop effective care is to keep up to date with nursing literature. For example, a nurse caring for a patient with a decubitus ulcer would not use a textbook that was 10 years old to find ideas for nursing interventions. The thinking nurse would find a more current text, consult with more experienced nurses, do a computer search of the literature, or better yet, do all of the above. The thinking nurse tries to keep current with the latest nursing research findings. Nursing research refines nursing interventions. Periodical literature (journals) provide the most current reports on nursing research.

When nursing interventions are effective they save time, money, and energy for the nurse, the patient, and the health care delivery system. Effective care also is cost effective.

EFFICIENCY

The third principle, providing efficient care, calls for making the best use of the nurse's time, which results in the best use of the patient's time. Efficiency sounds like common sense. The faster care is provided, the sooner the patient's problems are resolved and the more time the nurse has for other problems and other patients. Again, thinking is required to find the proper balance to attain efficiency as well as provide great nursing care. Efficient, poor nursing care or efficient, adequate nursing care are not acceptable goals for most nurses. The key to efficient, great nursing care is time management.

Time management includes issues of delegation of activities to other licensed and non-licensed personnel. Learning how to effectively delegate requires another textbook and hands-on experience. What the beginning nursing student needs to know is that delegation is a critical skill that can mean the difference between safe, effective, and efficient care and poor to dangerous care.

Time management is a complex efficiency issue. Dealing with this complexity is one of the great challenges of implementing care, and it requires planning—not just the type of planning done for the written care plan, but day-to-day planning embedded in the implementation process.

Each day when nurses start work, they make some sort of time-line or plan for the day that includes their own work as well as the work of those to whom they will delegate tasks. If 10 nurses were asked how they did this, it is likely that 10 different responses would be given. Such differences are largely related to differences in nurses' organizing styles, thinking styles, and working styles, as well as differences in what they believe is important in their work environments. Some nurses do schedules in their heads; others write them down. Beginning nurses generally need to write them down because they are less familiar with the routines. Reading, listening, watching, asking questions, and keeping those thinking caps on are equally useful. To learn about some real-life examples, complete Action Learning #50.

⟩Action Learning #50: Finding Safe, Effective, and Efficient Ways to Implement Nursing Care

Ask a practicing registered nurse the following questions and write a short summary of your findings to share with a classmate.

1. What things do you do routinely to provide for safe patient care?

2. What things do you do routinely to provide effective patient care?

3. What things do you do routinely to provide efficient patient care?

4. What do you think are the three most important things to remember when implementing care?

5. What tips do you have for me on good time management?

6. What tips do you have for me about delegating responsibility?

THINK ABOUT THIS ■ How did the responses of "your nurse" compare with the responses of your "classmate's nurse?" What words of wisdom will you take with you as you develop your practice of implementing safe, effective, and efficient nursing care? What kinds of things might affect a nurse's responses (eg, type of nursing education, years in practice, and job description)?

NURSING INTERVENTIONS

With the principles of the implementation (DOING) component of the nursing process locked firmly in your TOTAL RECALL, we can proceed to the last two phases of planning, determining nursing interventions and identifying sound rationales for those interventions.

Nursing interventions are those things the nurse does to help the patient to (1) achieve outcomes, (2) meet goals, and (3) resolve problems.

THINKing Through Nursing Interventions

Determining the best nursing interventions for each patient requires all modes of T.H.I.N.K. TOTAL RECALL draws on memory of information or where to find information in books, journals, policy and procedure manuals, and so forth. HABITS allow the use of shortcuts and techniques that save time. INQUIRY asks key questions about how standard ideas can be adapted to fit with individual needs. NEW IDEAS AND CREATIVITY encourages developing interventions that are oriented toward each patient's unique needs and strengths. KNOWING HOW YOU THINK provides insight into how to do all of this safely, efficiently, and effectively.

Resources Needed

Experienced nurses who know their area of clinical practice well can design appropriate nursing interventions based on their experience and their expanding knowledge base. However, beginning nurses and nursing students, who have less experience and a less developed knowledge base, generally rely more on external resources. These external resources include, but are not limited to, textbooks, journal articles, nursing diagnosis manuals, standardized care plans, mentors, preceptors, instructors, and other nurses.

In some textbooks and institutions, nursing interventions are also called "nursing actions" or "nursing orders." Similar to the work described earlier on the Classification of Nursing Outcomes (NOC), there is a Nursing Interventions Classification (NIC). The NIC, which was also mentioned in Chapter 3, is a classification of standardized intervention terms. This classification includes both direct care and indirect care activities. In other words, it is a classification of those things that nurses do. For the purposes of this discussion of care planning, we focus on the direct care activities that help patients meet their outcomes.

There are multiple ways of determining appropriate nursing interventions. When using NIC, nurses can focus their thinking on choosing from the list of interventions those that are appropriate for each specific patient situation. Nurses also can determine interventions from their experience (knowledge base) and use textbooks to augment their knowledge. Remember that the words and language used to describe interventions will vary from text to text. When documenting, however, it is desirable to use standardized terms for the interventions so that others can more easily understand what you have done.

The nurse who develops interventions must keep in mind that his or her plan, in most health care settings, will be used by other nurses. Therefore, nursing interventions should be written with enough specificity that all nurses involved can understand and implement the plan. Keeping the purposes of continuity of care and clarity of communication in mind will help the nurse develop or select interventions that are clear, specific, concise, and focused on what the nurse will do. Obviously, these interventions must be based on sound principles of nursing care that maintain patient safety. The classifications systems of NANDA, NIC, and NOC were developed to enhance nurse communication within and across settings by providing a common set of terms (standardized) that all nurses could use to communicate with one another about care.

Regardless of which source of knowledge a nurse uses, it is essential that each outcome have a set of nursing interventions to go along with it. In the following example there are several interventions for one outcome.

Outcomes	Nursing Interventions
1. Explaining how to self-administer insulin safely by the end of 1 week.	1a. Ask pt. to share what he already knows about insulin injections.
	1b. Add to current knowledge by teaching pt. about proper technique for holding equipment, maintaining sterility, selecting and rotating sites and injecting and storing insulin.
	1c. Demonstrate for pt. and ask pt. to repeat back what he learned, providing positive reinforcement, and correcting misunderstandings before he does own injection.

For more examples, refer back to the Sample Care Plan in Chapter 4 or forward to the plans in Chapter 14.

Standardized Plans Used to Trigger Thinking

Standardized care plans are commonplace in health care today. Nurses may use computer programs with such plans that address problems for which patients commonly are treated in a particular setting. For nursing care in hospitals, "clinical pathways" or "critical pathways" have become commonplace as well. These guides cite usual interventions for specific patient populations and often are unit-specific. Where computers are less available or less sophisticated, standardized plans may be sheets of paper that are taken from a file and added to the patient's record as the care plan.

Using standardized plans does not mean copying the care plan from a book onto a sheet of paper and writing the patient's name at the top. Nor does it mean pulling a preprinted standardized form out of a drawer and writing a patient's name on it before inserting it in the patient's chart. It means using only the parts of the plan that fit a particular patient's needs, and using the rest as a guide to trigger INQUIRY and NEW IDEAS AND CREATIVITY to identify additional nursing interventions. For example, most standardized approaches to the care of a patient with a nursing diagnosis of "Constipation" recommend that the nurse encourage the patient to increase intake of raw vegetables. This is good, safe care in most cases—but suppose the patient has renal problems and is on a low-potassium diet?

The nurse in this case must individualize nursing interventions to specify which vegetables or foods would help with the constipation *and* to maintain a low potassium intake to avoid making the patient's renal problems worse.

This example illustrates how standardized plans and standardized nursing interventions, which are designed *only* to address the problem portion of the nursing diagnostic label, can be used as tools to individualize care. Standardized plans do not, and cannot be expected to, address the infinite number of related factors that make a problem unique for a particular patient. Standardized plans should be used only as guides to start the thinking required for selecting individualized nursing interventions. Standardized plans are a valuable tool if they are used appropriately, but they should not be used as cookbook solutions for all patients with similar problems.

⊃ACTION LEARNING #51: Individualizing a Standardized Care Plan

Find a book with some standardized care plans for nursing diagnoses. Review Mrs. Partridge's case in Action Learning #44 in Chapter 9 and, for the nursing diagnosis "Diversional Activity Deficit related to fatigue and time demands of new mother role," find a standardized plan and individualize it to Mrs. Partridge. Explain to a classmate how you changed the standardized plan and why.

THINK ABOUT THIS ■ What was the biggest challenge to doing this? Did you find that the standard plan helped or hindered your thinking about what Mrs. Partridge needed? Do you see how easy it is to just transfer plans from a book to a patient situation without giving it much thought? What are the benefits of individualizing a plan? If you were the patient, what would you want?

Using Nursing Interventions Classification (NIC) to Trigger Thinking

The NIC, although similar to standardized care plans, is slightly different in that it provides many options for interventions in a variety of categories. A nurse can look at the entire list of interventions and choose those that are appropriate for a particular patient; rarely will the nurse use all of the possible interventions for one patient. There are several advantages to using NIC as a guide for interventions. First, the NIC language for interventions was developed and validated by practicing nurses. Nurse educators, clinicians, and researchers across the country worked together to create the comprehensive sets of standardized terms included in the NIC and also in the NANDA and NOC systems. The refinement of these classifications continues today through the ongoing feedback and collaboration of practicing nurses. This is in contrast to a variety of texts written independently about interventions that are based primarily on their authors' experience or a literature review. These texts use non-standardized terms to describe nursing care. The language of NIC is standardized, and the NIC interventions are comprehensive. There is a list of almost all possible interventions in many categories, from which the best ones can be chosen. Sometimes seeing the choices will assist the nurse's thinking; perhaps some of those listed would not have entered the nurse's mind without that "jogging" of the memory.

Let's look at an example under the intervention of "exercise therapy: ambulation," which might be used to determine the activities for a patient whose outcome is independent ambulation (McCloskey & Bulechek, 1996, p. 265). As you can see from the list in Display 10-1, 20 activities are listed.

A nurse using this classification would have to make choices about which interventions and activities to use in a plan for a given patient. Some choices would be immediately obvious; others might not be. The list may cause some nurses to remember activities under the interventions label they might not have considered otherwise. Look at the first activity on the list, for example, "Dress the patient in nonrestrictive clothing." This might significantly affect the range of motion of a patient and therefore benefit ambulation, but it is not something that would necessarily come to mind as important.

Putting Interventions Back Together With Outcomes

In Chapter 9 patient goals and outcomes were described as the first part of a nursing plan. Interventions must be tailored to fit the outcomes. However, there are many "fuzzy areas" between adequate and great planned interventions. To check your learning thus far, do the following Action Learning #52.

⊃ACTION LEARNING #52: What's Missing in This Written Plan?

Study the following abbreviated care plan and circle the things that do not follow the guidelines discussed above. Explain to a classmate why they are a problem. If you really want a challenge, try to fix the plan's problems and identify rationales for the appropriate nursing orders.

> **Nursing Diagnosis:** Fatigue R/T anemia, depression, and sleep pattern disturbance.
>
> **Goal:** The patient will feel better.

DISPLAY 10–1.   Exercise Therapy: Ambulation

DEFINITION: Promotion and assistance with walking to maintain or restore autonomic and voluntary body functions during treatment and recovery from illness or injury

ACTIVITIES:

Dress patient in nonrestrictive clothing
Assist patient to use footwear that facilitates walking and prevents injury
Provide low-height bed, as appropriate
Place bed-positioning switch within easy reach
Encourage to sit in bed, on side of bed ("dangle"), or in chair, as tolerated
Assist patient to sit on side of bed to facilitate postural adjustments
Consult physical therapist about ambulation plan, as needed
Instruct in availability of assistive devices, if appropriate
Instruct patient how to position self throughout the transfer process
Use a gait belt to assist with transfer and ambulation, as needed
Assist patient to transfer, as needed
Provide cueing card(s) at head of bed to facilitate learning to transfer
Apply/provide assistive device (cane, walker, or wheelchair) for ambulation, if the patient is unsteady
Assist patient with initial ambulation and as needed
Instruct patient/caregiver about safe transfer and ambulation techniques
Monitor patient's use of crutches or other walking aids
Assist patient to stand and ambulate specified distance and with specified number of staff
Assist patient to establish realistic increments in distance for ambulation
Encourage independent ambulation within safe limits
Encourage patient to be "up ad lib," if appropriate

BACKGROUND READINGS:
Alora, J. (1981). Exercise and skeletal health. *Journal of the American Geriatric Society, 29*(3), 104–107.
Donohue, K., Miller, C., & Craig, B. (1988). Chronic alterations in mobility. In P.H. Mitchell, L.C. Hodges, M. Muwaswes et al. (Eds.). *AANN's neuroscience nursing: Phenomena and practice* (pp. 319–343). Norwalk, CT: Appleton & Lange.
Glick, O.J. (1992). Interventions related to activity and movement. In G.M. Bulechek & J.C. McCloskey (Eds.), Symposium on nursing interventions. *Nursing Clinics of North America, 27*(2), 541–568.
Lubkin, I. (1990). *Chronic illness: impact and interventions* (2nd ed.). Boston: Jones & Bartlett.
McFarland, G.K., & McFarlane, E.A. (1989). *Nursing diagnosis and intervention*. St. Louis: Mosby.
Moorhouse, M., Geissler, A., & Doenges, M. (1987). *Critical care plans, guidelines for patient care*. Philadelphia: F.A. Davis.
Smith, E.L., & Gillian, C. (1983). Physical activity prescription for the older adult. *The Physician & Sports Medicine, 11*(8), 91–182.
Snyder, M. (1992). Exercise. In M. Snyder (Ed.). *Independent nursing interventions* (2nd ed.) (pp. 67–77). Albany: Delmar Publishers.

(McCloskey, J.C. & Bulechek, B.M. (1996). *Nursing interventions classification (NIC)*. St. Louis: Mosby.)

Outcomes	Nursing Interventions
Pt. will experience less anemia in 1 wk.	Pt. will follow doctor's orders and take iron pills.
Pt. will be less depressed	Develop trust with patient to encourage him to talk about his depression.
	Encourage pt. to identify things that help him feel good and feel depressed.
	Help pt. structure day to avoid long periods of isolation.

THINK ABOUT THIS ■ How many less-than-ideal things did you find? How easy was it to fix those areas? Would it have been easier to start from scratch? What is the best way to remember all these criteria for developing planning for nursing diagnoses?

[Authors' note: Our students have found that "fixing" care plans is an excellent way to increase understanding of care plans in terms of both content and format. Additional activities might include looking at old plans of yours or someone else's and "fixing" them. Be sure that you and your classmates feel free to make constructive criticism and suggestions without hurting one another's feelings.]

✔ *Thinking-Learning Check*

Pause here for a thinking-learning check. You should be able to elaborate on these ideas:

- ✔ Nursing interventions assist the patient in achieving the outcomes necessary to meet a goal and resolve a problem.
- ✔ *Doing* (Implementing) involves interventions taken with the principles of safety, effectiveness, and efficiency in mind.
- ✔ Effective time management produces efficient nursing care.
- ✔ Standardized plans trigger thinking for developing individualized nursing interventions.
- ✔ NIC triggers thinking for developing individualized nursing interventions and activities.

IDENTIFYING SOUND RATIONALES

Identifying sound rationales for nursing interventions and activities is a part of planning that is particularly important to beginning nurses. This is the process by which the knowledge learned in the "theory" classes is put to practical use. Whenever a nurse develops or chooses an intervention, it is vital that a sound reason for that intervention be identified. Why, for example, should a patient be given at least 1500 mL of fluid each day? Why this amount and not 2500 mL or 1000 mL?

It is tempting to choose interventions that are "always" done "on this unit" but that have no other rationale for doing them. This is one of those times when HABIT thinking becomes a problem. Such choices are potentially dangerous because they indicate that interventions are being planned and carried out without thinking. One way to avoid slipping into this habit is to beef up your INQUIRY mode and ask "why" very frequently. Why am I doing this? If the only answer you come up with is "because this is the way we do it," then you have a problem. "This is the way we do it" is NOT SOUND RATIONALE. This kind of answer usually means that the nurse did not take the time to think about the sound rationale or does not know the rationale. It is a signal to fire up the INQUIRY mode and re-learn the rationale, search for new information, or consult some nursing experts.

Where to find those answers may be a challenge for beginners, but nurses who have been practicing for a while tend to have a ready repertoire of sources that they check. For beginners, texts are a starting place. Some texts are dedicated to specific topics (eg, chronic obstructive lung disease or substance abuse disorders). In general texts (eg, medical-surgical texts or psychiatric texts), the nurse can look for a chapter heading or in the index in the back of the book.

Following is an example of how a beginning nursing student might demonstrate the ability to document rationale:

Nursing Diagnosis: Risk for Impaired Home Maintenance Management related to fractured hip, living alone in older home.

Goal: Patient will be able to maintain self safely in own home after discharge.

Outcome #1: Patient will identify potential barriers to care at home by end of week.

Nursing Intervention/ Activity:	**Rationale with Documentation:**
Assess home environment for barriers to ambulation.	Physical barriers (especially stairs, bathrooms) may limit patient's ability to ambulate and care for self at home (Smeltzer & Bare, 1992, p. 1815)

This is a good time to briefly review and summarize all the parts of traditionally written nursing care plans. Although not all nursing schools and health care organizations use the traditional nursing care plan, it is still helpful to recognize the components and the criteria for each component. You never know when you may have to draw on this knowledge. Display 10-2 provides an overview for developing written plans of care.

DISPLAY **10–2.   Overview for Developing Written Plans of Care**

Care Plan Component	**Basic Things to Think About**
I. Conclusions of Assessment	
A. Strengths	Compare with population norms and validate with patient or significant other. Strengths can be used in planning.
B. Health concerns	
1. Nursing diagnosis	Problem label for Actual or Potential problem or Wellness condition that is clearly supported by data that has been compared with both population and patient norms; the concern is treatable by a nurse.
	ALL related factors are connected to the first part of the diagnostic statement with the phrase "related to" or "R/T."
2. Interdisciplinary problems	Problems that require interventions in collaboration with other health care professionals, but maintain involvement of nursing as well
3. Problems for referral	Problems that require interventions outside the expertise of nursing
II. Conclusions of Planning & Implementing	
A. Set priorities	Follow guidelines on p. 183 (eg, immediately life threatening, safety, pt's priority, nurse's priority)
B. Establish nursing-sensitive patient outcomes	
1. Goals	Patient centered
	Designates direction for change: restore; maintain; improve
	Focuses on the problem part of the diagnostic statement
	Includes a time frame for completion
2. Outcome indicators and outcome measures	Patient centered
	Measurable
	Focuses on reversing or eliminating the related factors when possible
	Focuses on patient behaviors such as affective, cognitive, psychomotor, or patient physiologic conditions
	Includes a time frame for completion
C. Develop nursing interventions with sound rationales	Nurse focused; providing specific directions for nursing care
	Specifically addresses each outcome with one or more interventions
	Based on sound rationale

DESIGNING CARE FOR INTERDISCIPLINARY PROBLEMS AND PROBLEMS FOR REFERRAL

So far the discussion of plans has centered on plans the nurse develops for nursing diagnosis-type conclusions. It also is necessary to plan for other conclusions. With interdisciplinary problems, it may be the nurse, the collaborator, or both people together who design the plan. How this collaboration is achieved often depends on the setting and the usual types of problems addressed. Generally speaking, however, most disciplines take the same approach to planning that nurses take in designing plans for nursing diagnoses. There usually is a goal or outcomes and interventions to be taken by health care providers. In some settings, such as mental health, these are called Interdisciplinary Treatment or Master Treatment Plans.

Planning for problems for referral may sound easy, but it requires skill in several areas, including:

1. Knowing what resources are available for making referrals
2. Knowing who to contact to be sure the referral is appropriate
3. Making sure the patient and/or family members make the connection with the organization to which they have been referred
4. Following up to evaluate the effectiveness of the referral

The nurse usually refers the patient to another health care provider for the identified problem(s). The other provider either plans the care or returns to the nurse to design an interdisciplinary plan. Documentation indicating that the nurse made the referral and explaining why is important. Where this information is documented depends on the agency or institution; generally, it is recorded in the progress note. The key is to remember to record it somewhere.

It also is important that, as priorities are set, nurses look at all conclusions collectively. It may be that an interdisciplinary problem or a problem for referral has a higher priority than a nursing diagnosis. Thinking and keeping the "big picture" in focus is of utmost importance in planning care.

Designing care for any health concern is no small undertaking if it done well. Although there are minor variations among schools of nursing and health care agencies, the major issues addressed in this chapter can be found in most well designed care plans.

A BRIEF RETURN TO IMPLEMENTING

With the phases of planning complete (for the moment, anyway—remember, plans change constantly; we will be discussing modified plans shortly), we will assume that the nurse is ready and able to implement care. When this implementation occurs it becomes the visible behavior of the nurse. This behavior typically is labeled "real nursing care." The nurse teaches, the nurse administers medication, the nurse counsels a patient, and the nurse DOES nursing.

Think for a moment about what it took for the nurse to get to this point. It has taken us the majority of 10 book chapters and more than 200 pages to just begin to examine the thinking needed to get to the point of DOING. If it took nurses this long to DO nursing care, most patients would have been discharged long ago, become significantly sicker, or just given up and walked home.

Obviously an experienced nurse can get to the point of DOING in much less time. Sometimes the thinking behind that DOING occurs in microseconds; sometimes more detailed planning requires a few hours. This is said not to discourage you, but to help you appreciate the depth and the magnitude of the high-level thinking that goes on and is not visible. The only evidence of this level of thinking is in the quality of the care provided.

And at this point, the nurse's thinking in the nursing process is not even finished! Now the nurse and the patient have to collaborate again. They have to use their thinking to determine the quality of care through the final component of the process, evaluating.

DETERMINING QUALITY OF CARE (EVALUATING)

Evaluation is the "checking" part of any activity that provides feedback as to how well the activity worked and whether the desired results were achieved. In daily life, evaluation occurs informally. If you are doing a load of wash with extra stains, you might try a new stain-removing product that came in the mail. After the wash cycle, you check to see whether the stains are gone. That's evaluation.

In nursing, evaluation is done in more formal ways. The classic method includes evaluation of structure, process, and outcome. Most nurses are not regularly involved in structure evaluation because it includes evaluation of the physical building (eg, room sizes, classroom space), the physical environment (eg, ventilation, room temperature), and resources that support direct care (eg, equipment, supplies, computer terminals). When these structural elements directly affect care, however, they become necessary areas for all nurses to evaluate.

Process evaluation focuses on what and how things are done. In nursing, that generally means how nursing interventions are carried out. Policy and procedure manuals describe ideal nursing interventions and may be used as a standard for process evaluation. Employment evaluations for pay raises and promotions also fit in this category. Some process evaluation occurs with the nursing process. Look at the example that follows to see how process evaluation is used in documenting nursing interventions. First, look at the sample portion of the care plan, and then look at the note a nurse might put in the patient's record. The note is an example of process evaluation. (Note: Outcomes and interventions are not based on the NIC and NOC standardized languages.)

Example of Process and Outcome Nursing Evaluation Notes

Nursing Diagnosis: Social isolation R/T forgetting to wear hearing aid.

> **Goal:** In 2 weeks patient will have improved socialization.
> **Outcome:** Patient will insert hearing aid before breakfast every day and leave it in until bed time.
> **Nursing Intervention:** Remind patient to insert hearing aid before going to the dining room in the morning; assist as necessary to insert and adjust volume.
> **Process Evaluation Note documented in patient's record:** "Patient needed help inserting aid due to stiffness in fingers today. Best volume setting for her is at high."

Outcome evaluation focuses on what it is about the patient that has changed over time. Does it fit with the outcome that was pre-planned? The following note reflects outcome evaluation of the patient situation just described.

> **Outcome Evaluation Note documented in patient's record:** "Patient accepted help putting in hearing aid before breakfast. Said her arthritis in her fingers usually prevented her from doing it so early in the morning. She took her hearing aid out after breakfast, saying it was uncomfortable. Outcome not met."

The key difference between the process note and the outcome note is that the latter focuses on the actual change in the patient in contrast to the expected change (identified in the outcome). Both notes have some information about what happened, but the first note is just that—a report of what happened without a focus on the relationship to an expected outcome or goal. The second note tells what happened, but in the form of an "explanation" of circumstances surrounding the patient outcome—a set of reasons why the expected outcome was not met. Following is a more detailed discussion of the definition and purpose of outcome evaluation, along with guidelines and discussion on how to modify plans.

Definition and Purpose of Outcome Evaluation

Outcome evaluation is just as it sounds, a determination of whether or not a desired result has occurred. It is a time when the nurse's thinking and the patient's thinking again work together. The task this time is to determine how close the patient's present situation/status matches what both of them agreed should happen (the outcomes established in the early phases of planning).

Evaluating often is seen as an end point, but in actuality it is a way of constantly updating nursing care. Outcome evaluation, commonly called "evaluation" within the nursing process, is the way to measure whether or not the patient is meeting the goals and objectives of the care plan.

To see the purposes of evaluation clearly, think of what nursing is all about. Nurses try to help improve patient responses to their health conditions; there must be a way to determine whether that is happening. Evaluation is the nurse's ever-present, internal quality control device. Because of the need for professional accountability, evidence of evaluation must be written in a patient's record. Written documentation is discussed in greater detail in Chapter 11.

Guidelines for Outcome Evaluation

Outcome evaluation consists of a series of steps and questions. It starts with the establishment, in the planning stage, of the expected outcomes as evaluation criteria. Remember that in Chapter 9 we emphasized how important it was for both the nurse and the patient to collaborate and think together about the outcomes.

Another word for expected outcomes and evaluation criteria is "indicators." Indicators or expected outcomes become the measurement tools to determine whether or not patients have achieved their goals.

Outcome evaluation is the fourth component of the nursing process that makes use of previously established outcomes. A formal evaluation of outcomes must be documented (written) in a patient's record. This is particularly important for quality assurance, which is discussed in Chapter 11.

Although it is very important to document the nurse's conclusions about the quality of care (evaluation) this is one aspect of nursing care that continues to require more attention and focus. Nurses, however, are improving their ability to document outcomes. Reimbursement for care seems to have become a major incentive to do a better job of documentation.

The action learning activity that follows is designed to help beginning students recognize outcome and process evaluation notes in the real world.

⊃Action Learning #53: The Hunt for Process and Outcome Evaluation in Medical Records

Look at one or two patient charts. Write down three examples of the following (remember to maintain confidentiality and use only patient initials if you find real names in the progress notes):

PROCESS EVALUATION STATEMENTS:

1.

2.

3.

OUTCOME EVALUATION STATEMENTS:

1.

2.

3.

THINK ABOUT THIS ■ How easy was this to do? Did the evaluation statements
give you a clear picture of what the nurse did? Of what the patient did? How
would you have improved on the evaluation statements?

Evaluation becomes an ongoing process as nurses assess patients to determine whether outcomes are met within the designated time frames. Evaluation is a dynamic process of moving back and forth among the parts of the whole nursing process. If needed, modifications are made and evaluations continue until a patient problem is resolved or discontinued. Figure 10-1 illustrates the outcome evaluation process (a process within the nursing process).

The outcomes planned for each health concern are continually evaluated. The first question to ask is: did the patient meet the expected outcomes? If so, the patient achieved what was expected. The nurse can assume that data collection for that issue was complete, the analysis was accurate, the goals and outcomes were realistic, and the nursing interventions were sound and well implemented. If the patient outcomes were not met, the nurse must go back through the steps of the process until the point of breakdown is found. That backtracking process requires INQUIRY thinking, in which all phases of the nursing process are examined. That is where outcome evaluation becomes a process evaluation.

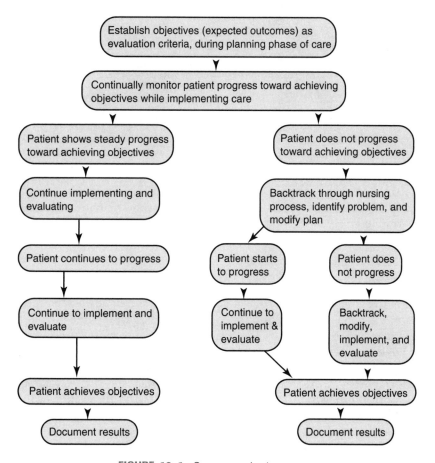

FIGURE 10–1   Outcome evaluation process.

DISPLAY **10–3.**   **Evaluation Tracking Patterns**

TRACK #1: PATIENT RESPONSES FIT WITH EXPECTED OUTCOMES

Evaluation Question Sequence	Answers
1. Patient objectives met?	Yes
2. Patient goal(s) met?	Yes
3. Problem or issue resolved?	Yes

TRACK #2: PATIENT RESPONSES DO NOT FIT WITH EXPECTED OUTCOMES

Evaluation Question Sequence	Additional Questions
1. Objectives not met? or partially met?	Were they realistic? Was time frame OK? Complete (all related factors addressed)?
2. Goal(s) not met? or partially met?	Were they realistic? Time frame OK? Linked to problem (conclusion or Dx)?
3. Problem or issue not resolved?	Did it change? Was it validated or not validated by the patient? Priority or not?
4. Implemented actions done fully? or partially?	Reasons why not done as planned?
5. Planned actions	Sound? Realistic? Fit with objectives and goals? Complete?
6. Analysis of data and clusters	Accurate (conclusions fit with data)? Complete (all possible conclusions considered)? Clusters of data logical?
7. Data	Complete? Accurate?

Study the tracking patterns shown in Display 10-3. The first is the ideal situation in which everything works as planned. The second provides the questions to ask along the way to find the point of breakdown. That point is where the nurse should start to revise the process. This revision process is called modifying.

Modifying Plans

Modifying plans is a significant part of evaluating. If outcomes are not achieved by their designated time frames, this often is an indication that some part of the nursing process was not completed—something broke down during thinking and doing. The hunt begins to locate the process "breakdown." The hunt involves methodically backtracking through the process to find the problem or problems. Once these are discovered, the breakdown can be corrected. Sometimes the "fix" is simple, such as when a time frame needs to be adjusted. Sometimes the fix is more complicated, such as when the nurse discovers that he or she did not validate a problem with the patient but proceeded to plan care anyway.

Consider the following situation. A nurse concludes that a patient is overweight and needs a reducing diet. The nurse develops a goal and an expected outcome that the patient will lose 2 pounds by the end of 1 month. The nurse teaches a new diet and helps the patient develop meal plans for 2 weeks. The nurse evaluates to see whether the patient is halfway toward achieving the objective by the end of the 2 weeks of meal plans (it is a good idea to do interim checks). The patient is not progressing toward achieving this objective; in fact, he has gained 3 pounds. What happened? The expected outcomes (goals and objectives) were not achieved, even though they were realistic, had appropriate time frames, and addressed all of the related factors identified as contributing to the problem (numbers 1 and 2 of the evaluation checking sequence). What about number 3 on the evaluation checking sequence? Bingo, there's the breakdown—validation of the problem with the patient. The patient did not see his weight as a problem. What the nurse needs to do in this case is explore why the patient does not think it is a problem. By revisiting assessment and collecting more data, the nurse may discover that the patient has a culturally related desire to be overweight and sees no reason to change; he was just being "polite" when he agreed to the plan initially.

Evaluation may be humbling at times, especially when nurses find that they were off target in their conclusions. The purpose of evaluation, however, is not to place blame, but rather to ensure that the patient is getting the best care possible and is moving toward healthy responses. No one—nurse or patient—is perfect. Both can learn much from each other in the process of achieving great nursing.

✔ *Thinking-Learning Check*

Pause here for a thinking-learning check. You should be able to elaborate on these ideas:

✔ All nursing interventions must be supported by a rationale.

✔ Care must be planned for all conclusions of assessment.

✔ Determining quality of care (Evaluating) works best when its value is appreciated and it is completed with systematic INQUIRY.

THINKING WITH PLANNING, IMPLEMENTING, AND EVALUATING

Throughout this chapter, there have been many references to the importance of the thinking of both the nurse and the patient. Actually, it is just about impossible to plan, implement, and evaluate care without high-level thinking from both nurse and patient. It is, however, possible to "go along" and do a minimum level of nursing without great thought—to carry out medical orders and do the routine nursing tasks without accepting the responsibility to help patients get better, prevent their problems, or reach their highest potential. Such behavior is potentially dangerous to patients and is certainly not professional. Accepting the professional responsibility for consistently thinking must become firmly implanted in the nurse's brain as a good HABIT; otherwise, nursing becomes a cookbook routine.

One way to develop the good habit of high-level thinking is, again, to put one-self in the patient's situation. If you were the patient, what would you want? Would you want a nurse who pulls a standardized plan out of a file drawer, puts it on your chart, routinely implements only predetermined care, and occasionally checks to see whether you are progressing? When the question is put that way, just about everyone would say, "Of course not." Most people want a nurse who uses high-level thinking, and that means using all thinking modes.

Throughout the earlier discussions, TOTAL RECALL was shown to be neces-sary—to use knowledge and resources for planning, to know how to implement a variety of nursing interventions, and to recognize reasonable expectations for evaluation. Several thinking HABITS were important—putting patient safety first, including the patient in all planning, respecting the individuality of each patient, and habitually using INQUIRY. INQUIRY was the key to the continual ques-tioning of what was best in each situation—determining how each health issue af-fected others, how priorities were set, how realistic goals and objectives were estab-lished, how the best ways to promote patient strengths were developed, how constant evaluation of the patient's progress was achieved, and which were the best ways to manage time. In short, INQUIRY forces the nurse to ask, "Is there a better way to accomplish the task at hand?" NEW IDEAS AND CREATIVITY was described as the driving force of individualized care; creative nurses expand the standardized approaches and make each patient feel unique. The final mode, KNOWING HOW YOU THINK, merits a bit more consideration as this chapter draws to a close because it brings thinking back to its core for each individual nurse.

Accomplishing the simultaneous tasks of designing and doing care and deter-mining its quality can be seen as an insurmountable obstacle or an exciting chal-lenge. Choosing the obstacle or challenge option depends on the quality of the nurse's thinking in all five modes, but especially in the KNOWING HOW YOU THINK mode. Three areas in particular are critical to successfully accepting the challenge. The first area involves the environment for thinking, the second area covers skill in convergent thinking, and the third returns to the concepts of dualis-tic and relativistic thinking that were addressed in Chapter 1.

The working environment of nurses frequently includes noise, confusion, con-stant interruptions, time pressures, and downright chaos. Yet thinking and deci-sion making still must occur. Identifying which environmental factors help and hinder thinking is an important step in KNOWING HOW YOU THINK and apply-ing the nursing process. If the environment itself cannot be altered to enhance thinking, certain parts of the environment, or the nurse's ability to cope with the environment, must change.

Convergent thinking is the ability to bring pieces of information together to create a whole. It is like putting a puzzle together with all the separate pieces. In nursing, effective convergent thinking allows the nurse to bring all the phases of the nursing process together to make sense out of the patient's health response puzzle. It is the dynamic blending of assessing, planning, implementing, and evalu-ating all rolled into one. KNOWING HOW YOU THINK with regard to convergent thinking will give you some clues about how to see the big picture, and will show whether this aspect of thinking needs enhancing.

Relativistic thinking is the ability to accept the fact that most things in this world are not simply "right" or "wrong," nor do they fit in neat little boxes. In nursing, relativistic thinking is accepting the fact that patients, their health responses, and the solutions to those responses do not usually fit into those well-defined boxes. KNOWING HOW YOU THINK relativistically provides understanding and guidance for growth in this area of thinking.

To get a better idea about your "KNOWING HOW YOU THINK" mode regarding the environment, convergent thinking, and relativistic thinking, answer the following questions about your thinking in general:

Are you a person who needs absolute quiet to think through a problem?
Does your thinking become energized in the midst of chaos, excitement, noise, and confusion?
Do you like to talk things through with others before making decisions?
Do you prefer thinking things through privately before involving others?
Can you think on your feet quickly or do you like to mull things over?
Does chocolate help you think?
How threatening is it to share ideas with others before you are "sure" of your ideas?
How do you feel if you can't find the "right" answer?
Does lack of time pressure you into decisions you might not make otherwise?

This very brief self-evaluation of your thinking is designed only to trigger your further exploration. You may want to return to the T.H.I.N.K. Inventory in Chapter 1 for some similar queries. It is very important for beginning nurses to return continually to this thinking mode. Regular attention to KNOWING HOW YOU THINK allows beginning nurses to recognize the "hindrances" and identify the "helps" of putting together the planning, implementing, and evaluating phases of the "big picture."

Here are some suggestions for dealing with one major hindrance (chaos and confusion) to effective thinking about planning, implementation, and evaluating.

Find a quiet room to work.
Jot down ideas before working with patients.
Identify a trusted colleague with whom to talk things over.
Develop and write care plans at less chaotic times, such as at the beginning of a shift.
Eat chocolate (or popcorn, for those who are more diet conscious) if it helps.
Practice saying, "I need time to think about this," and then say it.
Think out loud and tell patients and other staff what you are doing (you'll be a great role model for other nurses).
Keep paper and pencil handy for jotting down ideas and organizing thoughts.
Monitor your behavior, your thinking, and your communication style when you feel pressured.

Try to select a work environment that is suited to your thinking style (ie, busy, fast-paced, quick-changing; or slower, in-depth, long-ranging).

Unfortunately, nursing has been portrayed as an action-oriented rather than a thinking- *and* action-oriented profession. This misconception makes it very difficult for beginning nurses who do not always "think on their feet" as quickly as they would like. This situation also promotes less useful thinking HABITS that hinder great nursing. If beginning nurses learn to value higher-level thinking, especially KNOWING HOW YOU THINK, *and* build "think time" into their practice, the results are inevitable: great nursing through simultaneously designing and doing care, and determining its quality.

CLOSING COMMENTS

First of all, congratulations; mastering the concepts presented in the last two chapters required high-level thinking and concentration. Designing care, doing it, and determining its quality are all essential components of great nursing care. They must be appreciated for their own unique contributions to the nursing process. However, it is only when designing, doing, and determining quality are applied as a dynamic whole, in conjunction with assessing and in collaboration with the patient, that great nursing is possible.

TOTAL RECALL and HABITS will instill the knowledge gained from these chapters in memory, but all five thinking modes must be used to apply the principles of designing, doing, and determining quality of care in practice. The remaining chapters provide more guidance and practice activities to continue to nurture your thinking skills as you incorporate planning, implementing, and evaluating skills into your repertoire of great nursing.

THINKING LOG #10 ➤ The first nine chapters of this text have been full of many ideas about nursing and thinking. It is very likely that your thinking has been modified to accommodate all this learning. To illustrate the changes that have occurred, redraw your Thinking Cap. Describe to a classmate the changes that have occurred since the first drawing, and write out a brief description of how your thinking has changed.

References

McCloskey, J.C. & Bulechek, B.M. (1996). *Nursing interventions classification (NIC)*. St. Louis: Mosby

3

Communicating Thinking and the Nursing Process

11

Written and Verbal Communication of Thinking and Doing

✻ *Learning Outcomes*

After reading and doing the activities in this chapter you will be able to:

Appreciate the importance of clear verbal and written communication.

Document the results of thinking and care during assessing, planning, implementing, and evaluating.

Describe several methods of documentation.

Explore the finer points of clear communication.

Thinking and doing great nursing are not enough—the thinking and doing must be communicated to others. Because the doing can be seen, but the thinking cannot, it is especially important that the thinking be communicated. Nurses often are, and need to be, more skilled communicators than other people. The information communicated by nurses can be significant to the well-being—even the life—of patients. To add to the challenge of communication, nurses often have to organize their thoughts and communicate them clearly in the midst of busy schedules, overwhelming demands, and, sometimes, even chaos.

In this chapter you will examine your present written and verbal communication style and judge how well it works in nursing situations. Methods to enhance communication are explored. Selected methods of written communication in nursing and how they are used in various phases of the nursing process are examined. Finally, this chapter will whet your appetite for some of the finer points of written communication.

DESCRIPTION OF CLEAR COMMUNICATION

Clarity of communication is not automatic. It requires thinking. In all communication, there is a sender and a receiver of information, each of whom exchange roles throughout an interaction. The receiver must listen, see, read, or sense the message. Hopefully, the receiver gets the message from the sender in the way the sender meant it to be. There is a better chance of that occurring if the sender is clear about what the message is and how the message is communicated.

This chapter focuses on the sender role and the importance of clarity. "Clarity" means that the message is descriptive of what is in the sender's mind. It is organized, specific, and to the point. In nursing, it also means that the communication is professional, which is different from social communication. Professional communication portrays respect for the receiver and for the person who is the subject of the communication (usually the patient) and for that person's privacy.

PURPOSES OF CLEAR COMMUNICATION

There are several purposes of clear communication, some of which are quite obvious. The first is to promote continuity and consistent quality of care. Nurses must coordinate their care with that of others. If care issues are not well communicated, patients get disjointed, sporadic care. Accurate and specific verbal and written reports from one nurse to another or between nurses and other health care providers will decrease duplication of efforts, ensure that important issues are not missed, and save time, energy, and resources.

A second purpose of clear communication is to provide evidence of the thinking that accompanies the nursing process. All parts of the nursing process must be communicated verbally or in written form. Notes and oral reports reflect the thinking that guided data collection and analysis, which resulted in well designed and implemented care, and the thinking that judged changes in a patient's conditions.

A third purpose of clear communication is to establish credibility and legal accountability for care. Nurses are legally accountable for the care they do *and* do not provide. Written communication, in particular, is a tangible way to validate that legal responsibility. Records are legal documents, and as such, may be called into court. What a nurse writes in a patient record can make the difference between winning or losing a lawsuit. The legal issues are discussed more fully in Chapter 12.

There also are some less obvious but equally important purposes of clear communication. Effective verbal communication with patients and their significant others enables the nurse to obtain information that might otherwise remain unknown. Clear verbal communication also plays a major role in developing the nurse–patient relationship, which is based on trust. Studies conducted more than a decade ago have shown that health care providers who are classified as "good communicators" are less likely to be sued by patients and more likely to have their treatment plans followed (Northouse & Northouse, 1985).

Clear written communications in the forms of well worded nursing diagnoses and well worded goals and outcomes go a long way toward streamlining nursing care and achieving successful outcomes. Developing these finer points of written communication requires great thinking, and is explored at the end of this chapter.

VERBAL COMMUNICATION

Personal Styles of Verbal Communication

It is often said that no matter how smart you are, if you cannot communicate well, the world will not see you as smart. Regardless of the truth of that statement, it is worth some consideration. Great thinkers without great communication skills may make great eccentric hermits, but they do not make great nurses. Great nurses must be able to communicate their thinking.

Clear communication requires practice and thought. People vary widely in their abilities to communicate verbally. Verbal communication is affected by self-image, self-confidence, thinking styles, language background, and so many other personal factors that it often is difficult to pin down where each person's strengths and weaknesses are. Because of the personal nature of communication skills, it is worthwhile for nursing students to do some self-assessment or thinking about their communication abilities.

⊃Action Learning #54: Evaluating Your Verbal Communication

Tape-record yourself giving a 5-minute report on a topic about which you are well versed. (If you have access to a video recorder, videotape yourself.) Do not rehearse what you will say ahead of time or write it out; rather, mentally map your thoughts and main points. Then, listen (or watch, if you used video) to the tape and analyze your verbal skills. Answer these questions:

- Was I clear?

- Did I make my main point?

- Did I develop my ideas in a logical manner?

- Did I sound as if I knew as much about this subject as I really do?

- How often did I use speech hesitation mechanisms such as "er," "ah," "you know," "like," or "well"?

- Was my voice too loud or too soft?

- Did I vary the pace and tone?

THINK ABOUT THIS ■ So, are you a clear communicator? Did you like what you heard? If you found things you did not like, what can you do about them? Based on listening to that tape, what do you think others would think of you, of your communication skills, of your thinking skills? Keep in mind that the point of this exercise is not to decrease your self-esteem, but to increase awareness so that you can identify what works, what does not work, and what you want to change. Some people have more skill in this area than others, but effective communication is learned; no one is born with it.

Verbal Communication in Nursing

Nurses, of course, communicate with patients and their significant others as they assess, plan, implement, and evaluate care. "Therapeutic communication" is a term used in a variety of ways in nursing. Some refer to all nurse–patient communication as therapeutic, because it is focused on nurses helping patients deal with health needs. At other times, such as in the specialty area of psychiatric nursing, therapeutic communication is used to mean specific communication techniques. It is beyond the scope of this book to describe in detail the elements of the varying definitions of therapeutic communication. To avoid confusion over terms, the focus here will be on clarity of communication.

Clear verbal communication by a nurse will put patients at ease and help them open up and share information with the nurse during assessment. Nurses who communicate well with patients during planning will design the most individualized care. During implementation of care, nurses who communicate clearly find that patients are more cooperative. During evaluation, patients provide the most useful feedback on how their care is going when nurses are open and clear in their interactions. In all of these situations, clarity of expression is vital.

In addition to communication with patients and their significant others, nurses also communicate daily with other health care providers. Some of these interactions are preplanned; many others occur spontaneously. Change-of-shift reports and conference reports are two common preplanned events. Reports on changes in patients' conditions are examples of spontaneous interactions.

It often is easier to recognize unclear communication techniques than to practice clear ones. The example of an end-of-shift report that follows illustrates the problems with unclear, ineffective communication. An end-of-shift report was chosen as an example because such reports are a good test of clarity and concision. Also, these reports are a type of communication that beginning students must practice early in their nursing programs. In these short reports, nurses highlight important information but do not have time to fill in large amounts of detail. They must be organized, specific, and clear in their directions to others and they must address the components of the nursing process they have used—and do all of this in a professional manner.

⊃Action Learning #55: Evaluating Nurse Elie Norman's Communication

Read this script of a taped end-of-shift report by a nurse, Elie Norman, RN. After reading it, make a list of things that you think are problematic with this communication.

> Hiya guys. This is Elie reporting on the new patient in 51. He was admitted before lunch but I'm just now getting his stuff together. I'm so tired today, I'm just dragging around. Must be the late hours last night. Ah, well, let's

see, this patient was in the ER for a few hours before coming up here. His family is floating around the hospital somewhere. They are quite the tribe; watch out for them. Let's see, his diagnosis is diabetes insipidus and he goes to the bathroom every time you turn around. I think we're supposed to watch his intake and output really carefully. I started assessing him and got some things written on the intake form, but I only have a few hunches yet. No one knows why he has this disease; the docs from urology are working him up. They wrote some orders that I think were processed; the lab should be getting his blood by now. One thing I do know is that he is scared. I filled in one column of a care plan dealing with his fears, but I don't have it finished yet. I'll try to get that done before I leave.

PROBLEMS WITH ELIE'S COMMUNICATION:

THINK ABOUT THIS ■   What is interfering with clarity here? If you are appalled and unable to imagine a nurse communicating like this, think about having a hectic day at work after a busy night of socialization and ask yourself, honestly, would you do and say some of the same things that Elie did? Do you think Elie gave this patient good care? How can you tell? Does Elie give any evidence of her thinking about this patient and his needs? Giving Elie another chance, here is how she could have given the same verbal report:

Mr. Packer was admitted to Room 51 from the ER at 11 AM, accompanied by his family, who went to the cafeteria at 2:30. His admitting medical diagnosis is diabetes insipidus of unknown origin. He is being worked up and should have his lab work completed by now. Drs. Jones and Brown from urology have written orders, including a request for strict intake and output records. Mr. Packer has been urinating every hour since his arrival. From my assessment, which is still incomplete, I have found him to be fearful of this mysterious illness. My care plan includes some strategies to decrease his fears. My other conclusions are possible problems with fluid volume deficits, nutritional problems, and family conflicts. Please see my notes for details on these and for suggestions for further assessment today.

Strategies for Clear Verbal Communication

Unlike Elie's first report, the revised one is characterized by organization, specificity, clarity of direction to others, evidence of the nurse's thinking and use of the nursing process, and professionalism—or the omission of social chit-chat and value judgments (Fig. 11-1A,B). Even though the second report included much of the same information as the first, it was professional and exemplified the work of a thinking nurse—someone in whom one could put trust. Given the choice, which report would the next shift's nurses prefer? Now there's an easy answer. To develop the kind of style seen in the revised report, study and practice the following parameters of effective communication.

FIGURE 11–1A   Elie at her worst.

FIGURE 11–1B   Elie at her best.

Organization

Speaking in an organized manner requires organizing one's thoughts first. There are many ways to do that; most people have a personal approach that works for them. Some folks write notes to themselves; others use a scheme such as thinking about the who, what, where, when, why, and how of subjects. Whatever the method, INQUIRY thinking is needed to decide what is important and what is relevant. The actual method used to organize one's thoughts needs to become a HABIT. The method is less important than finding something that works and sticking with it. KNOWING HOW YOU THINK will help you find a system that works.

Specificity

Vague communication is both frustrating and potentially unsafe, not to mention a waste of time. In Elie's first report, although she had assessed the patient and made some preliminary conclusions, she was so vague about them that the nurse on the next shift would have had to redo what had already been done. Decisions about which areas need to be communicated specifically and which ones can be mentioned casually or omitted are not easy to make. A good report is not necessarily a long one that provides detail about everything. Listeners start to ignore a report when it is overdone. As with organization, the nurse needs INQUIRY thinking to make decisions about the relative importance of details.

Clarity of Direction to Others

Many verbal reports that nurses give are meant to let the next nurse caring for the patient know what needs to be done next. Without clear directions, the next nurse has to second-guess the first one. In the revised report, the nurse hearing the report would know that directed data collection was needed to verify Elie's hunches that Mr. Packer had fluid, nutrition, and family problems. The second nurse could pick up where Elie left off with the nursing process. The revised report specified the need for accurate intake and output records, an interdependent nursing activity critical to the patient's medical care. Elie's flippant comment in the first report ("I think we're supposed to . . .") lacked clear direction and could have caused harm to the patient or, at the very least, would have delayed his care.

Evidence of Thinking and Using the Nursing Process

It was unclear in the first report what Elie's thinking was and how it fit with her assessing, planning, implementing, and evaluating. Because the patient had been recently admitted, other nurses could guess that some assessment had been completed, but how much of it was completed was not clear at all. In the revised report, Elie showed that she had collected data, had some hunches, and knew that other data were needed to verify those hunches. Others could tell that she had been thinking. In the first scenario, she was not focused on the data as much as she was on filling out the intake form, or getting things written in the right place. Likewise with the plan, it appeared that she was more focused on what was written in the columns of the plan than she was on the significance of the whole approach. The revised report showed her thinking within the framework of the nursing process much more clearly. She was focused on thinking about the significance of data rather than on filling out forms.

Professionalism: Omitting Social Chit-Chat and Value Judgments

Nurses are educated to appreciate diversity and the uniqueness of each person; however, nurses are people just as prone to value judgments and biases, as others. The difference is that nurses do not act on those value judgments or communicate them to others. Nurses also are social people, but they need to keep their social lives separate from their professional lives. That doesn't mean that Elie should not have told other nurses about her socialization the night before. It's just that she should not include it in a report about a patient. When referring to other health care providers, she should identify them by their names, not as "the docs from urology."

Patients have the right to be respected and identified accurately in reports. Their names, rather than some other designation (eg, a room number or a medical diagnosis), should be used. In the revised report, Elie called the patient by name, not by a room number designation.

Clear communication takes practice and should not be taken lightly. A good rule of thumb for deciding what constitutes a professional report is this: If you would be comfortable with the patient and significant others hearing the report, then it probably is appropriate. Another guideline for deciding whether a report is organized, specific, and clear is to ask yourself this: If I were hearing this report, would I know the important aspects of care for this patient, and would I know what needs should be addressed next?

✔ *Thinking-Learning Check*

Pause here for a thinking-learning check. You should be able to elaborate on these ideas:

- ✔ The importance of clear communication: promotes continuity and consistent quality of care, provides evidence of thinking, establishes credibility and legal accountability, and enhances rapport and trust with patients.
- ✔ Personal verbal communication styles: analyzing them for clarity.
- ✔ Verbal communication in nursing occurs with patients and significant others, other nurses, and other health care providers.
- ✔ Strategies for effective verbal communication include organization, specificity, clarity of directions to others, evidence of thinking and use of the nursing process, and professionalism.

WRITTEN COMMUNICATION: DOCUMENTATION

There are many forms of written communication in nursing. Nurses write policies, procedures, letters, reports, self-evaluations, articles, chapters, and books, among other forms of communication. This chapter, however, focuses on one type of written communication—documentation of nursing care in a patient's record. Next to verbal communication, written documentation may seem a more daunting task; however, the same principles of organization, specificity, clarity, thinking, and professionalism that apply to verbal communication also apply to written communication.

Written documentation is a necessary part of nursing because storing information in one's head is neither safe nor practical. In many professions, as in nursing, writing notes in a patient's record is referred to as "documentation." As the term implies, documenting is a formal recording of events. A patient's record, or chart, is a formal, legal record of health care.

Today, documentation must be interpreted to include computerized "writing." With computer programs, the nurse gets some assistance with organization because certain things can be entered only in certain ways. Computer programs also help with wording because multiple-choice options are available to describe what is being reported. Computers are organized, logic-oriented machines. Their programs provide basic patterns for recording data in preestablished, organized ways. This can be very helpful and time saving. But computers do not think. (Some might argue that "artificial intelligence" is approaching some degree of thinking, but systems used for daily documentation in most health care settings are not that sophisticated.) Because computers don't think, nurses must continue to decide which information is important, what it means, and what to do about it. Whether entered into a computer or written on paper, it is the nurse's thinking that must get communicated to promote good patient care. Because handwritten communication will continue in many settings even with computerization, the traditional issues of documentation continue to be relevant.

Parts of a Patient Record

The specific information in a record may vary from setting to setting, but, generally, records contain progress notes, assessment forms, care plans, critical paths, physician order sheets, laboratory results, consultation records, and graphic sheets. Nurses need to be familiar with everything in a patient's record.

Sometimes records are divided by discipline, with nurses writing on one section of the chart, physicians on another, social workers elsewhere, and so forth. That format is less common today than it once was, especially in acute care settings. Today, for example, rather than having a section for the nurses's notes, there is a section for multidisciplinary progress notes. All health care providers write their progress notes in this newer style in the same section of the patient's chart. They identify their disciplines at the beginning of their note or with the credentials after their names, so that those reading the notes can see who the provider was.

The way a record is organized and how a progress note is written usually are stated in an institution's policies. After a preliminary discussion of other elements of documentation, some examples of progress note styles are presented.

Documentation Rules

There are certain universal "dos and don'ts," or rules of documentation. These rules, when used properly, provide consistency and clarity in documentation as well as legal protection. There also are some generally accepted "rules" that are important but not quite so critical. The "dos" include the following: all entries should be legibly written in pen and accompanied by a date, time, signature, and professional title; when mistakes are made, one line should be drawn through the entry, and it should be signed and dated. The "don'ts" include recording unsupported value judgments or inferences; obliterating or trying to erase errors; and using pencils. Other generally accepted rules for documentation include using phrases instead of full sentences and making entries compact with no blank lines inside the entry or between the entry and the nurse's signature.

Computers have added a few dos and don'ts and eliminated a few. They replace the pen with an electronic entry system (keyboard, light pen, touchpad) and printer. The date and time may be recorded automatically, or the nurse may need to type them in. The nurse's signature often is coded into the computer. The rule of computer signatures is never to share one's code or chart under someone else's code. Computer programs have a method for correcting errors that eliminates the need to cross things out.

⊃Action Learning #56: Finding the Documentation Errors in a Progress Note

Examine the following documentation entry in Mrs. Blake's record. Identify where documentation rules were not followed and discuss with a classmate how to fix them. Rewrite the entry and correct the problems.

> Pt. looks terrible today. I sat with her for 30 minutes trying to get her to talk to no avail. B/P 220/80, 124/70; P 80; R 16. Refused lunch. Slept. Stayed in room all afternoon with the lights out and covers pulled over her head. I. Smith, RN

Think about this ■ How many errors did you find? How easy was it to fix the problems? Did the note reflect any thinking or use of the nursing process?

Documenting the Nursing Process

Parts of a record can be linked to the phases of the nursing process. This is more evident in the record systems some agencies use than it is in others. For example, first-encounter assessment data are recorded on assessment tools, nursing histories, and data bases. Planning is recorded on care plans or critical paths and kardexes. Implementation is recorded on progress notes, graphic sheets, flow sheets, and critical paths. Evaluation is recorded on care plans, progress notes, and discharge summaries. These places are not mutually exclusive, however. For example, after initial encounters, assessment data may be recorded as evaluation data. Documentation of implementation, once it includes conclusions about how a patient is progressing, becomes documentation of evaluation rather than implementation.

The complexity of documentation is the reason why nurses must continually use their T.H.I.N.K. modes. Documentation is more than merely writing things down; thought must go into deciding the best place to record things, the best things to record, and how to word what is to be recorded.

Documenting Assessment

In some settings, assessment data are written in narrative form on blank sheets of paper. More often, initial assessment data are recorded on assessment forms (usually a form with blank spaces for specific data collection identified, sometimes as checklists). The assessment tool in Chapter 13 is an example of this type of form. These forms are used to record a first assessment or the baseline data on a patient. These data provide the basis for initial conclusions of assessment and for care plans. As such, these forms should include only raw data, not inferences or conclusions, unless there are designated sections labeled "conclusions or impressions." These sections usually are at the end of the forms.

In acute care settings, data and conclusions from the second, third, and fourth encounters with a patient usually are recorded in the progress notes, rather than on the assessment tool. The progress notes are just what they sound like—a record of the patient's progress. As a patient's condition changes, new assessment data become significant for showing progress. Sometimes, new problems are discovered; sometimes, the previous problems change. Data discovered through ongoing assessment may actually become evaluation data and are recorded as such. These methods of documenting assessment data are noted in the following sections, which describe documentation in the other phases of the nursing process.

In long-term care and community health settings, initial data collection tools may be used differently. In nursing homes, for example, a patient receives a complete nursing assessment at least once a year in an effort to track over longer periods of time changing patient health status and needs. In community health, where the data base typically includes a whole family unit, data are added to the form over time. Because the amount of data required for family care is extensive, it cannot all be collected at one time. This continual adding to the initial assessment allows for historical data, growth and development data, and similar information to be analyzed in the ongoing plan of care for the family.

Overall, what is important during documentation of assessment is that data are raw data and conclusions are judgments based on the data. There should *never* be any conclusions recorded on a patient's chart that cannot be tracked to their supporting data.

Documenting Planning

The nursing plan that is written on the patient's record (chart) is the result of much complex thinking on the nurse's part; the better the thinking, the better the plan. In reality, it is often the written plan and not the thinking behind the plan that is equated with the process of planning. As with many things in nursing and elsewhere, what gets written down takes on special significance because it is what everyone can *see*. Unfortunately, this gives beginning nurses a false impression about where to focus their energy. Great plans do not write themselves or get copied out of books; they require great thinking. A well-written, great plan, therefore, should be seen for what it truly is—clear evidence of the great thinking behind the written words.

Written formats for nursing care plans vary somewhat from institution to institution. Most settings use some type of column format similar to that used for care plans in this book. There usually is a place for the nursing diagnosis or interdisciplinary problem, goals or outcomes, and nursing interventions. Some plans have a column for evaluation comments; some do not. All entries on a plan are dated and signed, either with the nurse's full signature or with initials that can be linked with a name elsewhere on the record.

With the increasing use of computers in health care, many institutions have computer programs for nursing care plans. Sometimes standard plans for commonly found problems can be "pulled up" by indicating that the patient has one of these problems. These standard plans then can be adapted to the patient, just as preprinted standard plans are adapted. Computer software also is available for health care organizations. This software includes the NIC and NOC information for assisting in care planning and coding of nursing interventions and outcomes, and ultimately has the capability of assisting with billing specifically for nursing care (McCloskey & Bulechek, 1996).

Other parts of the patient record devoted to planning are flow sheets, critical paths, graphic sheets, and kardexes. These are shorthand plans that give direction for parts of the plan that are usually done repetitively. Part of a plan for a patient with diabetes might be to track the patient's blood glucose levels. A kardex might say "BS QID," (blood sugar four times a day) or a flow sheet might be put on the record as a reminder to do this. Likewise, these quick references might be used for parts of the plan that cross over many problem areas. For example, if a patient does not communicate verbally, but uses an alphabet board to spell words, "Use alphabet board for communication" might be written on a kardex. That piece of information, then, does not need to be rewritten on all parts of the plan; it is automatically assumed in all other parts of the plan where communication is necessary.

Documenting Implementation

The documentation of implementation is the recording of interventions and activities performed for or with a patient. When a conclusion about how a patient is progressing is included in a written note, the nurse is documenting evaluation as well. Because nurses are expected to record actions and their effect on a patient's progress, intervention documentation is more often than not incorporated into evaluation notes. There are, however, some interventions that are documented solely as interventions and that need no comments about evaluation. The administration of medications, one of nursing's interdependent functions, is a common example.

Generally speaking, independent nursing actions are more often documented as evaluation notes, and interdependent actions are more often written as intervention notes. For example, many interdependent nursing actions are part of the medical plan of care. It makes sense that physicians would be doing most of the evaluation of the medical plan and that nurses would be communicating that their part of the plan had been implemented. Likewise, nurses are the primary evaluators of their independent plans. Their implementation notes also include an evaluation of the patient's progress in the areas of nursing care. These are only general rules, with many exceptions.

Documenting Evaluation

Documenting evaluation probably comprises most of the recording a nurse does because nurses must constantly monitor and record changes in patient conditions. Some conclusions or judgments need to be made about those changes, and, when judgments are made, evaluation has occurred.

Evaluation notes usually are written in the progress notes section on a patient's record, although some care plan formats are set up with evaluation columns. Most documentation formats for progress notes have some element of evaluation built into them. The many formats for documenting evaluation are too numerous to explain in detail here; other nursing textbooks may be used to explore other methods. Three methods will be discussed here—narrative notes, SOAP (**S**ubjective and **O**bjective data, **A**ssessment, and **P**lan) notes, and DAR (**D**ata, **A**ction, **R**esponse) notes. Of these three, SOAP and DAR have evaluation built in, so a well-written note will contain some judgments about the patient's progress. Narrative notes do not have this built-in mechanism, but they often include judgments about patient progress.

Documentation Formats

Most institutions or units adopt a documentation format that is expected to be followed by all care providers in that setting. This format is shared with new employees during orientation. One of the purposes of newer documentation formats is to reflect thinking in all phases of the nursing process. When used appropriately, the newer formats are triggers for thinking.

With the advent of computer charting, the formats may be adapted to computer capabilities, or the usual format can be kept, with the staff simply typing in their notes rather than writing them by hand.

As already mentioned, three formats used for progress notes are described in this chapter—narrative notes, SOAP notes, and DAR notes. Each of these requires a different sort of organization of information. Depending on how you organize information in your mind, you may find one of these is easier or harder than the others. Most people remember events chronologically. If they tell a story, it usually is reported in the order of events. Think about that. Have you had a conversation recently with someone who told you about a particular event? "I ran into Sue the other day. She told me she recently got engaged. I was so surprised that I told her I was shocked. You should have seen her face. She said she was insulted. I felt bad and apologized and then things were OK between us." This story is told chronologically. The story-teller could have rearranged the story and told it differently. It could have gone like this: "I need to be more careful about how I word things. The other day, when I saw Sue, I had to apologize to her because I insulted her by blurting out that I was shocked that she got engaged." In the second example, it is not the chronology as much as the "lesson" learned from the events that drives the organization of the report. However, the story-teller had to think about the information differently before reporting it. She had to reorganize it around the central theme of her communication style.

With nursing documentation, the documentation format provides some of the organizational scheme. The remainder of the organizational plan comes from the central theme or purpose of the note itself. Of the three formats, narrative notes probably lend themselves to chronological reporting more than the others. The other two formats force a sorting of information into categories such as patient data, nursing actions, results or progress, and so forth.

Whichever format is used, the nurse must decide on the right amount of detail to record. This is not an easy decision to make but there are some general guidelines. First, one has to put oneself in the shoes of the reader and ask, "What would I need to know to understand what is going on here?" Second, one must remember that everyone in health care is pressed for time, so conciseness is critical. A note that is too long and wordy will not get read carefully because readers will skip through things to save time. Third, one needs to have enough detail so that any conclusions can be justified. Balancing conciseness with enough details for full understanding by the reader is one of the keys to successful written communication and a mark of great nursing.

Narrative Notes

A narrative note is just what it sounds like—a narrative of what has occurred. This is the oldest format for charting and its effectiveness is highly dependent on the nurse's skill in writing clear, organized information. The order of recording generally is the chronological order in which events occurred. For example:

11/20/98 1300 Ambulated with walker 20 feet once in AM and once in PM. Vital signs stable during ambulation. Complained of back pain after walking, relieved with massage and sitting with pillow at back for 30 minutes. Dry dressing changed over hip staples. Incision site clear, no signs of infection. Pt. states she is anxious to start physical therapy so she can get home before the holidays.

J. Gold, RN

In this example, there is evidence of the nurse's data collection and conclusions about the data, implementation, and evaluation. There is not much about planning. This type of note allows a nurse to record all of the nursing process in any order desired. A problem with this format is that the parts of the nursing process are not automatically evident. Nurses who write narrative notes must give extra thought to the flow of ideas and to wording that reflects both thinking and use of the nursing process. What will make sense to the person reading the note? There are many individual styles of narrative notes, some of which work better than others.

⊃ACTION LEARNING #57: Writing a Narrative Note

Read the following case study. Write a narrative note to report the information on today's visit. Compare your note with that of a classmate and discuss your different styles.

Case Study

Ms. Jacob is a 48-year-old lawyer. She had polio at the age of 10 years. Two years ago she suffered from post-polio syndrome (a recurrence of some of the symptoms of the earlier disease). She was hospitalized for 6 months with progressive paralysis. After a respiratory arrest, a permanent tracheostomy was performed (a tracheostomy is a special tube inserted into the trachea through which a person breathes). Ms. Jacob is now home. She has had to quit her job but is financially comfortable. She lives alone in a one-floor apartment and has a community health nurse visit twice a week to help her manage her tracheostomy care. She is a fast learner and is performing the care with no problems. Today the nurse watched her performing the tracheostomy care and only had to remind her of one thing—to wipe with strokes rather than in a back-and-forth motion. During today's visit (1 month after hospitalization) she has puffy, red eyes, avoids eye contact with the nurse, and finally admits she feels very alone. She says, "I hate going out in public; I can talk if I cover up the trach but people seem so uncomfortable around me and I don't like to make people uncomfortable. Even my friends don't visit very much; they're so busy, but really I think they don't know what to say or do. I can deal with the trach myself and I don't mind using the cane to walk, but I feel so isolated, I'm going crazy."

NARRATIVE NOTE:

THINK ABOUT THIS ■ Was this an easy type of note to write? Did you remember to use the "rules" of documentation? Do you think another person would have a good picture of the day's events by reading the note? On which part or parts of the nursing process was your note primarily focused?

SOAP Notes

SOAP notes are used with problem-oriented medical records, which have a central list of problems identified by the health care team. That problem list includes the conclusions reached by the whole health care team—medical diagnoses (eg, L. CVA, tuberculosis), interdisciplinary problems (eg, decubitus ulcers), nursing diagnoses (eg, Self-Care Deficit ..., Social Isolation ...), and diagnoses made by other providers (eg, recreational deficit). Each problem has a number and a plan of care. All progress notes refer to a problem by number.

SOAP notes are used to document all parts of the nursing process, but they are primarily focused on assessment *or* evaluation. Understanding this distinction makes learning the SOAP format much easier. In the following description, "A" designates how each component of SOAP is used to write an assessment note, and "E" designates how the components are used for evaluation notes.

SOAP stands for Subjective, Objective, Assessment, and Plan. If this sounds strangely like the nursing process, that's because it is. Here is a closer look at the parts of a SOAP note:

Subjective: What the patient (or significant others) said (A and E).

Objective: What was observed or measured (A and E) **and** what the nurse did (E). "What the nurse did" does not obviously fit with the word "objective," so it is important to think of some way to remember this piece of SOAP.

Assessment: This is the tricky part. When nurses hear the word "assessment," they automatically think, "First phase of the nursing process, which includes data collection, data analysis, and conclusions." The only part of that traditional meaning that works with a SOAP note is the "conclusions" part. Other nurses think of the "A" in SOAP as meaning "analysis." This also is confusing and results in inaccurate SOAP notes. What is important here is that the "A" of "assessment" in SOAP stands **only** for one of two types of conclusions in the nursing process—assessment conclusions or evaluation conclusions. Assessment conclusions are judgments about patient strengths and health concerns. Evaluation conclusions focus on whether the goals and outcomes were met, not met, or partially met. Therefore, **when writing the "A" part of a SOAP note, the nurse either makes an assessment conclusion about the strengths and health concerns (A) or makes an evaluation conclusion about how the patient is progressing toward meeting the plan's goals and outcomes (E).**

Plan: This is just what it sounds like. It is what the nurse is going to do about the conclusions (A and E). Given the subjective and objective data and the conclusions reached based on those data, what is the plan for the **future**? The difference between plans made after assessment and those made after evaluation is that plans are first developed after assessment, and they already exist and need to be continued or modified after evaluation. If, as is typically the case, the plan is written on the care plan part of the record, the nurse may refer to the plan in the SOAP note. "See plan" or "see plan for changes" may be written at the "P" part of the notes. The actual plan changes may be written in the note, but this should be done only if it does not duplicate what is written elsewhere.

See Table 11-1 for a summary of what you have just read.

Here are some examples of both kinds of SOAP notes:

EXAMPLE 1. EVALUATION NOTE

11/20/98, 0900: #3, Pain:

S: "My back really hurts today. The pain is about a 6 (on a scale of 10). I barely slept last night. I feel better now" (1/2 hour after massage and medication).

Table 11–1   **Similarities and Differences Between an Assessment SOAP Note and an Evaluation SOAP Note**

	ASSESSMENT SOAP NOTE	EVALUATION SOAP NOTE
S.	What the patient or significant other told you	What the patient or significant other told you
O.	What was observed or measured	What was observed or measured **WHAT THE NURSE DID**
A.	**ASSESSMENT CONCLUSIONS** (Judgments about pt. strengths or health concerns, eg, N. Dx., Interdisciplinary problems, Problems for referral)	**EVALUATION CONCLUSIONS** (Judgments about whether the Goals and Outcomes were met.)
P.	Statement about what the nurse is going to do about the **conclusions of assessment**	Statement about what the nurse is going to do about the **conclusions of evaluation**

O: Pt.'s face in a grimace. Lying on side with pillows behind back. Heating pad applied to lower back. Medicated with Darvocet. Area massaged. 1/2 hour after interventions, pt.'s face and body in relaxed position.

A: Pt. progressing toward goal of pain relief, but continues to need narcotic medication.

P: See additions to plan to offer heating pad and massage more frequently. G. Blakely, RN

EXAMPLE 2. FIRST ENCOUNTER WITH PATIENT (ASSESSMENT NOTE)

11/20/98, 1500: #1, Skin impairment:

S: "I know I shouldn't lie in one position so long; it makes my skin break down. I've had dry skin all my life."

O: Skin warm, dry, 4-cm circular, reddened, unbroken area on coccyx; right heel cracked, peeling in a 3-cm area. Pt. turned and sheepskin pads applied to heels.

A: Impaired Skin Integrity related to immobility and bed pressure.

P: See care plan #1. G. Blakely, RN

Notice how the "A" parts of the notes differ. The evaluation note "A" addresses how the patient is progressing toward the goal. The "P" comment mentions *additions* to the plan. In the assessment note, the "A" is a nursing diagnosis and the "P" refers only to the plan, without any changes (because the plan was just written).

In both notes, the date and time are recorded and the note starts with a reference to a numbered problem. Identifying the problem allows everyone reading the note to know exactly which aspect of patient care is being discussed. Reading a series of notes on one problem allows a person to track the progress of a health concern.

⮧ACTION LEARNING #58: Sorting the Parts of a SOAP Note

Examine the following pieces of data and sort them into the proper SOAP note categories. Indicate for each situation whether it is an evaluation note or an assessment note.

SITUATION A:

See new objective and action on care plan.
"I'm walking much better."
Goal met.
Patient walked 30 feet independently with walker.
"I think I can walk further by myself."

Steady gait.
11/15/98, 3 PM, #3, Impaired Mobility
S.

O.

A.

P.

SITUATION B:

High Risk for Injury: falls R/T unsteady gait, use of area rugs in home, and dim
 lighting.
Patient 93, CVA 3 months ago, lives alone, small apartment, hardwood floors
 with area rugs at entrance and in kitchen.
Recently ambulating with quad cane.
No overhead lights, table lamps in each room with 25-watt light bulbs (patient
 states to save energy and money).
"But I love my Oriental rugs, they're family heirlooms."
Patient stated she has had her rugs a long time and never had problems before.
Patient encouraged to purchase rug adhesive to stabilize rugs and keep the
 edges flat.

Taught patient importance of good lighting. Brochure from the Center for Independent Living on methods of improving indoor lighting given to patient.
#2 High Risk for Injury
11/18/98, 1400
Follow-up visit arranged for next week to check on status.

S.

O.

A.

P.

DAR Notes

Notes that are organized by Data, Action, and Response are used with a system of "focus" charting. Similar to problem-oriented records using SOAP, in which a problem is identified for each note, the "focus" is the problem or health concern that is being addressed each time a DAR note is written. The note can be organized into columns—one for the patient data, one for the action taken by the nurse or other health care provider, and one for the patient response. Some agencies write out the DAR running down the page just as the SOAP note is written. This form of documentation, like SOAP, has evaluation built in. Making a judgment about a patient's response focuses on the outcome of the care or changes in the patient's condition.

Example of column format DAR note:

Focus: Reflex Incontinence: Self-Catheterization

Data	Action	Response
11/10/93 2100	Assisted pt. to try positioning knees; set up cath. equip.; reviewed importance of cleaning meatus thoroughly. Plan to review this next time.	Objective of self-cath not met yet, but pt. making progress.
Pt. reports she is still having difficulty finding meatus using mirror. After 3 position changes, pt. did cath. Urine clear; yellow, odorless.		

G. Blakely, RN

⊃**ACTION LEARNING #59: Writing a DAR Note**

Sort the following information into a DAR note:

11/16/98, 1300
"I enjoyed the Bingo game, especially because I could sit next to Mr. Jones."
Objective of attending one recreation program/day being met most days.
After some prompting, patient went to recreation room after Bingo game had started.
Prompt patient half hour before recreation program in future.
Patient returned to room, smiling.
Diversional Activity Deficit: Increase recreation activities
Helped patient choose recreation program from the day's schedule.

Focus:

Data	Action	Response

✔ *Thinking-Learning Check*

Pause here for a thinking-learning check. You should be able to elaborate on these ideas:

- ✔ Documentation: must be organized, specific, clear, and professionally done to represent great thinking.

- ✔ Documentation follows several rules and can be done on computer or through handwritten records.

- ✔ Documentation must reflect all phases of the nursing process: assessing, planning, implementing, and evaluating.

- ✔ Documentation formats: three examples and how they trigger thinking to address all phases of the nursing process.

- ✔ The "A" in a SOAP note represents a "conclusion" in either the assessment phase or the evaluation phase of the nursing process.

THE FINER POINTS OF WRITTEN COMMUNICATION

So far, this chapter has focused on the basic issues of communication that every nurse must master. As beginning students gain proficiency in these basic verbal and written communication skills, they will be able to move their focus to some of the finer points of communication. These finer points require even more thinking about the subtleties of word selection. The more clearly and concisely the patient's health condition is described with words, the better the chance of designing and implementing the best individualized care. Well-written plans of nursing care can increase the efficiency and accuracy of nurses' work and the quality of patient care.

As you probably have deduced by now, there are few all right or all wrong answers to most nursing issues, but there are qualitative differences—adequate, good, better, and best. The following pages illustrate how the wording of the nursing diagnosis and the wording of outcomes result in qualitative differences in a plan and thus in nursing care.

Well-Worded Nursing Diagnoses

In earlier chapters, descriptions of differential diagnoses showed how important it was to consider alternative options as labels for nursing conclusions. Some of the work of differential diagnosis has to do with making decisions about wording. A well-worded nursing diagnosis can make care planning much easier. What, then, is a well-worded nursing diagnosis? Look back to Action Learning #57 and Ms. Jacob's situation. There are several nursing diagnoses that could be equally valid as conclusions, based on the data. There is a definite data cluster reflecting her emotional response pattern.

Data Cluster

Has tracheostomy
Lives alone
Quit her job
Puffy, red eyes
Avoids eye contact with nurse
Admits to feeling alone
"I hate going out in public; I can talk if I cover up the trach but people
     seem so uncomfortable around me and I don't like to make people un-
     comfortable."
"Even my friends don't visit very much; they're so busy, but really I think
     they don't know what to say or do."
"I can deal with the trach myself and I don't mind using the cane to walk,
     but I feel so isolated, I'm going crazy."

From these data, there are several possible nursing diagnosis conclusions
that could be reached, each seemingly equally valid.

Possible Nursing Diagnosis Conclusions (Differential Diagnoses)

A. Social Isolation related to living alone, recently quitting job, and perception
     that friends are uncomfortable with her.
B. Body Image Disturbance related to tracheostomy and mobility changes.
C. Diversional Activity Deficit related to excess time alone, recently quitting
     job, dislike of going out in public, and perceived discomfort of friends.
D. Impaired Social Interaction related to decreased contact with friends, per-
     ceived discomfort of friends, changed verbal skills with tracheostomy, living
     alone, and recently quitting job.
E. Ineffective Individual Coping related to situational crisis of illness (tra-
     cheostomy, impaired mobility) and change in roles.

These are five possible nursing diagnoses that are supported by the data
in the cluster; there could be others as well. A nurse whose thinking led to
these conclusions would need to decide which of these diagnoses was the
most accurate label for the patient's situation. By focusing on the finer
points of written communication, the nurse would be able to make the conclusion that is the most accurate, precise picture of the situation and the
one that points toward realistic interventions that would improve the patient's situation. By using INQUIRY thinking, a nurse might ask and find
answers to several questions. Answers to each question, some of which are
found through TOTAL RECALL of nursing knowledge, will assist the
nurse in making the final conclusion.

> *Question #1*:
> Which conclusions best reflect the data fully?
> *Answer*:

Dx. A, C, and D

Rationale: B may be a less accurate label for the cluster because the patient stated she could deal with the tracheostomy and didn't mind using the cane. The body image issue may need to be addressed, but the patient is not primarily focused on that. E focuses on her inability to cope, but it is a very broad label. She is coping well with caring for the tracheostomy and using a cane, but she may not be coping with being alone. Therefore, ineffective coping is too broad to reflect best the specifics of the data.

Question #2: Of diagnoses A, C, and D, which ones reflect critical subjective data? In other words, what is the patient most focused on?

Answer: Dx. A and D

Rationale: The patient doesn't actually say she doesn't have enough to occupy her free time, and C is focused on activities. She specifically said, "I hate going out in public"; "My friends don't visit much"; "I feel isolated." She admits to feeling alone. Each of these comments is focused on aloneness and social interaction more than on not having enough diversional activities in general.

Question #3: Of diagnoses A and D, considering the difference between "Social Isolation" and "Impaired Social Interaction," which one is a better label?

Answer: Dx. A is better

Rationale: The North American Nursing Diagnosis Association (NANDA) definition of "Social Isolation" is "Aloneness experienced by the individual and perceived as imposed by others and as a negative or threatened state" (NANDA, 1996, p. 38). "Impaired Social Interaction" is defined as "The state in which an individual participates in an insufficient or excessive quantity or ineffective quality of social exchange" (NANDA, 1996, p. 37). The patient is focused on aloneness and she perceives it as imposed by others. Therefore, Social Isolation most closely matches this patient situation.

This fine-tuned level of thinking for selecting the best words to describe a health concern is not reached overnight. Beginning students have many things to think about; they may not develop this finer level of thinking and communicating for quite some time; however, it is an ideal toward which nursing students should aim. Before these skills get well tuned, an acceptance of their importance will trigger the nurse's thinking each time a conclusion is written in a patient's chart. The nurse will remember to ask, "Are these the most descriptive words for what I want to convey?"

This fine-tuned thinking about the wording of nursing diagnoses will deter nurses from overusing HABIT thinking about written communication. Excessive HABIT thinking occurs when the first label that comes to mind is the one that is recorded on the patient's record. Questioning those first words and thinking about how they can be refined will trigger the INQUIRY mode and promote more accurate documentation, and, ultimately, more efficient nursing care. The best-worded nursing diagnosis will almost literally lead to a great plan for care. In Ms. Jacob's case, the chosen diagnostic statement points to a goal of increased socialization as evidenced by such things as the patient considering alternatives to living alone, considering finding something to do with her time that has a social component, and openly discussing with her friends her perception of their discomfort. If these outcomes were achieved, the problem would very likely be resolved. If one of the other diagnoses had been chosen, the path to those outcomes might be more circuitous. Another diagnosis might not be wrong; it might even turn out to be just as helpful as the chosen path. The precision of the recorded label for Ms. Jacob's health concern, however, diminishes the chances for confusion among other providers, and ensures a more direct line from the problem to the resolution.

How Well-Worded Outcomes Affect Implementation and Evaluation

Chapter 10 provided extensive descriptions of how to formulate outcomes for care plans. Many of the directions focused on wording issues—including specificity, measurability, and clarity. Review that part of Chapter 10 if you need a refresher. Now, bearing in mind this chapter's focus on clear communication, think about the actual written words of the outcomes (Note: many outcomes currently are standardized with NOC but until the NOC language is used consistently throughout nursing, it is still important to create outcomes that are well worded.) A well-worded outcome will simplify evaluation and clearly guide the way to developing great nursing interventions; conversely, poorly worded outcomes create confusion and result in sloppy evaluations. For an example, go back again to Ms. Jacob's situation and the final nursing diagnosis that was chosen, "Social Isolation Related to living alone, recently quitting job, and perception that friends are uncomfortable with her." Because Social Isolation was used as an example in an earlier chapter, it should be a familiar nursing conclusion by now, one to which the finer points of communication can be applied.

The goal for care would be for Ms. Jacob to increase her socialization within a month. (A month probably is realistic considering that she is at home and needs to do several things to meet that goal.) Using the general guidelines for formulating outcomes, the nurse would look at the factors related to the isolation—living alone, recently quitting her job, and her perception of her friends' discomfort.

Assuming the patient has been a partner in the planning process, how would the nurse decide which were the best-worded outcomes? Because nurses ideally try to address all factors related to a problem, one can assume that at least three outcomes are needed for a start because there are three related factors. There certainly

Options for Outcomes for Ms. Jacob	Rationale for Selecting the Best Outcomes
1. Outcome options related to her living alone: Ms. Jacob will:	
A. Describe how she can compensate socially for living alone.	A is measurable (the nurse can hear the patient describe something); it seems automatically to show that nursing interventions should be directed toward helping the patient explore options, and it involves the patient very directly. Keep this one.
B. Consider living with someone else.	B is narrow and may be too disruptive; because the patient has been managing on her own, there is no reason to ask patient to consider this. Not easily measured. Discard this one.
C. Accept how her living arrangements contribute to her isolation.	C is OK but it doesn't help her progress from where she is now. Consider discarding unless patient seems unrealistic about her living arrangements. Not easily measured either.
D. Increase her socialization at home.	D is too vague and hard to measure. What would constitute an increase? Discard this one.
2. Outcome options related to her recently quitting her job: Ms. Jacob will:	
E. Describe her feelings about quitting her job.	E is probably a necessary first step, considering she quit her job recently and very little is known about her feelings about that. It is measurable and "points" to nursing care focused on feelings. Keep this one.
F. Think of options for jobs to increase socialization.	F is not measurable because one cannot see or measure another person's thinking. Discard this one.
G. Know her job options.	G is not measurable; how would anyone evaluate someone "knowing"? Unless the verb is changed to "describe," "explain," "list," or something equally measurable, discard this one.
3. Outcome options related to her perception of her friends' discomfort with her: Ms. Jacob will:	
H. Understand her friends' discomfort.	H is not measurable. "Understand" is like "know"; one needs a measurable sign to evaluate it. Also, Ms. Jacob seems to understand her friends' discomfort already; she was able to describe their behavior. Discard this one.
I. Increase her friends' comfort with her.	I is too vague. What would the nurse do to help? The nurse would need to work with the friends to know whether this outcome occurred, and Ms. Jacob is the person of focus here. Discard this one.
J. Role-play how she will confront her friends with her perceptions of their discomfort.	J is very specific and leads directly to the nurse participating in role-playing. This outcome specifies a tangible intervention for the patient and allows her to explore a potentially uncomfortable situation in a safe environment. Keep this one.

FIGURE 11–2   Examining the wording of patient outcomes.

K. Describe how she will deal with her friends' discomfort.	K is OK but not as good as **J** because it requires less involvement by the patient. This would also be a necessary part of **J** for **J** to work well. Would keep if **J** weren't better.
L. Tell her friends how she feels.	L does not help the patient in any specific direction. There is very little nursing care that automatically comes to mind with this outcome. Discard because **J** is better and will accomplish the same thing and more.
M. Invite at least two friends over to her house.	M is very specific and measurable; it is a reasonable start, but it is not focused on the discomfort per se. Could keep it, but it is not very dynamic.

FIGURE 11–2   Examining the wording of patient outcomes. (continued)

could be more than that, however. Stop for a moment and review the options in the left column of Figure 11-2, or develop some of your own. As you will see, you have several choices for wording outcomes that correspond to one of the related factors.

Now look at the right column of Figure 11-2. This column describes the nurse's thinking and why he or she would or would not select one of the options listed in the left column.

The nurse is left with A, E, and J as the best-worded objectives. These are measurable, specific, relevant to the patient situation, and they logically lead the nurse to specific nursing actions that would be individualized to Ms. Jacob. The final selection of wording would be as follows:

> **Nursing Diagnosis:** Social Isolation R/T living alone, recently quitting job, and perception that friends are uncomfortable with her.
> **Goal:** By the end of 1 month, Ms. Jacob will increase her socialization A.E.B.:
> 1. Describing how she can compensate socially for living alone.
> 2. Describing her feelings about quitting her job.
> 3. Role-playing how she will confront her friends with her perceptions of their discomfort.

Obviously, to complete this plan, clear nursing interventions are needed. Students generally have fewer problems wording nursing interventions because there are many suggestions provided by textbooks and the Nursing Interventions Classifications (NIC) reference book. However, without clear nursing diagnoses and patient outcomes, the wording of nursing interventions can be more difficult. When learning written communication, beginners can best use their time honing their diagnoses and patient outcome wording skills; then the nursing interventions will fall into place.

CLOSING COMMENTS

It is hoped that this chapter has provided an appreciation of the thinking that must occur for clear verbal and written communication. It is easy, when learning communication, to focus on the structure, or the "how" of talking and writing. Nursing students may, for example, try to learn documentation formats by memorizing what goes where. Although that know-how can be learned and converted to HABITS, it will not help with deciding what should be recorded when, where, in what way, and in what order of importance. Nor will it help with verbal communication. Communicating the complexities and interrelationships of all parts of the nursing process requires the use of TOTAL RECALL, INQUIRY, NEW IDEAS AND CREATIVITY, and, most of all, KNOWING HOW YOU THINK.

THINKING LOG #11 ➤

If you are in a clinical area, examine several medical records. List several questions that you have about the documentation. Then look at three nursing progress notes and evaluate them with regard to what you have learned in this chapter. Note: It is not appropriate to inform the staff verbally of any errors you perceive in the notes; these can be shared confidentially with your instructor, who will also be able to explain the documentation for that particular agency in greater detail.

If you are not in a clinical area, ask a practicing nurse what he or she believes are the most helpful aspects of nursing progress notes. For example: Which format provides the most information and why? How much detail is needed? How are thinking and the nursing process best reflected in written nursing communication?

References

McCloskey, J.C., & Bulechek, G. M. (1996). *Nursing interventions classification (NIC)* (2nd ed.). St. Louis: Mosby.

North American Nursing Diagnosis Association. (1996). *NANDA nursing diagnoses: Definitions and classification 1997–1998.* Philadelphia: Author.

Northouse, P.G. & Northouse, L.L. (1985). *Health communication: A handbook for health professionals.* Englewood Cliffs, NJ: Prentice-Hall.

Consequences of Thinking and Not Thinking When Documenting

❋ *Learning Outcomes*

After reading and doing the activities in this chapter you will be able to:

Discuss the relationships among the nursing process, thinking, documentation, quality assurance, and legal issues.

Identify errors and problems within several documentation examples.

Appreciate the value of documentation as a reflection of thinking and doing in nursing practice.

In Chapter 11, the purposes of clear communication, including documentation, were discussed. These purposes included promoting continuity and consistent quality of care, providing evidence of thinking, and establishing legal accountability for nursing care. When communication is unclear, the quality of patient care is severely compromised, nurses do not show their thinking, and they become vulnerable to legal action against them.

In this chapter, the nursing process and the documentation process are explored as sequential processes. Several case studies are used to illustrate how the nurse's thinking is reflected in documentation. The relationship between documentation and quality assurance is discussed, as well as the use of incident reports and the legal ramifications of documentation.

RELATIONSHIP OF THE NURSING PROCESS TO THE PROCESS OF DOCUMENTATION

Remember, the nursing process and the documentation process are true processes. A process is a *continuous series* of thinking and actions that arrives at an *end result*. The nursing process is a series of thinking and actions—assessing, planning, implementing, and evaluating. The nursing process also is continuous; the nurse must constantly reassess, replan, reimplement, and reevaluate as the patient's condition changes. The end result is reached when the patient's goals and outcomes are met. Figure 12-1 is a schematic drawing of the nursing process.

Now, superimpose the word "documentation" over each word in the nursing process diagram, and the documentation process emerges. Every aspect of the nursing process must be documented; otherwise, the sequence of the process breaks down and thinking is not reflected.

Process Characteristics of Nursing and Documentation

Because both nursing and documentation are processes, they work best when completed. If the process stops, nursing care stops, or looks like it stops. Compare this with making a car, which is called an "assembly process." If the assembly line stops, does the car get built? No, the car remains in whatever state it is until the assembly line starts up again. The same problem occurs when the nursing process stops. If a nurse collects a data base but fails to make conclusions about the strengths and health concerns of a patient, how can a plan of care be developed or action be taken? The nursing process stopped short. Until the nurse identifies the patient's needs (makes conclusions as part of assessment), a safe, effective, and ef-

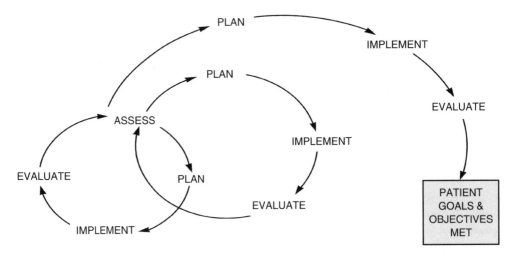

FIGURE 12–1 Nursing process.

ficient plan cannot be formulated. In another situation, the nurse may assess, develop, and document a wonderful plan, but if the plan is never implemented, the nursing process stops at planning. If nothing is done for the patient, there are no outcomes to evaluate and the nursing process is incomplete.

Again, add the word "documentation" to the preceding paragraph. If documentation does not accompany each part of the nursing process, there can be no high-quality nursing care except for very short-term interventions by one nurse. If one nurse does not communicate to other health care providers what has been done or what needs follow-up, the next person must start the process all over again. This results in sporadic care and inefficient use of the nurse's and the patient's time and energy.

Sequential Characteristics of the Nursing and Documentation Processes

Both the nursing process and the documentation process are sequential. "Sequential" does not mean strictly linear. The nurse constantly goes back and forth among the phases of the process many times before all the phases are completed. Sequence is important, however, in that some things must be done before others. For example, to change a flat tire on a car, one would first get the jack and tire iron out of the trunk, then remove the hubcap, loosen the lug nuts, raise the car on the jack, and so forth. The lug nuts cannot be loosened without first removing the hubcap, but they must be loosened before the car is jacked up. The tire-changing process illustrates the importance of certain things being done first. Examine the tire-changing process in relation to the components of the nursing process:

Assessing: Recognizing the car doesn't steer quite right: "Oh, no, I've got a flat tire! I'll be late for class."

Planning: Thinking through what needs to be done efficiently and safely: "I guess I'd better change tires! What do I do first? Do I have everything I need? Do I remember how to do it safely? Will I need outside help? Should I have kept up my road service insurance? Where is the nearest phone? I need to get out the right equipment and do this in the right sequence."

Implementing: Changing the tire: Getting the jack and tire iron out of the trunk, removing the hubcap, loosening the lug nuts, raising the car on the jack, and so forth ... until the tire is changed.

Evaluating: Determining whether desired outcome was met and making changes in plan: "I did it; I changed the tire; good thing I had a spare with air. I'm going to have to buy some lubricant for those lug nuts so that if I get a flat again, I'll have something to help me loosen them. I'll also put a rag in here to wipe my hands when I'm done."

The point here is that one has to follow a reasonable, logical sequence of steps and document them (in the case of nursing care) along the way to achieve the desired purpose, whether it is changing a tire or caring for a patient's needs. Otherwise, safe, efficient outcomes have a very low probability of occurring.

Problems That Arise When Process and Sequence are Ignored

When the nursing process is not used in a sequential manner, the patient does not receive high-quality nursing care. This can result in prolonged hospitalization. Even worse, a problem may go unrecognized and untreated, which could result in serious complications or death for the patient. Consider the following examples of "partially processed nursing."

⊃ACTION LEARNING #60: Mr. Schultz's Missing Care

Read this case and answer the questions that follow:

Case Study

Mr. Schultz had his gallbladder removed today and is now complaining of incisional pain. The nurse writes " Patient states pain is a 9 on a scale of 10. Patient is grimacing and holding abdomen." The nurse takes no action, however. She walks out of the room because she got paged for a phone call. Later, she comes back into Mr. Schultz's room and asks, "So, how are you doing?"

How do you think Mr. Schultz might respond?

If you were Mr. Schultz, how would you feel?

Which nursing process component(s) did the nurse complete?
(Circle one or more.)
Assessing   Planning   Implementing   Evaluating
What should have happened to complete the nursing process for Mr. Schultz?

What else should the nurse have *assessed* in this case?

What should the nurse have *planned* to do?

What should the nurse have *done* (implemented) for Mr. Schultz?

How should the nurse have *evaluated* the care?

THINK ABOUT THIS ■ Clearly, this nurse began to assess Mr. Schultz's complaints of pain; however, there was no plan to do anything about his pain. Thus, poor Mr. Schultz continued having postoperative pain of uncertain origin.

⊃ACTION LEARNING #61: Mr. Fodler's Missing Care

Read about Mr. Fodler and answer the following questions:

Case Study

Mr. Fodler had a CVA (cerebral vascular accident, or stroke) and has right-sided paralysis. The nurse enters Mr. Fodler's room and starts feeding him breakfast. Mr. Fodler tries to interrupt the nurse but, because he has difficulty speaking, he has trouble making his wishes known. The nurse speaks in a very loud voice to Mr. Fodler, telling him, "You must rest; you've had a stroke. Now let me do this for you." The nurse then proceeds to bathe and shave him, brush his teeth, and dress him. Mr. Fodler simply gives up in disgust. The nurse finishes and can't understand why Mr. Fodler is so disgruntled.

Which component(s) of the nursing process did the nurse complete while caring for Mr. Fodler?

Assessing   Planning   Implementing   Evaluating

How do you think Mr. Fodler felt having this nurse care for him?

Which component(s) of the nursing process should have occurred *first* in Mr. Fodler's care?

THINK ABOUT THIS ■ You probably said the nurse needed to do some further assessment of Mr. Fodler's abilities to do his own care. Had the nurse done this, it would have become apparent that Mr. Fodler was able to feed, dress, and bathe himself. With a little more investigation, the nurse may have discovered that Mr. Fodler owns a business and has been self-sufficient since his early 20s, when he lost both parents. He is a very proud man and likes to do things for himself. He had made great strides in rehabilitation and adapting to his paralysis, but his strengths were being ignored.

With this additional information about Mr. Fodler, what more appropriate interventions could the nurse have tried? How would this additional information have saved the nurse a lot of unnecessary work and Mr. Fodler a lot of unnecessary frustration? What do you think of the efficiency and quality of nursing care this nurse delivered to Mr. Fodler?

In the last two examples, great nursing care was not given to these patients. The nurses did not demonstrate evidence of *thinking*. In the case of Mr. Schultz, the nurse assessed his pain, but did not seem to think about the patient's answers; hence, nothing was done to relieve his pain. In the case of Mr. Fodler, the nurse did not even assess his needs. Implementing nursing care that did not fit the patient's needs reflected a lack of thinking on the nurse's part. Thus, Mr. Fodler's strengths—being capable of performing some of his own activities of daily living—were not identified, and he was treated as an invalid unnecessarily.

CASE STUDIES ILLUSTRATING APPROPRIATE AND INAPPROPRIATE DOCUMENTATION

Not only is it important to think to provide high-quality care to patients, it is equally important to document the care to reflect the thinking that occurred. The following case studies are from actual nursing malpractice suits (the names and cases have been altered to protect the privacy of those involved). Study the nursing care that was documented and analyze the documentation for evidence of thinking during use of the nursing process.

Case Study

CASE STUDY #1: MRS. HENDRICKS

Mrs. Hendricks was admitted through the emergency room with a history of vaginal bleeding for several weeks. Her hemoglobin at that time was 4.0 (normal is 12 to 16). Her vital signs were stable and her only complaints were of being a little tired and cold (due to the low hemoglobin). She was admitted to the surgical unit where an IV line was started and blood transfusions were administered. The following narrative-style nurses' notes were recorded in her chart.

3/21/98
1300 The first unit of blood started to infuse into the right hand IV.—B. Smith, RN
1400 The right hand and fingernails became bluish in color. Radial pulse is palpable. Patient complains the hand feels numb and cold.—B. Smith, RN
1500 The right hand is purplish in color, but is not swollen.—B. Smith, RN
1600 Blood transfusion in progress infusing into right hand. The right hand is dark purple in color and swollen, the skin is cold, and the hand is painful. Radial pulse is palpable. The IV was discontinued from the right hand and restarted in the left arm with an 18-gauge angiocath. The right hand was ele-

vated on pillows and warm compresses were applied. Dr. Doyle was notified regarding the patient's hand. He states he will be in to see the patient as soon as possible.—J. Jones, RN

1800 Dr. Doyle in to examine patient's hand at 1630. See care plan for frequency of circulation checks and warm compresses. Continued to keep hand elevated on pillows. Medicated patient with 50 mg Demerol for pain, patient now states relief of pain. Hand remains swollen, purple in color, cool to touch with a palpable radial pulse.—J. Jones, RN

⊃Action Learning #62: Analyzing Documentation for Mrs. Hendricks

Examine the care B. Smith, RN (the first nurse) delivered to Mrs. Hendricks and answer this question: Which components of the nursing process did B. Smith complete, beginning at 1400? It may be helpful to ask yourself the following: what did she assess, what did she plan, what did she do, and what did she evaluate?

Now, look at the notes written by J. Jones, RN beginning at 1600. Which components of the nursing process did she complete while caring for Mrs. Hendricks? Again, ask: what did she assess, what did she plan, what did she do, and what did she evaluate?

How were the approaches of the two nurses different?

THINK ABOUT THIS ■ If you were a nurse–lawyer reading this record, what would you think of these nurses? How would you feel about defending their ability to use the nursing process?

Case Study

Now, for the rest of the story. When B. Smith noticed that Mrs. Hendricks' right hand became blue, cold, and painful at 1400, those signs and symptoms should have indicated to the nurse that the IV was no longer in the vein but was leaking into the subcutaneous tissues. The nurse should have been thinking about the relationship between pieces of data by using TOTAL RECALL of population norms for color, comfort level, and temperature of hands, along with signs and symptoms of IV infiltration. She should have used INQUIRY to ask herself whether this situation was normal and what might be happening. When an IV leaks into subcutaneous tissue, it is necessary to discontinue the IV and restart it in another vein. However, Ms. Smith failed to do this. Instead, at 1500, the hand remained discolored; in fact, by then it was purple in color, and the IV blood transfusion continued into it.

At 1600, when J. Jones took over the care of Mrs. Hendricks, she assessed the hand, recognized the signs and symptoms as a problem, planned, and took action. She discontinued the IV, elevated the hand on a pillow, applied warm compresses to help reduce the swelling, and contacted the physician, who ordered pain medication. Ms. Jones treated Mrs. Hendricks' pain and swelling and, at 1800, she reassessed and evaluated her previous care.

Because B. Smith did not discontinue the IV at 1400 (she did not plan and implement) when the first signs of infiltration occurred, and because it wasn't until 1600 (2 hours later) that the IV was finally discontinued, Mrs. Hendricks' hand became very swollen and gangrene eventually developed. Unfortunately, Mrs. Hendricks had to undergo surgery to amputate part of her index finger, as well as all of the other three fingers. She then had a second surgery to revise the stumps for possible placement of artificial fingers (prostheses). She had a third surgery to place the prostheses. To make matters worse, Mrs. Hendricks was right handed.

CASE STUDY #2: MS. ROSE

26-year-old Ms. Rose was admitted to the hospital for treatment of an abscess on the right side of her neck. She was treated with IV antibiotics and pain medications. Ms. Rose had a history of Raynaud's disease (poor circulation to the hands and feet). Her doctor, Dr. Bell, also diagnosed a clotting disorder. To treat the clotting problem, Dr. Bell prescribed a medication, Konyne, which contains clotting factors V, VII, and IX. These notes were recorded on the third day of Ms. Rose's hospitalization. Study this narrative documentation and look for evidence of the nurses' thinking during use of the nursing process.

2/22/98

1600 IV was restarted in the left thumb. Patient was given Tylenol grains X for
     complaint of left arm pain.—H. Hannon, RN
2000 Patient complains of tingling of left hand and fingers, IV is patent, no
     swelling is noted.—H. Hannon, RN

2200 Patient complains of pain in the left hand and arm, IV patent. Slight swelling of the entire arm is noted. It is cool to touch and firm, slightly discolored. Radial pulse is present.—H. Hannon, RN

2230 Dr. Bell was called regarding patient's left arm complaints. Ordered 3 inches of Nitropaste to be applied to the left arm. Paste was applied and the patient was given Percocet 5, two tablets, for pain. The IV was removed from the left thumb.—H. Hannon, RN

2/23/98

0045 Patient continued to complain of arm pain. Arm continues to be dusky in color. Lower arm and hand are swollen. IV was restarted in the right hand with 22-gauge angiocath.—T. Rizer, RN

0300 Percocet 5, two tablets were given for left arm pain.—T. Rizer, RN

0400 Left arm and hand continue to be swollen and painful, elevated on pillow.—T. Rizer, RN

0800 Left arm edematous, hand highly swollen. Finger joints highly swollen and spongelike. Skin cool, color dusky. Unable to palpate radial pulse due to edema.—D. Davis, RN

1000 Patient crying, complaining of much pain in left arm and hand. Demerol and Vistaril IM given.—D. Davis, RN

1130 Some relief noted, but pain not completely gone.—D. Davis, RN

1200 Dr. Bell in to see patient. Ordered venous Doppler study and morphine for pain management.—D. Davis, RN

1400 Morphine 5 mg IV for complaints of severe pain. Left arm is the same. Patient to vascular lab for Doppler study.—D. Davis, RN

1600 Returned from vascular lab. Left arm, shoulder to hand, has major edema, firm, appears twice the size of the right arm. From elbow to fingers, pale purple-blue in color, cool and very painful to touch. —D. Davis, RN

⊃ACTION LEARNING #63: Part A. Analyzing Documentation for Ms. Rose

Study the documentation by H. Hannon, RN from 1600 to 2230. Which components of the nursing process did Mr. Hannon complete when caring for Ms. Rose? Did he assess? Plan? Implement? Evaluate? Write the appropriate component label next to each part of the documentation that it reflects.

THINK ABOUT THIS ■ You might have said, "There is documented evidence that he identified all components as being performed except evaluation." The documentation reflects only assessing, planning, and implementing. After Mr. Hannon described the condition of the hand and arm to Dr. Bell, the physician thought Ms. Rose was having a Raynaud's disease attack (of poor circulation, causing the discoloration and pain). The nurse applied Nitropaste to the arm. Nitropaste is a vasodilator and, if this were a Raynaud's disease attack, one would expect to see the circulation in the arm improve. This would be evident by the arm returning to its natural pink color, the temperature becoming warm to the touch, and the patient having no further pain. Unfortunately, there is no documentation that anyone evaluated the results of applying the Nitropaste to the arm. The documentation indicates that only partially processed nursing was given.

⊃ACTION LEARNING #63: Part B. Further Analysis of Documentation for Ms. Rose

Study the documentation by T. Rizer, RN on the midnight shift. Which components of the nursing process did she document?

Was the patient still having problems with the hand and arm?

What could Ms. Rizer have done for Ms. Rose?

THINK ABOUT THIS ■ Ms. Rizer's documentation shows that she assessed, planned, implemented, and evaluated her care. Unfortunately, her interventions were not effective. The patient's arm was getting worse; she required stronger pain medication (Percocet is stronger than Tylenol), and the pain was not being controlled. As of 0400, the patient was still complaining of pain.

⊃**ACTION LEARNING #63: Part C. Even Further Analysis of Documentation for Ms. Rose**

Study the documentation of the day-shift nurse, Ms. Davis. Which components of the nursing process did Ms. Davis complete, as demonstrated by her documentation?

THINK ABOUT THIS ■ Ms. Davis also assessed, planned, implemented, and evaluated, but was there still a problem? There certainly was! Look at her assessment of Ms. Rose's arm at 0800. The arm was getting worse instead of better. At 1000, she gave Ms. Rose a Demerol and Vistaril injection for pain (Demerol and Vistaril are stronger pain medications than Percocet).

The 1600 assessment showed the arm to be worse even after the patient was given more medication (morphine) for pain management. Obviously, there was something seriously wrong with this arm that was not being dealt with effectively by stronger and stronger pain medication.

Case Study

CONTINUATION OF CASE STUDY FOR MS. ROSE

At 1400, Ms. Rose had a venous Doppler study done that showed a large blood clot in the left subclavian vein. This clot was causing the poor circulation to the arm. The clot was caused by the Konyne (the medication with clotting factors) that Dr. Bell had prescribed. Dr. Bell had made an error in diagnosing the clotting problem from the beginning. Ms. Rose never should have received this medication and, in fact, it made her blood clot too much. (Dr. Bell was sued for misdiagnosing the clotting problem.) The patient was eventually transferred to another hospital, where many efforts were made to save her left arm. Unfortunately, the arm had to be amputated because it became gangrenous.

This scenario about Ms. Rose illustrates what can happen when all phases of the nursing process are not used well or are not documented. Continual evaluation of patient care is extremely important. If a patient's condition does not improve or if there is little progress toward goals and objectives, the nurse must reassess, re-plan, reimplement, and reevaluate. Nurses must communicate clearly all aspects of care with other health care providers. Without such communication, each nurse works without knowing what previous nurses assessed, planned, implemented, and evaluated. There is no continuity of care, patients suffer, and time is wasted.

Both written and verbal communication are needed to achieve continuity of care. In the preceding scenario, both written and verbal communication obviously were lacking. For example, if Mr. Hannon had said to Ms. Rizer: "I put some Ni-tropaste on Ms. Rose's arm and haven't had a chance to see whether it did any good. Please be sure to check on that, and if it's not better, call Dr. Bell," the out-come might have been entirely different for this patient. Because Ms. Rizer's notes show no continuation of the work that Mr. Hannon started, one can assume that Mr. Hannon did not communicate his plan or his thinking processes to the next nurse.

Clarity and Specificity of Documentation

In the preceding case studies, the nurses not only did not document safe nursing, they apparently did not provide it either. What about nurses who provide safe care yet do not document that care? Unclear or missing documentation of care can cause as many problems as not providing the care. Notes must be clear and specific so that the care is fully communicated. It is not enough, however, merely to list what was done for a patient. The patient's response to care (evaluation) also must be noted so that patient progress can be tracked. Without that, the patient's condition may worsen without anyone noticing the change.

⊃ACTION LEARNING #64: Charting Patient Responses and Nursing Care

Compare the following two examples of nurses' notes on the same patient. Ex-plain why the second one is better than the first.

Note #1: Assessment completed, AM care completed, medications given as or-dered, tube feeding maintained and decubitus ulcer dressings changed per protocol.—I. Root, RN

Note #2: See Assessment Sheet and Care Flowsheet for details of assessment and routine care. Patient shows good response to morning dose of furosemide with 600 cc urine output and less edema present in his ankles. Tolerating tube feedings at 100 cc per hour, without evidence of aspiration; residuals are less than 5 cc. Decubitus ulcer dressings changed after the pa-tient was premedicated with Demerol and Vistaril. Lesion on coccyx, 4 cm by 6 cm and 1/2 cm deep, has pink granulation tissue present, no drainage noted. The right heel ulcer, 2 cm by 2 cm, covered with black eschar. Travase ointment is beginning to debride the outer edge of lesion area. See nursing care plan for updated dressing protocol. Patient tolerated procedure with minimal discomfort.—B. Greenwald, RN

The second note is better because:

THINK ABOUT THIS ■ Does the first note tell you anything about the patient or how the patient is responding to treatments? The only thing you can deduce from this note is that the patient is receiving tube feedings and has a problem with pressure sores (decubitus ulcers).

Nurses are expected to assess their patients. In fact, in some institutions, a written assessment at specified intervals, such as every 8 hours, is required. It also is expected that patients receive proper attention to hygiene. Often this routine type of care is recorded on a flowsheet rather than in note format. Ms. Root's note is focused on routine things that were done, rather than on the actual data found through assessment. Actually, the statement about the routine, "medications given as ordered," is worrisome. Would a nurse give medications as *not* ordered? That would be practicing medicine without a license! The statement as recorded is redundant.

In contrast to Ms. Root's note, Ms. Greenwald's note gives a clear picture of the patient's responses. For example, the medication furosemide is a diuretic, which causes the patient to remove excess fluid from his body by making more urine. The note clearly identifies how well this drug is working. The patient also is receiving tube feedings at 100 cc per hour. Problems that can occur with tube feedings include abdominal distention as the feeding sits in the stomach, diarrhea if too much is given, or aspiration of the feeding into the lungs if the patient vomits. The note tells how the patient is responding to the tube feeding so that the reader would know that none of those potential problems had occurred.

There also is a clear description of the status of the decubitus ulcers. The nurse noted the size of the lesions and that granulation tissue was present. (Granulation is healthy tissue that fills in the wound. Eventually, skin will grow to cover the granulation tissue.) She also described a black eschar on one of the wounds. Eschar is dark, dead tissue, which must be removed (debrided) before the remainder of the wound will heal. These facts would let readers know exactly how the lesions looked on that day, so that nurses caring for this patient in the future would be able to judge how things have changed.

Note that the nurse in the second example did not simply repeat the nursing care plan; nor did she say that she had done this and that. By recording the results of what she did, she let others know she did these things. For example, there was no need to say, "Checked tube feeding residuals every shift." This appears on the care plan. Because she recorded, "Tube feeding residuals are less than 5 cc," one knows she executed her plan. Notes should be as brief as possible, because no one wants to read pages and pages of unnecessary information. Recording the results of one's actions lets the reader know the plan was executed and how the patient responded to the actions.

✔ *Thinking-Learning Check*

Pause here for a thinking-learning check. You should be able to elaborate on these ideas:

- ✔ Nursing and documentation are both processes.
- ✔ The nursing process and the process of documentation both follow a sequential pattern.
- ✔ Illustrations of what can happen when those patterns are not followed show how dangerous poor-quality nursing care can be.
- ✔ Clarity in documenting care is as important as the care itself.

DOCUMENTATION AS PART OF QUALITY ASSURANCE

It is essential that patients have an assurance of high-quality health care. High-quality health care is not only cost effective in the long run ("Do it right the first time and you do not have to do it again," or "A stitch in time saves nine"), it is a matter of safety or even of life and death.

Who Assures Quality, and How?

High-quality care is the individual responsibility of each nurse, but there also are formal professional and institutional mechanisms to ensure that high-quality care is provided. High-quality nursing is defined and standards for that quality are set forth in such guidelines as State Nurse Practice Acts and Standards of Practice developed by the American Nurses Association. Health care institutions also have formal programs for assuring high-quality care. Often there are representatives from all branches of health care delivery, including nursing, who serve on committees to oversee quality in an institution. There also are external agencies, such as the Joint Commission on Accreditation of Health Care Organizations, that send auditors to institutions to ensure that quality, as defined by specific criteria, is being maintained.

How nurses use and document the nursing process plays an important role in quality assurance. This role is played out in many ways, even in the specific parts of a documented plan of care. Look at the following example of a patient outcome found on a nursing care plan. "Patient will independently administer the correct dose of insulin subcutaneously using aseptic technique." If the nurse or an auditor were assessing for the quality of care related to this outcome, that person would look for some documentation that the patient could or did achieve this outcome. One way to document this would be to see whether the outcome was measurable and realistic for this patient, and, later, whether the patient achieved this outcome.

The outcome statement is measurable but because the patient is partially blind and has severe arthritis in his hands, it is not realistic. This patient would not be able to achieve this outcome. If the statement is revised, however, it can become realistic. A revised patient outcome statement for this particular patient might be as follows: "The patient's wife will independently administer the correct dose of insulin to the patient, subcutaneously using aseptic technique."

If the nurse had pursued the first outcome, the patient never would have achieved it. High-quality care would not have been attained. The nurse would have wasted valuable time and money while frustrating the patient and preventing him from receiving his insulin correctly once he was discharged home. With his insulin being given incorrectly, the patient's diabetes would have been uncontrolled, and severe diabetic complications ultimately would have developed that would have necessitated future hospitalizations and diminished his quality of life.

By pursuing the second outcome statement (having the wife learn to give the injection), however, the nurse allows a much better chance of success. The second outcome statement is both measurable and realistic for this patient. With it, the nurse would not waste time and money; the patient, his wife, and the nurse would not become frustrated, and the patient's diabetes would be managed. Documentation of the second outcome statement reflects planning of high-quality care. Later, when the outcome is evaluated, documentation of that evaluation can reflect high-quality care as well.

Quality Assurance Audits

Nursing documentation often is audited (reviewed and evaluated) through quality assurance programs. Auditors use preset criteria that are closely related to the policies of an institution or agency. The records are reviewed to make sure everything that should be documented is indeed being documented. The person doing the auditing may be a staff nurse or a nurse specifically assigned to auditing duties. Here are some examples of policies that could serve as criteria for a medical record audit in an acute care setting. The auditor would search records to ensure that these policies were being followed.

Nurses' notes:

1. Are written every 8 hours.
2. Reflect the patient's or family's response to nursing intervention.
3. Are signed with the appropriate nursing signature.

Nursing care plan interventions:

1. Reflect interventions specific to each patient problem.
2. Are written in measurable, behavioral terms so staff know exactly what is to be done for a patient.
3. Are updated as the patient's condition changes.

⊃ACTION LEARNING #65: Mr. Smock's Missing Details

Assume you are a nurse quality assurance auditor. Read the following case study and documentation. Audit the notes by answering the questions, using the criteria provided.

Case Study

Mr. Smock, 56 years old, was admitted for complaints of shortness of breath with any activity and a blood glucose level of 265 mg/dL (normal is 60 to 120) on November 23rd at 8 AM. He has a history of congestive heart failure and insulin-dependent diabetes mellitus. He was placed on 2 L of oxygen. At home he took insulin, Lasix, and digoxin, but said that the doctor told him his medications needed to be adjusted. The following admission note was found on his chart:

> 11/24/98
> 1600
> 56-year-old male admitted to bed 42B on 11/23/98 at 0800. Resting in bed with call light within reach, watching television.—BW, RN

Audit the above admission note using the following criteria.
Admission notes:

1. Address each patient problem within 12 hours of admission
2. Are accurately timed and dated
3. Are signed with the appropriate signature and title

Does the admission note meet criterion #1? Why or why not?

Does the admission note meet criterion #2? Why or why not?

Does the admission note meet criterion #3? Why or why not?

Practice writing a better admission note for Mr. Smock; then have a class-mate audit your note to see whether you meet the criteria.

THINK ABOUT THIS ■ In the example given here, but hopefully not in your own, criterion #1 was not met because the nurse did not address Mr. Smock's problems. He had two medical problems—congestive heart failure and diabetes mellitus. The nurse did not record anything about those issues. Remember, monitoring medical problems is part of the interdependent function of nurses. The nurse did not record anything about independent nursing functions, so no one knows which nursing diagnoses exist. Even with the limited information known, it was highly likely that the nursing diagnosis, "Activity Intolerance related to shortness of breath and congestive heart failure" should have been a conclusion.

Criterion #1 also was not met because the note was not written until 11/24 at 4 PM, 32 hours after the patient was admitted!

Assuming the date and time recorded were accurate, criterion #2 was met in this example.

Criterion #3 was not met. An appropriate signature is first initial, last name, and title. Initials and title do not constitute an appropriate signature. An appropriate signature would be "B. Walton, RN."

DOCUMENTATION AND INCIDENT REPORTS

Even for great nurses, there are occasions when something happens to a patient that should not happen; the patient may be given the wrong medication or may fall out of bed. When something of this nature occurs, it is called an *incident*. It is important to document the incident because the patient may require follow-up medical and nursing care, and the health care institution must know the incident occurred to prevent the same type of incident from occurring again. For these two reasons, it is necessary to describe the situation in the medical record as well as in an *incident report*. The note in the record will allow other care providers to follow up on any care, and the incident report allows the institution to monitor such risks. There are specific "Risk Management" committees or departments in most health care institutions that monitor incidents and plan actions to prevent them from recurring.

In documenting an incident, the following five basic guidelines should be followed:

1. The person who discovers the incident, even if he or she is not the person who was involved in the incident, should write the report.
2. In the medical record, nursing documentation should reflect the nursing process. In other words, what did the nurse assess, plan, do, and evaluate with regard to the patient and relative to the incident?
3. The incident report form must be completed according to the institution's policy and procedures (these vary from institution to institution).
4. *Never* make reference to an **incident report itself** in the patient's medical record. The incident report is *not* part of the patient's medical record. The incident report belongs to the hospital and is used for internal tracking of incidents. You only describe the situation in the record, not that an incident report was made.
5. In the section of the incident report that calls for a description of the patient's condition and what the nurse assessed, simply copy the nurse's note from the medical record onto the incident report form.

⊃ ACTION LEARNING #66: Tracking an Incident: Mr. Katz's IV

Read the case study and documentation. Then evaluate the documentation according to the guidelines for documenting an incident. You will be able to use numbers 1, 2, and 4 of the guidelines. For numbers 3 and 5, if possible, obtain a blank incident form from an agency where you practice and fill it out using the information in the case study and note.

Case Study

The physician ordered an IV of 5% dextrose and water (D5W) at a rate of 20 cc per hour for Mr. Katz, who has a history of congestive heart failure. When Sally Tower, RN entered Mr. Katz's room on her initial rounds, she noticed that Mr. Katz's IV was 0.9% saline infusing at a rate of 100 cc per hour. Sally slowed the IV rate, left the room, and obtained a bag of D5W. She returned to Mr. Katz's room, discontinued the 0.9% saline, and hung the bag of D5W. She double-checked the rate of infusion, making sure it was at 20 cc per hour, and auscultated Mr. Katz's lungs, noting that his lungs sounded clear. She also noted that Mr. Katz had no sacral or pedal edema, and asked him whether he felt short of breath. She then called Mr. Katz's physician and informed him that Mr. Katz had received approximately 700 cc of 0.9% saline and reported her other findings. Then Sally documented the following in Mr. Katz's chart:

11/30/98
1630
IV of 0.9% NS infusing at rate of 100 cc/hr. 0.9% NS discontinued. D5W at 20 cc/hr IV initiated. Patient's lung sounds are clear, no sacral or pedal edema noted. Patient has no complaints of dyspnea. Dr. Butler notified of patient's current status. Will continue to monitor patient for fluid overload.—Sally Tower, RN.

THINK ABOUT THIS ■ Based on Sally's note, one can see that she assessed (wrong IV solution and rate), planned ("I need to correct this situation"), intervened (hung the correct solution, adjusted the infusion rate, and called the physician), and evaluated (the patient's lungs were clear, and he had no edema or difficulty breathing). After Sally documented the situation in the patient's medical record, she was able to copy her note directly from the record onto the separate incident report form for the hospital's use.

LEGAL RAMIFICATIONS OF DOCUMENTATION

The medical record is the only legal record of the care a patient receives and of the patient's response to that care. Documentation is a professional responsibility and is as important as delivering care. If a patient receives care, but no one documents it, there is no way that other caregivers, auditors, or lawyers can know what was done and how the patient responded. How is a hospital to be reimbursed for the care provided to patients if there is no documented evidence of care? Documentation is a *must* (Marrelli, 1992).

If a patient decides to sue because of care received or not received, one of the first documents the attorney representing the patient will request is the medical record. The attorney can request parts or all of a medical record as well as billing statements. Nurses' notes are part of the medical record and will be requested by the attorney.

If nurses' documentation reflects the nursing process and appropriate actions taken, chances are the documentation will stand up very well in a malpractice suit. In addition, the documentation will serve to remind nurses of the care they gave to a particular patient. By the time a suit is brought to court and nurses are questioned by attorneys about their practice, 2 or more years may have elapsed. It is possible, indeed likely, that the nurses involved would not remember the patient, let alone what they assessed and what they did for the patient. Documentation is what nurses have to rely on to refresh their memories. Documentation completed today that reflects the nursing process will be a welcome sight to the nurse who is facing a possible malpractice claim tomorrow.

NOT THINKING AND LITIGATION

One of the serious consequences of not thinking when documenting or delivering care is litigation against the nurse. Over the years, litigation has become an increasingly important issue for nurses. Nurses more often are being held accountable for their professional actions and as a result, can find themselves out of the hospital and in the court room involved in litigation. Thus, it is important to think about minimizing one's risk of becoming involved in a malpractice action. "An ounce of prevention is worth a pound of cure," is another one of those sayings that fits well here.

Delivering great nursing care with quality documentation is essential to avoiding litigation but what else can the nurse do to avoid problems with litigation? Communication is the number one risk management tool a nurse possesses. (Risk management is the terminology used in health care institutions these days to think ahead about where potential liability problems may occur, implement a plan to avoid problems, and deal with the ones that do occur.)

As discussed in Chapter 11, documentation is the written portion of communication. (By the way, documentation that cannot be read and/or interpreted correctly has no communication value whatsoever!) Verbal and non-verbal communications also are essential. Whether the nurse is communicating with a colleague, another healthcare professional, the patient, or the family members, opening and maintaining lines of communication is essential to professional practice.

Failure to communicate, either in writing or verbally, can lead to disastrous results for the patient, not to mention the embarrassment one would suffer in front of a jury. At this point in your education you have many opportunities to seek help with documentation from your instructors. After graduation, you may want to do some spot checks with colleagues to be sure you don't fall into some poor documentation HABITS that would not accurately reflect your thinking and doing.

The following are resources available for nurses interested in gaining a better understanding of malpractice and litigation issues.

- American Association of Legal Nurse Consultants
  4700 W. Lake Ave.
  Glenview, IL 60025-1485
  Phone: 847-375-4713
  FAX: 847-375-4777
- Medical-Legal Consulting Institute, Inc.
  2476 Bolsover
  Suite 632
  Houston, TX 77005
  Internet Web Site: http://www.legalnurse.com
  E-mail: MedLegCons@aol.com

CLOSING COMMENTS: THE IMPORTANCE OF THINKING AND DOCUMENTING

The nursing process and the documentation process both require thinking. Thinking that occurs during the use of the nursing process allows the nurse effectively and efficiently to assess, plan, implement, and evaluate care. If thinking continues to be used in the documentation process, anyone reading the documentation will quickly recognize the quality of thinking and care provided. Thinking and great nursing care are most easily measured by great documentation of care and patient outcomes. The phrase, "If it's not documented, it didn't happen," is a useful reminder to both beginning and experienced nurses to dedicate time and energy to high-quality documentation.

THINKING LOG #12 ➤

Think of a recent note you wrote in a patient's medical record. Recreate that note as accurately as possible. (*Remember* not to use the patient's name for the sake of confidentiality.) Describe how the note would help or hinder you if you had to defend your actions in court. Evaluate your note to see whether it reflects the nursing process. Are all four components present? If not, what should be added to this note so that it does reflect the nursing process?

Reference

Marrelli, T.M. (1992). *Nursing documentation handbook*. St. Louis: Mosby–Year Book.

Thinking Through a Complex Patient Situation

13

Assessing a Complex
Patient Situation

✳ *Learning Outcomes*

After reading and doing the activities in this chapter you will be able to:

Track the thinking skills and content knowledge used to complete the assessment phase of the nursing process in a complex patient situation.

Set priorities for care in a complex patient situation.

The final section of this workbook, Chapters 13 through 17, is designed to pull all the pieces of thinking and doing back together and into the "big picture" of great nursing. Looking at the big picture is an important theme that was introduced in Chapters 3 and 4, but the view from now on will be different. This time, the view will be enhanced because of the reader's growing sophistication in thinking about the nursing process and personal thinking abilities.

This section provides an opportunity to work with and think through a complex patient situation, from data collection and analysis (assessment) to determining the quality of care (evaluation). Even though this is a complex situation, the nurse uses the same thinking skills and nursing process that are used with simpler nursing situations. Such skills, however, evolve with experience. The primary purpose of this section is to continue to acknowledge and nurture the reader's existing thinking skills as those skills grow toward achieving the goal of providing great nursing. A "Tracking Nursing Thinking" checklist is provided in Appendix D to aid this continuing learning process, and will be used throughout these last chapters.

This chapter briefly reviews the equation for great nursing that was introduced in Chapter 3, and then focuses on the case study of a woman named Betty. Her data base is presented on a Nursing Assessment Tool and Data Base (see Figure 13-1). The nurse's thinking, from the initial analysis to setting priorities for the assessment conclusions, is highlighted throughout this chapter.

Name _Betty_   Age _46_   Sex _F_   Admit Date _10/98_

Medical Diagnosis _ALS, Iron deficiency Anemia, Irritable bowel syndrome_

Allergies _None known_

Medications _Estrogen 0.625 mg QD, Baclofen 10 mg TID, Nortriptyline 75 mg Qhs, Metamucil 1pkt. prn.,_
Ferrous Sulfate 325 mg. QD

Persons/groups involved in care _Dep't. of Social Services, Methodist Church, County Hospice anticipated; Hannah Jones_
and Rhonda Smith (church friends)

COMMUNICATING: Sending messages
[Nsg. Dx.: Impaired Verbal Communication]

English (circle) (read) (write) (understand)

Other languages _Spanish (fluent)_

Speech impairments _Low, hoarse, monotone voice "its getting worse"_

Alternate form of communication _____

VALUING: Assigning relative worth
[Nsg. Dx.: Spiritual Distress]

Spiritual orientation _Methodist_

Important religious practices _None_

Cultural orientation _Mother is Greek, father from southern U.S._

Cultural practices _Likes southern cooking_

RELATING: Establishing bonds
Role
[Nsg. Dx.: Altered Role Performance, Altered Parenting, High Risk for Altered Parenting*, Sexual Dysfunction, Altered Family Processes, Caregiver Role Strain, High Risk For Caregiver Role Strain, Parental Role Conflict, Altered Sexuality Patterns]

Marital status or significant relationship _Divorced 15 years (mother in Ohio, father deceased)_

Age and health of significant other _N/A_

Number of children _2 sons_   Ages _20 & 16_

Role in home _16 yr. old son at home & in school; 20 yr. old son lives in same apt. complex_

Financial support _No income, but apt. rent & utilities paid by former employer; Appl. for SSI & Medicare completed_

Occupation _Retired (10/29/98) Apartment manager_

Job satisfaction/concerns _N/A_

Recent losses _job, independence, self care, ability to walk, some parenting activities_

Sexual habits _Celibate_

Relationships (satisfactory/unsatisfactory)

  Effects of illness on relationship _N/A_

  Sexual Concerns _N/A_

Socialization
[Nsg. Dx.: Impaired Social Interaction*, Social isolation]

Relationships with others _Close to Hannah & Rhonda "I have talked with ex-husband about caring for our son."_

  Patient's description _"My sons & friends are very helpful, I miss working."_

  Significant others' descriptions _per Hannah, pt's relationship with mother strained_

  Staff observations _Positive, open relationships_

KNOWING: Meaning associated with information
[Nsg. Dx.: Knowledge Deficit (Specify)*, Altered Thought Processes]

Perception of current health issues _"I've written my eulogy. I've come to accept the fact that I will die soon, probably this_
coming year. I have made plans for my funeral, talked with my minister, lawyer, ex-husband & sons about death."

Perception/knowledge of medications, treatments, procedures _Reported clearly what meds for. Said Nortriptyline for_
outbursts of laughing. Resists moving bed to first floor.

Previous illnesses/hospitalizations/surgeries _Perforated uterus during D&C (1979), Ruptured ovarian cyst (1983)_
Hysterectomy (1997) Several episodes of pneumonia & bronchitis (most recent 4 yrs. ago)

FIGURE 13–1 Nursing assessment tool and data base.

KNOWING (cont.)
History of the following:

	Patient	Family		Patient	Family
Anemia/Blood disorder	✓	____	Kidney Disease	____	____
Cancer	____	____	Stroke	____	____
Diabetes	____	____	Tuberculosis	____	____
Heart Disease	____	_Father_	Alcohol/Substance Abuse	____	_Uncle_
Hypertension	____	_Father, Mother_	Smoking	____	_Parents_
Peripheral Vascular	____	____	Other	____	____

Readiness to learn _Open, asks questions, listens attentively_
   Requests information about _Hospice, ALS_
   Education level _Business School Degree_
   Learning impediments _Fatigue & decreased vision ("difficult to read")_
Orientation
[Nsg. Dx.: High Risk for Injury]
Level of alertness _Alert_
Orientation: Person_____✓_____Place_____✓_____Time____✓____
Appropriate behavior/communication _Yes_

Memory
Memory intact: ⟨yes⟩/no Recent _____✓_____Remote_____✓_____

Feeling: Subjective awareness of information
Physical Comfort
[Nsg. Dx.: Pain*, Chronic Pain]
Pain/discomfort: ⟨yes⟩/no If yes:
Date of onset/course _Yesterday, fell on kitchen floor, flat onto face_
Exact location _Teeth (broken front tooth), Lip (lacerated top lip), arm (left arm near elbow)_
Terms for quality and quantity _"My lip feels sore and puffy; my arm aches."_
Aggravating and alleviating factors _"Eating and chewing hot and cold liquids hurts my mouth, Tylenol helps dull the pain."_
Inter-system connections _Headache & nausea (Pt. went to Emergency Dep't. for this)_
Labeled by patient as: _"Frustrating," "Discouraging," "I should wear shoes more."_
Emotional Comfort
[Nsg. Dx.: Dysfunctional Grieving, Anticipatory Grieving, High Risk for Violence: Self directed or directed at others, High Risk for Self-Mutilation, Post-Trauma Response, Rape Trauma Syndrome, (Compound Reaction, Silent Reaction), Anxiety*, Fear*]
Recent stressful life events _Forced early retirement 2° ALS. Fall yesterday._
Many "hassles filling out forms for Social Security."
Verbalization of feelings of: _Frustration, anxiety about finances. "It's not death itself that I fear,_
but the interim time before I die."
Physical manifestations of emotions _None obvious_
Fears or concerns _" I've talked to my sons about how they will cope with my death and to my ex-husband about his caring for_
our youngest son." "I fear having to spend my final days with my mother."

MOVING: Activity
Activity
[Nsg. Dx.: Impaired Physical Mobility*, High Risk for Peripheral Neurovascular Dysfunction*, Activity* Intolerance, Fatigue*,
High Risk for Activity Intolerance]
History of physical disability _ALS diagnosed 10/96_
Use of device _(cane, ⟨walker⟩ artificial limb) wheelchair ordered last week_
Limitations in daily activities _"I can walk short distances; it's hard to go up and down stairs, my son has to be behind me. I_
can't drive, cook, clean. My son does laundry and grocery shopping and drives me to my appointments."

FIGURE 13–1   Nursing assessment tool and data base. (continued)

MOVING (cont.)

Exercise habits *"I don't do any exercise at all"*

Physical symptoms with activity *Shortness of breath, fatigue, increased pulse, unsteadiness*

Rest

[Nsg. Dx.: Sleep Pattern Disturbance]

Hours slept/night *8-9*   Feels rested (yes)/no   Sleeps alone: (yes)/no

Position preference *Flat*   Naps during the day *None usually*

Sleep interruptions (number and type) *1-2 per night "I've always done this — just thinking"*

Sleep aids (pillows, meds, food) *"Just one pillow is fine"*

Difficulty falling/remaining asleep *None*

Recreation

[Nsg. Dx.: Diversional Activity Deficit]★

Usual leisure activities *"Shopping, going to movies and plays. I used to write poetry & read a lot."*

Usual social activities *Job had much social contact, lunch outings with Hannah and Rhonda*

Illness-related changes *Home alone; difficulty going to restaurants, ("smoke bothers me") "I get bored, I can go out only if someone takes me. I've worked all my life; I'm not used to so much free time."*

Home Maintenance

[Nsg. Dx.: Impaired Home Maintenance Management]

Size & arrangement of home ((stairs)/bathroom) *2-floor apt; 2 bathrooms - full bath upstairs, & 1/2 bath downstairs, 2 steps to enter apt, kitchen floor tiled & slippery, carpets in other rooms*

Safety issues *Cluttered rooms, no safety bars in bathrooms. Safe neighborhood. Pt wearing socks.*

Ability to maintain home *"I can't do housework." Sons & friends clean; sons do laundry and grocery shopping.*

Health Maintenance

[Nsg. Dx.: Altered Health Maintenance]

Health insurance *HMO, Appl. for Medicare, SSI completed*

Schedule of health exams *MD seen monthly, Dentist every 6 months*

Access to health care *Friends, son must provide transportation*

Self exams (breast, testicular) *"I used to do self breast exams, but not as often as I should."*

Self Care

[Nsg. Dx.: Feeding Self Care Deficit★, Impaired Swallowing★, Ineffective Breastfeeding, Interrupted Breastfeeding, Effective Breastfeeding, Ineffective Infant Feeding Pattern, Bathing/Hygiene Self Care★ Deficit, Dressing/Grooming Self Care Deficit★, Toileting Self Care Deficit]

Ability to perform ADLs (Indicate I for independent, D for dependent)

Feeding *I*, Infant feeding (as applicable) *N/A*, Bathing/Hygiene *D*, Dressing/(Grooming) *D* Toileting *I*

Specific deficits *Feeding: Chew slowly, eat small amounts, swallowing difficulties; Bathing: can't sit in tub, uses chair, can shower when someone in the house; Grooming: "I can't shampoo my hair well, It's too much trouble to put my shoes on so I just usually wear socks."*

Types of assistance needed *Stand-by for bathing; minimal for grooming*

Growth and Development

[Nsg. Dx.: Altered Growth and Development★]

Developmental stage *Middle adulthood (but preparing for death)*

Ability to meet developmental responsibilities *Talks of death and funeral plans easily. "I had pictures taken while I still looked healthy (family & individual). Some parenting responsibilities can't be met."*

Relocation

[Nsg. Dx.: Relocation Stress Syndrome]

Recent move: yes/(no) description_____

Adjustment to move_____

FIGURE 13–1   Nursing assessment tool and data base. (continued)

PERCEIVING: Reception of information
Self-Concept
[Nsg. Dx.: Body Image Disturbance, Self-Esteem Disturbance, Chronic Low Self-Esteem, Situational Low Self-Esteem, Personal Identity Disturbance]
Presenting appearance *Casually groomed, no make-up, no body odor*
Patient's description of self *"I've always been organized and logical. I liked to maintain control when I worked. I'm quiet around people I don't know. I like to be happy, I joke a lot."*
Effects of illness *"I can't do my hair well anymore. I'm surprised how many people have helped and brought food."*
Meaningfulness
[Nsg. Dx.: Hopelessness, Powerlessness]
Verbalization of hope/hopelessness *No specific comments*
Verbalization of control/loss of control *"I'm just frustrated with the system—all the red tape."*
Nonverbal cues about hope/control *None*
Sensory/Perception
[Nsg. Dx.: Sensory/Perception Alterations (Specify) (Visual*, auditory, kinesthetic, gustatory, tactile, olfactory), Unilateral Neglect]
History of restrictive environment *Confined to apt. due to weakness*
Vision deficits *I have trouble reading. I'm getting farsighted* Glasses *None*
Hearing deficits *None* Hearing Aid
Other Sensory/Perceptual changes *"I seem to have an exaggerated smell for things like perfumes and smoke."*

EXCHANGING: Mutual giving and receiving
Circulation
[Nsg. Dx.: Altered (Specify Type) Tissue Perfusion (Renal, cerebral, cardiopulmonary, gastrointestinal, peripheral), Fluid Volume Excess, Fluid Volume Deficit, High Risk for Fluid Volume Deficit, Decreased Cardiac Output]
Cerebral:
Neurological changes/symptoms *Dx ALS, weakness of arms & legs, esp. left side. Respiratory muscles and swallowing muscles weak*
Verbal response *Voice weak, hoarse, esp. in A.M.*
Motor response *Unsteady gait, balance, weakness, weak grip, fine motor control (worse on left)*
Cardiac:
Heart rate and rhythm *86 Reg.* Blood pressure: R *118/78* L *110/72* Position *sitting*
Peripheral
Pulses *All palpable and equal bilaterally* Skin temp. *Cool*
Color *Pale* Moisture *Dry* Capillary refill *Rapid* Edema *L. & in ankles & feet*
Physical Integrity
[Nsg. Dx.: Altered Protection, Impaired Tissue Integrity, Altered Oral Mucous Membrane, Impaired Skin* Integrity, High Risk for Impaired Skin Integrity]
Tissue Integrity *Changes 2° fall yesterday* Turgor *Adequate* Rashes *None*
Lesions: *Lip: 1cm. cut with sutures* Petechiae *None* Bruises *L. arm — 8cm, circle above elbow*
Other (specify) *None*
Past history/treatment of skin breakdown *None*
Pressure sores (site/grade) *None*
Treatment *Keep lip clean, watch for infection. "I get stitches out in four days."*
Oxygenation
[Nsg. Dx.: Impaired Gas Exchange, Ineffective Airway Clearance, Ineffective Breathing Pattern*, Inability to Sustain Spontaneous Ventilation, Dysfunctional Ventilatory Weaning Response (DVWR)]
Complaints of Dyspnea *Yes* Precipitated by *Activity, smoke, cold air, aerosol sprays*
History of pulmonary problems *Pneumonia & Bronchitis — last episode 4 yrs. ago*
Smoking: Y/Ⓝ Pk Yrs. Respiratory rate *16* Rhythm *Regular* Depth *Shallow*
Ⓛabored/unlabored; use of accessory muscles *During activity*
Cough: (Productive/Ⓝonproductive) *"occasionally"*

FIGURE 13–1 Nursing assessment tool and data base. (continued)

EXCHANGING: Oxygenation (cont.)

Sputum: Color _N/A_ Amount _____ Consistency_____

Need for suction (frequency) _N/A_ Breath sounds _Decreased at bases_ _____

Oxygen percent and device _N/A_

Physical Regulation and Protection

[Nsg. Dx.: High Risk for Infection*, High Risk for Altered Body Temperature, Hypothermia, Hyperthermia, Ineffective Thermoregulation, Dysreflexia, High Risk for Injury*, High Risk for Suffocation, High risk for Poisoning, High Risk for Trauma, High Risk for Aspiration*, High Risk for Disuse Syndrome, Alt. Protection]

Temperature _98._ Route _Oral_ _____

Menstrual Period: Last _1997_ Frequency _N/A_ Duration _Hysterectomy, 1997._ _____

Immune Status _Not affected yet_ _____

White blood count _7200_ Differential _Not available_ _____

Clotting: PT _N/A_ PTT _N/A_ Platelets _Not available_ _____

Intermittent unusual sensations _None, "But I worry about choking. I don't know how to do the Heimlich maneuver,_
neither do my sons." _____

Immunizations up-to-date _Yes (Flu shot & Tetanus October 1998)_ _____

Alcohol/caffeine/narcotic use _None except for occasional cola_ _____

Environmental/personal safety conditions _House cluttered, pt. rarely wears shoes. Kitchen floor slippery, showers alone_
(someone in house, not in BR) No railings in BR, no use of transfer belt when walking upstairs _____

Nutrition

[Nsg. Dx.: Altered Nutrition: More than body requirements, *Altered Nutrition: Less than body requirements, Altered Nutrition: Potential for more than body requirements, Impaired Swallowing*, High Risk for Aspiration]*

Eating patterns:

Number of meals/day: Usual _2-3_ Current _2-3, plus snacks_ _____

Special diet _Soft–Dinners prepared and brought in by friends and neighbors 3-5 times per week_ _____

Food preferences/intolerances _Dislikes bananas & cottage cheese (too "sticky"), likes jello, mashed potatoes & pudding_

24-hour recall of food intake _Granola bar, applesauce, yogurt, meatloaf, potato, green beans, milk, 1 can pop_

Fluid intake/Type _water, pop_ Amount _1-2 glasses/day_ Preferences _Pop_ _____

Appetite changes _"I seem to eat less at each meal."_ _____

Swallowing difficulty _"Yes, I have to chew well & eat smaller portions; it takes longer to swallow."_ _____

History of ulcers _No_ Indigestion _No (but history of irritable bowel syndrome)_ _____

Anorexia/nausea/vomiting _Some nausea after fall yesterday, but OK now._ _____

Condition of mouth/throat/teeth _1 broken front tooth, mouth dry_ _____

Height _5'2"_ Weight _100 lbs._ Ideal Weight _110-130_ _____

Current diet therapies _None_ _____

Lab values (place * by abnormal values):   (No recent values available)

Hemoglobin _11_ Hematocrit _32_ RBC _4.2_ Na_____ K_____ Cl_____

Glucose (fasting/not fasting) _____ Cholesterol _____ Triglycerides_____

Total protein _____ Albumin _____ Iron _____ Other_____

Elimination

[Nsg. Dx.: Constipation*, Perceived Constipation, Colonic Constipation, Diarrhea, Bowel Incontinence, Altered Urinary Elimination, Stress Incontinence, Reflex Incontinence, Urge Incontinence, Functional Incontinence, Total Incontinence, Urinary Retention]

Gastrointestinal/bowel:

Usual bowel habits _Every other day_ Changes from normal _"I get constipated easily"_ _____

Last BM _today_ Remedies used _Metamucil most days_ _____

Bowel sounds _Present 4 quds_ Abdominal examination _WNL_ _____

Stool Color _Brown_ Amount _Medium_ Consistency _Hard_ _____

Renal/Urinary:

Usual urinary patterns _2-3 times a day_ Changes from normal _"Perhaps a bit less"_ _____

Urine: Color _Amber_ Odor _No unusual_ Amount _Not measured_ per_____

Output for last 24 hours _Unknown_ Avg. hourly _____ Bladder distension: yes/no

Urinalysis _None available_ Urine C&S_____

FIGURE 13–1   Nursing assessment tool and data base. (continued)

CHOOSING: Selection of alternatives
Coping
[Nsg. Dx.: Ineffective Individual Coping, Impaired Adjustment, Defensive Coping, Ineffective Denial, Ineffective Family Coping Disabling, Ineffective Family Coping: Compromised, Family, Coping, Potential for Growth*]
Patient's usual problem-solving methods *"I try to be organized & logical."*

Family's usual problem-solving methods *"My son helps. We talk well."*

Patient's method of dealing with stress *"I talk to someone – often Hannah or Rhonda."*

Family's method of dealing with stress *"We talk"*

Patient's affect *Flat (probably related to muscle weakness of face 2° ALS)*
Physical manifestations of emotional state *None evident*
Support systems available *Church, friends, neighbors in apt. building. "My close friends from church help with negotiating the health care system to get services."*
Participation
[Nsg. Dx.: Ineffective Management of Therapeutic Regimen (Individuals), Noncompliance (Specify), Health Seeking Behaviors (Specify)]
Compliance with past/current health regimens *Usually, however stated, "I can't seem to decide to move my bed to the first floor."*
Willingness to comply with future health regimen *Yes*
Perceived barriers to compliance *"I feel bad about taking up so much of everyone's time. Every change seems to mean I'm more dependent on someone. For example, I need help to sort through things before the bed comes down, and this is such a busy time of year for my friends."*
Judgment
[Nsg. Dx.: Decisional Conflict* (Specify)]
Decision-making ability
Patient's perspective *"I make up my mind, but I change my mind often too. It's hard to accept all these changes."*
Others' perspectives *Betty has made realistic decisions about death, but she's prone to changing her mind about day to day decisions.*

PATIENT'S PRIORITIES FOR CARE

1. *Risks for aspiration, infection and injury*

2. *Self-care deficits*

3. *Constipation*

4. *"The decision about the bed"*

5.

6.

7.

8.

9.

10.

Tool adapted from: Guzzetta, C.E. Bunton, S.D., Prinkey, L.A., Sherer, A.P. & Seifert, P.C. (1989). Clinical assessment tools for use with nursing diagnosis. St. Louis, Mosby. (used with permission)

FIGURE 13–1   Nursing assessment tool and data base. (continued)

Chapters 14 through 16 illustrate how care is designed and revised over time for Betty. Planning, implementing, and evaluating relative to each health concern are described.

To promote an appreciation of the qualitative differences in thinking during the nursing process, alternative care plans are presented in Chapters 14 and 15. Some of these plans are of poor to mediocre quality, and are critiqued and improved to illustrate the contrast in quality. The improved plans for actual problems and potential (Risk for ...) problems illustrate not only increased quality but the different approaches to each of these types of problems. Planning for interdisciplinary problems, problems for referral, and wellness issues is discussed in Chapter 16.

As noted in the introduction to this book, these final five chapters can be read and used at any point during the course of study. Some may find it helpful to examine this more complex "big picture" even before starting Chapter 1.

RETURNING TO THE BIG PICTURE OF GREAT NURSING

The big picture, as described in Chapter 3, presented great nursing and its components. The components included the patient, the nurse (you), thinking skills, knowledge, and the nursing process. A linear equation was presented to illustrate how all these components added up to great nursing:

$$\text{Patient} + \text{You} + \frac{\text{Thinking}}{\text{Skills}} + \text{Knowledge} + \frac{\text{Nursing}}{\text{Process}} = \text{Great Nursing}$$

At that point this equation was sufficient, but by now most readers should be questioning its simplicity. As you proceed through the next four chapters, give some serious thought to this equation. Reexamine the components and their relationships to each other in greater depth. In Chapter 17, the final chapter of this text, the reader is asked to change this simple equation into something that better represents the dynamic qualities of the components.

TRACKING THINKING

Even with a deeper understanding of the concepts (components) contributing to great nursing and an increased awareness of individual thinking skills, it remains challenging for nurses to identify and track thinking because of its abstract nature. To assist the reader in systematically tracking the *thinking* and *doing* that occurred in the course of assessing, planning, implementing, and evaluating care for Betty, a simple checklist was developed. A checklist can never begin to measure the dynamic nature of thinking, but it can serve as a trigger to ensure that the basics are addressed.

The checklist, called "Tracking Nursing Thinking" (TNT), is given in Appendix D. The TNT serves two major purposes. For chapters 13 through 16, it helps the reader track the *thinking* and *doing* of the nurse who is caring for Betty. But, more important, the TNT can serve as a guide for students as they use the nursing process. The TNT also may serve as a guide for self-evaluation and instructor evaluation. Student nurses using the prototype of the TNT found it to be dynamite!

TRACKING THINKING THROUGH ASSESSMENT OF A COMPLEX PATIENT SITUATION

This section of the chapter examines a patient situation. Patient data are recorded on a Nursing Assessment Tool. The thinking that takes place from a point before data collection through to the major conclusions of assessment is studied. The final discussion of thinking focuses on working with the patient in prioritizing those conclusions.

The patient for this case study is Betty. Although Betty is not her real name, she is a real person with very real health concerns. High-level thinking is necessary to design individualized nursing care for her. Two years ago, Betty was told she had a progressive chronic disease affecting her motor neurons, amyotrophic lateral sclerosis (ALS). Betty currently is living at home in the northern part of the United States. The data were collected in late fall, as the first snows of winter were approaching.

ENGAGING THINKING SKILLS AND CONTENT KNOWLEDGE

A certain amount of knowledge is helpful before the nurse begins collecting patient data. That knowledge comes from school course work and experience; it helps the nurse collect the best data in the most efficient manner, and make sense of the data *during* collection.

Basic Knowledge Needed Before Initial Data Collection

In all patient situations, the nurse must use knowledge gained from TOTAL RECALL of information learned or from reference to some source of information. For beginning students who are gaining knowledge while they are simultaneously learning how to use that knowledge, there is that "cart before the horse" problem. It takes time to learn something and more time to learn how to apply that knowledge in a patient situation. What expert nurses take for granted, novices must learn. Novices must recognize that there are key areas of knowledge needed for each situation; there are points in the process where the knowledge is needed and there are good, better, and best ways to use that knowledge.

Knowledge about the usual or "normal" provides standards for population norms. Knowledge of population norms allows the nurse to compare a patient's response to what is usually seen and make decisions about the significance of data. But knowledge of population norms alone does not help the nurse to develop individualized care; it only guides standardized care. To achieve individualized care, the nurse must know about the patient's individual norms and strengths, as well as about caring. Individual norms are discovered by asking the patient about them; caring leads the nurse to recognize the need to collect that individual data.

There are three general categories of knowledge that are helpful before major data collection takes place:

- Demographic data
- Major health issues affecting the patient
- Typical patient response patterns to the major health issues and corresponding nursing care issues

The demographic data include age (chronologic as well as developmental), gender, marital status, and similar information. This basic information provides the nurse with a general starting point. With Betty, who is a 46-year-old, white, divorced woman with two sons (aged 16 and 20 years), knowing what is normal helps to identify relevant data (data different from the norm) as they are collected later. The nurse must look up or RECALL the norms associated with these demographic data. For example, 46-year-old women generally are healthy, productive people who may be experiencing early signs of menopause.

The major health issues affecting the patient include life stressors, situational or developmental crises, and medical diagnoses. In Betty's case these issues include a medical diagnosis of ALS and all the ramifications of having a chronic terminal disease. This knowledge guides the nurse's questions during data collection to focus on areas that typically are problems requiring nursing care.

The typical patient response patterns to these major health issues and corresponding nursing care issues include how Betty is responding to her ALS disease in terms of her eating patterns, sleeping patterns, elimination patterns, relationships with others, coping, and so forth. Understanding that all physiologic, psychological, social, cultural, and spiritual responses are affected by illness helps the nurse focus data collection on the "big picture." Applying this global understanding to assessment is the key to grasping the holistic nature of nursing. Nurses must obtain a large amount of data to determine the full range of a patient's responses.

Although these content areas are very important for the nurse to know to effectively ask questions and make comparisons with population norms, the nurse must be careful not to stereotype the patient by looking only for data that fit classic cases (population norms). INQUIRY is critical to keeping an open mind and going beyond the standards to also identify the patient's individual norms. For example, many patients with ALS become depressed and withdrawn as a way of coping with impending death. Data on Betty's emotional state do not indicate this typical coping response to ALS. Betty, therefore, does not fit into the population norm; she fits her own norm.

In most situations, the nurse will have this basic type of information either before working with the patient or at the very beginning of the interaction. For experienced nurses, with a great deal of stored knowledge and experience, the timing of learning this basic information about the patient is not a big issue. The experienced nurse can process it all very quickly and draw on it as he or she collects and analyzes data from the very start of the encounter.

For the beginning nurse, however, having this knowledge before meeting with the patient means "looking up" the necessary information. The beginning nurse can then plan ahead and know to assess for the most important information first, and not waste time on less relevant areas. For example, in Betty's situation, assessing her understanding of the safety precautions she can take to avoid respiratory infections is much more important than assessing her immunization status for DPT (diphtheria, pertussis, and tetanus) or her family history of breast cancer. A common problem for beginning nurses and students is to assume that a Nursing Assessment Tool needs to be filled out starting with the top of page one and ending with the bottom of the last page. If time permits, this is fine, but when time is limited, it is best to focus data collection and analysis on the critical areas first.

Basic Knowledge Needed About Betty's Situation Before Data Collection

Typically, healthy, independent, 46-year-old divorced women with two sons experience the common concerns of "middle age," with children starting to leave home and prepare for their separate lives. In Betty's case, stages of growth and development have been accelerated from those typical of middle age (generativity versus stagnation in terms of creativity, productivity, and work) to those more typical of old age, including integrity versus despair (Erikson, 1963). One son who had left home is returning to provide some care. Her younger son also is responsible for some caretaking, which is more typical of an adult role. Betty's role has changed from one of extreme independence to a fairly dependent one.

Knowledge about the disease and its course (how it progresses) also is critical. Amyotrophic lateral sclerosis is a neurologic disease of unknown cause in which the motor neurons of the spinal cord, medulla, and cortex degenerate. The primary problems are muscle weakness and the multisystem changes that go along with the progressive weakness. The course of this illness is highly individual, with most people living 3 to 5 years, but with some living 10 to 20 years; death often is the result of a respiratory infective process. There is no treatment for the disease itself, only for the symptoms of the disease. Betty was diagnosed exactly 2 years ago.

There are many risk factors associated with ALS that stem from muscle weakness. As the disease progresses, patients become increasingly immobile; immobility is associated with numerous hazards in almost all body areas. Gastric motility decreases, with concurrent nausea, indigestion, and constipation. Circulation is decreased, which can cause kidney problems, decreased urine output, edema, and decreased healing ability.

The respiratory system is affected in several ways. The muscles of the diaphragm and the chest may be weakened from the disease itself, so respirations become more shallow; secretions are not moved effectively. This is the most life-threatening problem; ultimately, patients with ALS may need tracheostomies and mechanical ventilation because they do not have the muscle power to breathe, or they get respiratory infections that they cannot overcome. Risk to the respiratory system is increased by swallowing difficulties that occur as muscles in the mouth and throat weaken. These swallowing difficulties increase the chance of choking and aspirating food or liquid into the lungs, which leads to either sudden death or aspiration pneumonia. Betty has experienced swallowing problems, but has not had problems with severe choking or pneumonia.

Knowledge regarding a chronic, terminal illness with its corresponding physiologic, psychological, social, cultural, and spiritual effects also is necessary preencounter information. The nurse must be knowledgeable and look for signs and symptoms of continually declining physical abilities to care for self and cope with the environment. How quickly patients experience the deterioration in functioning associated with chronic terminal illness is very individual, even for those with similar diseases. Nurses must be aware of the ranges of normal decline, and observe the degree and speed of change for each individual patient. Anticipating the patient's changing safety needs is particularly important with regard to declining functional abilities.

There also are several psychosocial concerns that accompany chronic terminal illnesses. Loss of independence and major role changes within the family and society are only two of the possible changes with which patients must cope. Some patients are anxious to know what to expect, and others prefer not to know. The nurse must assess the patient's readiness to learn about the illness and its ongoing impact on physical and psychosocial functioning. Grieving and impending death, which affect spiritual and cultural responses, are also paramount concerns that affect not only the individual but also the family and significant others.

⊃Action Learning #67: Identifying Possible Sources for the Knowledge Needed to Prepare for Data Collection With Betty

Make a list of at least three sources from which to gain the knowledge needed in Betty's situation. Follow the format below.

Area of Knowledge   **Sources of Information**

Think about this ■ How much of the knowledge did you already have? The more experienced you are, the more you will have already stored in your memory for instant retrieval. How much time did it take to find the proper sources? Most beginning students find the hunt for multiple sources of information to be a very time-consuming activity that requires perseverance. Did you identify the areas on the TNT checklist that correspond with knowledge?

The Thinking Needed to Put All the Pieces Together to Structure Data Collection Efficiently and Effectively

The following is a short example of the thinking used (combination of TOTAL RE-CALL and INQUIRY) to begin one small but very important segment of effective, efficient data collection:

> Betty has ALS.
> ALS causes the muscles of swallowing to weaken.
> Weakened swallowing muscles allow patients to aspirate food and liquids.
> Aspirated food and liquid can cause either immediate death or infections such as pneumonia.
>
> *Therefore*, the following are key pieces of data needed from Betty:
>
> How are her swallowing muscles right now?
> If they are weakened, what types of problems occur with swallowing? With certain types of foods or liquids? Saliva?
> Has she ever choked? How did she handle it?
> Does she know what to do for choking?
> Do her significant others know what to do for choking?
> What are her long-range plans for weakened swallowing muscles?
> Does she understand her high risk for aspiration?

This same process is used with all the available information about Betty. The more the nurse knows and *thinks* about before the initial encounter, the better prepared he or she will be for focusing data collection and data analysis on the most important areas first.

COMBINING THINKING SKILLS, KNOWLEDGE, THE NURSING PROCESS, THE PATIENT, AND YOU (THE NURSE)

This section draws on what was learned in Chapters 7 and 8 regarding data collection (finding clues) and data analysis (making sense of the clues and clusters of clues). After the nurse prepared for the assessment by reviewing the areas of knowledge that would be needed most, *thinking* about all the possible relationships and identifying key questions to address, data were collected and initially analyzed using a blank form of the Nursing Assessment Tool shown in Figure 13-1.

Read through the data on the completed tool to obtain an overall picture of Betty's health status. Remember that the recorded data are "objective" (what the nurse can see, touch, hear, and so forth), "subjective" (what the patient or significant others say), and necessary inferences (objective data for which there is no precise means of measurement). Interaction was the primary method of collection, but observation and measurement were necessary as well. The use of D.E.T.A.I.L. (see Chapter 7) was helpful in collecting information about Betty's discomfort after her fall.

As data were collected, initial hunches were developed. Those hunches are noted by stars the nurse placed next to the nursing diagnoses (listed for each response area) that *could* be assessment conclusions about the data. As you read, think about the reasoning behind these initial hunches. Also, write down any additional hunches you thought of that were not listed. Make a copy of the TNT checklist (streamlined) in Appendix E and keep it close by to track the thinking as it is described.

First Impressions

As the data are collected (or read about), *thinking* also occurs—initial hunches and preliminary conclusions are formulated.

⊃ACTION LEARNING #68: What Are Your First Impressions?

Briefly list your first impressions after having read the data. What do you think about Betty as a person? What do you think are her greatest concerns? What do you think are her nursing needs?

THINK ABOUT THIS ■ One of your first impressions probably is "Wow, that's a lot of information; where do I even begin?" It can be overwhelming if you do not begin to see relationships among the data; there is too much information to remember as single pieces. How did the tool help you initially to cluster pieces to show relationships? When did your thinking move you beyond seeing the basic clusters of data in the tool to seeing more complex relationships among the data? How will your first impressions affect the rest of your data collection?

Comparing Data With Norms and Standards to Identify Relevant Data

Some of the information on the tool is either "normal" for the general population or "normal" for Betty. How do you tell the difference? The answer is by using your knowledge to determine population norms, and asking the patient about her individual norms. Obviously, a medical diagnosis of ALS is not a population norm, and is relevant data. Examine the following pieces of data and judge whether they fit with population norms or with Betty's individual norms.

- Retired at age 46
- Alert and oriented to person, place, and time
- Sleeps 8 to 9 hours a night
- Needs help with bathing and grooming activities
- Difficulty with chewing and swallowing
- Pulse = 86

This preliminary thinking—comparing data with norms and standards—is a major factor in accurately identifying the patient's health concerns. This phase of thinking is extremely dependent on knowledge and experience, and thus presents a major challenge to beginning students. Beginners are expected to determine when they don't know something and be able to look it up so that they will know it. (Note the section on the first page of the TNT checklist, in which comparing data with norms is addressed.)

What is even more challenging is that looking something up does not complete the task. Even if the nurse has a "photographic memory" and can completely recall all the facts about ALS, that by itself is useless unless the T.H.I.N.K. modes are used to identify the relationships between those facts and this particular patient's responses to ALS.

Developing Initial Hunches

The nurse's first set of hunches was based on the diagnostic labels (from the NANDA taxonomy) presented at the top of each pattern or subpattern on the tool. These initial hunches illustrate how the tool can provide logical "preclustering" of data. The nurse placed a star in the margin of each area that seemed to have relevant data during the data collection. The star was a reminder of the thinking that took place during data collection. Remember, collection (finding clues) and analysis (making sense out of clues) occur simultaneously. The star also served as a reminder to do more with the data.

Many hunches come to mind as data are gathered. It is important to note them *and* keep an open mind to all possibilities. Many nurses jot down ideas in the margins or on separate paper as they use the assessment tool. Think about a system that works best for you to prevent you from narrowing your thinking too soon or forgetting an important hunch.

Initial hunches are triggers to further thinking (mainly more TOTAL RECALL and INQUIRY) about what additional data are needed (data gaps). Directed data collection fills in data gaps to rule in or rule out hunches. Below is a list of initial hunches. Some of them overlap and may be considered as differential diagnoses for the same patient response. Read through the list and think about whether there are any foundations for these hunches.

Impaired Verbal Communication
Impaired Social Interaction
Knowledge Deficit about stair climbing problems
Fear of loss of independence and need to live with mother

Impaired Physical Mobility
Activity Intolerance
Fatigue
Diversional Activity Deficit
Impaired Home Maintenance Management
Self-Care Deficits: bathing and grooming
Altered Growth and Development
Pain
Anxiety about finances
Risk for Peripheral Neurovascular Dysfunction
Ineffective Breathing Patterns
Risk for Infection
Risk for Injury
Risk for Disuse Syndrome
Risk for Altered Nutrition
Impaired Swallowing
Risk for Aspiration
Constipation
Family Coping: Potential for Growth
Decisional Conflicts

⟳ACTION LEARNING #69: Validating Hunches

Pick three of the above hunches.

#1 _____

#2 _____

#3 _____

Ask yourself the following questions for each hunch (you will need a nursing diagnosis reference book or nursing theory text to help you answer the questions):

Are there data on the assessment tool to support these conclusions?

#1 _____   #2 _____   #3 _____

Do the formal label definitions in a diagnostic manual fit with this patient's situation?

#1 _____   #2 _____   #3 _____

Are there defining characteristics in the data base that fit with the defining characteristics in a diagnostic manual?

#1 _____   #2 _____   #3 _____

What additional data, if available, would help support the label?

#1 _____   #2 _____   #3 _____

Which differential diagnoses need to be considered?

\#1 _____   \#2 _____   \#3 _____

THINK ABOUT THIS ■ What was the most challenging part of this task? Did it get any easier by the end? What shortcuts did you begin to develop to do this efficiently without sacrificing accuracy? What areas on the TNT checklist represent this activity of validating hunches?

Overview of the Nurse's Thinking to Determine Conclusions of Assessment

Examine the nurse's thinking about the hunch "constipation." The Nursing Assessment Tool helped to identify basic clusters of data. These clusters frequently led to the initial hunches. The following data cluster supporting the hunch "constipation" is found in the Nursing Assessment Tool.

Data Cluster

> BM every other day
> "I get constipated easily"
> Metamucil most days
> Drinks 1–2 glasses of water or pop/day
> Walks only short distances
> Medical Dx. of ALS
> Takes iron, baclofen, and nortriptyline

Basic knowledge and thinking needed to determine that the data in this cluster are relevant to constipation are as follows:

Most adults have a bowel movement every day, but every other day is not that unusual.

Patients who say they are constipated usually are constipated, but some also have "perceived constipation," so this will need to be ruled out.

Metamucil increases bulk in the gastrointestinal (GI) tract and helps diminish problems with constipation.

Water intake of one to two glasses per day usually is not adequate fluid for maintaining normal bowel movements.

Decreased physical activity (walking short distances) hinders GI motility and can lead to constipation.

A symptom of ALS is decreased GI motility, which can lead to constipation.

Iron, baclofen, and nortriptyline all have the side effect of constipation.

According to *NANDA nursing diagnoses: Definitions and classification 1997–1998* (NANDA, 1996, p. 18), the definition and defining characteristics for the diagnosis of constipation are as follows:

> *Definition:* A state in which an individual experiences a change in normal bowel habits characterized by a decrease in frequency and/or passage of hard dry stools.
>
> *Defining characteristics:* Decreased activity level; frequency less than usual pattern; hard formed stools; palpable mass; reported feeling of pressure in rectum; reported feeling of rectal fullness; straining at stool.
>
> *Other possible characteristics:* Abdominal pain: appetite impairment; back pain; headache; interference with daily living; use of laxatives.

What other data in Betty's case, if added to the cluster, would better support the conclusion of constipation? There were data gaps in these areas:

- The patient's normal bowel movement pattern before ALS
- The effects of the Metamucil on her bowel patterns
- Other signs or symptoms of constipation identified under defining characteristics or other possible characteristics

Another question the nurse had was, "What are the possible differential diagnoses to be considered?"

"Perceived constipation" and "colonic constipation" needed to be differentiated. The nurse examined the definitions and defining characteristics for these differential diagnoses in the same diagnostic manual. Because neither of these diagnoses fit this patient, the nurse made the decision to rule out these options and rule in her original hunch. This ruling-in process was the culmination of validating both the data and the diagnostic label. (Note the question on the TNT checklist about differential diagnoses.)

The nurse thought about all of the hunches in the same way. Most of the hunches were validated by definitions and defining characteristics. The next step was to consolidate the hunches into a manageable group for designing care. This required cluster analysis and a look at the big picture to determine which hunches were better dealt with as related factors to other problems. This task required that the nurse use INQUIRY and NEW IDEAS AND CREATIVITY to find the clusters best suited to becoming assessment conclusions. It also required that the nurse think ahead to planning by asking, "If I plan care for this problem, will it also cover that problem?" (Find the item on the TNT checklist that addresses this issue.)

This thinking is illustrated by the following example. Instead of writing three separate plans for Impaired Home Maintenance Management, Fatigue (weakness), and Impaired Physical Mobility (unsteady gait), the nurse recognized that all three issues could be handled in one diagnosis:

> Impaired Home Maintenance Management related to weakness, unsteady gait, and living in a two-floor apartment

This is an example of how clustering hunches that are related to each other can streamline the design of care. This example also illustrates how two nurses caring for the same patient could label their conclusions somewhat differently and yet be equally thorough in covering all concerns. Imagine the time it would take to write a plan for each of the original 24 hunches (or even half of them) if they were all valid. This would not be an efficient use of valuable nursing time. Thinking ahead and finding the best clusters results in much better time management and coordinated patient care.

⟲ACTION LEARNING #70: **Finding the Best Clusters**

Reexamine the initial hunches. Look for the clusters that will allow the nurse to consolidate those hunches. In other words, which hunches are related to each other? Write out a nursing diagnosis that illustrates the clustering of hunches. Don't hesitate to jot down ideas until you come up with the best cluster. Circle your final conclusion.

THINK ABOUT THIS ■ What was the most challenging aspect of this activity? What sources did you use to help guide your thinking as you were doing it? What will be the best way to validate your thinking and decisions?

MAJOR CONCLUSIONS OF ASSESSMENT

The next area of focus during assessment requires the nurse to select the best labels for all the major conclusions of assessment, and then share those conclusions with the patient. Those conclusions include the patient's:

A. Strengths
B. Health concerns categorized as:
  1. Nursing diagnoses
    a. Problem responses
      (1) Actual
      (2) Potential
    b. Wellness responses
  2. Interdisciplinary problems
  3. Problems for referral

Although the nurse already would have validated all conclusions with supporting data, for the sake of this discussion the supporting data are listed in Display 13-1.

DISPLAY **13-1. Summary of the Major Conclusions of Assessment for Betty**

STRENGTHS

High school graduate plus business college degree

Lives in a safe neighborhood with supportive neighbors who bring in meals three to five times a week

Twenty-year-old son lives in same apartment complex and provides transportation, shops for groceries, and does laundry

Close friends from church help in negotiating the health care system to get services she needs

Health and medical care coverage with HMO

Former employer (apartment management firm) is providing apartment and utilities at no cost to her now that she can no longer work for them

Making plans for her death with funeral home, minister, family, lawyer

Made arrangements with ex-husband to care for 16-year-old son after her death

Sixteen-year-old helps with laundry, meals, and getting up and down stairs to bedroom and full bathroom

Making arrangements with Department of Social Services for financial needs during extent of her illness

Sees MD regularly and dental checks every 6 months

Fairly well-balanced food intake

Bilingual

Alert and oriented ×3

Sleeps well

Likes to write poetry

Cares about personal appearance

Good sense of humor and good self-esteem

Vital signs stable

No smoking and no ETOH intake

Flu shot 10/98

Effective coping skills and problem-solving skills

HEALTH CONCERNS

Nursing Diagnoses

Actual Problems and Supporting Data

1. **Constipation related to inadequate fluid intake, side effects of medications, decreased mobility, decreased intestinal motility 2° ALS**

▼ **DATA CLUSTER**

Defining characteristics:	**Data supporting related factors:**
BM every other day	Drinks 1–2 glasses water or pop/day
Metamucil most days	Walks only short distances
"I get constipated easily."	Dx. of ALS
	Takes iron, baclofen, and nortriptyline (all of which can cause constipation)

2. Diversional Activity Deficit related to difficulty with reading, confinement to apartment, recently quitting job, limited energy 2° ALS

▼ **DATA CLUSTER**

Defining characteristics:
"I get bored."
"I've worked all my life and I'm not used to all this free time."
"I don't do any exercise at all."
Home alone

Data supporting related factors:
"I'm becoming far-sighted; I have trouble reading."
Quit job 1 month ago
Can go out only if someone takes her out
Can walk short distances only
Uses walker

3. Bathing and Grooming Self-Care Deficits related to weakness, shortness of breath, and unstable movement 2° ALS

▼ **DATA CLUSTER**

Defining characteristics:
Only takes shower when someone is there to help
"I can't shampoo my hair well anymore"

Data supporting related factors:
Unsteady gait
Weakness, esp. on left side
Can sit on chair, but not in tub itself
Gets short of breath and fatigued with activities
Dx. of ALS

4. Impaired Home Maintenance Management related to weakness, unsteady gait, and living in two-floor apartment

▼ **DATA CLUSTER**

Defining characteristics:
Home very cluttered
"I can't do housework."
"I can't drive, cook, or clean."

Data supporting related factors:
Unsteady gait
Weakness, esp. on left side
Uses walker for limited walking; wheelchair ordered
"It's hard to go up and down stairs"

5. Decisional Conflict about making changes in daily living activities and safety of home environment related to changes symbolizing decreased independence and reluctance to burden friends at holiday time.

▼ **DATA CLUSTER**

Defining characteristics:
"I can't seem to decide to move my bed to the first floor."
"I haven't started using the transfer belt."
"I'm still trying to manage the bath on my own."
"I make up my mind and then I change it."
Friends report patient is prone to changing her mind frequently about day-to-day decisions

Data supporting related factors:
"Every change seems to mean I am more dependent on someone."
"I need help to sort through things before the bed comes down, and this is such a busy time of year for my friends."
"I feel bad about taking up so much of everyone's time."

continued

DISPLAY 13-1. Summary of the Major Conclusions of Assessment for Betty

Wellness Nursing Diagnosis
Potential for enhanced effective preparation for death

▼ **DATA CLUSTER**

"I've talked to the minister and funeral home."

"I've come to accept the fact that I will die soon, probably this coming year."

"I had family and individual pictures taken while I still looked healthy."

"I've talked to my sons about how they will cope with my death."

"I talked to my ex-husband about caring for our youngest son."

"I wrote my eulogy."

"It's not death itself that I fear, but the interim time before I die."

"I've always been very organized and logical."

Potential (Risk for . . .) Problems

1. **Risk for Injury related to unsteady gait, weakness, living in two-floor apartment, spending much time alone, history of a fall, slippery kitchen floor, clutter on floors, and patient's usual pattern of wearing socks rather than shoes at home**

▼ **DATA CLUSTER OF RISK FACTORS**

Progressive weakness and unsteady gait 2° ALS

Weakness, esp. on left side

Bedroom and full bath on second floor of apartment

Lives with one son who is in school during the day

Son walks up stairs behind her but does not hold on to her or use a belt

Has not yet moved bed to first floor

No safety bars in bathroom

Kitchen floor tiled and slippery; carpeting in other rooms

"It's too much trouble to put shoes on so I usually just wear socks. I should wear shoes more."

Fell yesterday in kitchen and injured face

Clutter in many areas of apartment; patient unable to clean by herself

2. **Risk for Infection (especially respiratory and urinary) related to weakness of muscles of respiratory system, decreased mobility, swallowing difficulty 2° ALS, insufficient fluid intake, environmental irritants during cold weather, and exposure to many people bringing in food**

▼ **DATA CLUSTER OF RISK FACTORS**

Shallow respirations 2° ALS

Increased chance of aspiration of food and fluids because muscles used for swallowing weakened

"Cold air, aerosols, and smoke make it hard to breathe."

Food prepared and brought to patient by several different people

Drinks 1–2 glasses of fluid per day

3. Risk for aspiration related to swallowing difficulties due to weakened muscles 2° ALS

▼ **DATA CLUSTER OF RISK FACTORS**

"It takes a long time for me to swallow; I have to chew a long time and eat small amounts."

"I don't know how to do a Heimlich maneuver; neither do my sons."

"I worry about choking."

Drinks thin liquids

Interdisciplinary Problem

Altered Nutrition and Fluid Intake related to impaired swallowing and meal preparation by neighbors (Dietition and Speech Therapist)

▼ **DATA CLUSTER**

5' 2", 100 lbs

Increased weakness/fatigue with activities, including eating

"I seem to eat less at each meal."

Drinks 1–2 glasses of water or pop each day

Dinners prepared and brought in by friends three to five times per week

"I have to chew well and eat smaller portions; it takes longer to swallow."

Uses walker; wheelchair ordered

Homebound alone, except for 16-year-old son who goes to school

Dx. of ALS

No income since retirement

Problem for Referral

No income since retirement

The thinking behind these conclusions is discussed in greater detail in the following chapters as the plans of care are examined. How did you rate the nurse's thinking when using the TNT checklist?

The final validation of the conclusions listed in Display 13-1 will not take place until the plan is evaluated after implementation. An important validation at this stage, however, is for the nurse to confer with Betty and see whether she agrees with the nurse's decisions. A brief dialogue describing how this occurs, as well as how priorities are set, is presented in the next section.

SETTING PRIORITIES WITH THE PATIENT

Guidelines for setting priorities were discussed in Chapter 9. Briefly, the guidelines suggested the following order of priorities:

1. Immediately life-threatening issues
2. Safety issues
3. Patient identified priorities
4. Nurse identified priorities (based on the overall picture of each health concern in relation to other concerns and the patient as a whole person, and availability of time and resources)

Keeping these guidelines in mind, the nurse proceeded with the validation of her conclusions and worked with Betty to determine the best use of their time and energy to plan care. The conversation with Betty went something like this:

"Betty, I have asked you a lot of questions and found out a lot of information about you as a unique person with ALS. My job as a nurse is to determine what health care needs you have so we can decide what, if anything, you want to do about them.

"Nursing has developed some standardized labels for the different health care needs that people experience. We call these nursing diagnoses. I want to share with you my thinking about your health care needs and the resulting nursing diagnoses that I believe are appropriate to help us focus your care. There are also some conclusions about areas of need for which we can get help from others."

The list of conclusions was shared with Betty, and there was further discussion to explain and clarify any concerns she had. She agreed with all of the conclusions as stated above.

"Now we need to decide which are the most important things to work on first, keeping in mind that we can work on several issues simultaneously. One system for deciding how to start is to use the following guidelines."

The guidelines are shared and explained to Betty.

"Although you are not experiencing any immediately life-threatening issues, the risks for infection, injury, and aspiration definitely qualify as safety issues. I believe it would be best for you if we address these areas first."

Betty agrees. If she didn't agree, however, the nurse would need to help her recognize the consequences of her decision. First, the nurse would attempt to increase Betty's understanding of the seriousness of these issues. Sometimes, additional information is all that is needed. Other times, the patient uses the defense mechanism of denial and has difficulty accepting the life changes that are occurring. This requires patience and support on the part of the nurse. Still other times, the patient just has a different set of values and is not willing to be concerned about safety issues. In this case, the nurse must focus on other areas of care, especially when the patient is not hospitalized and is not in a health care-controlled environment.

With the life-threatening and safety parts of the guidelines addressed, the nurse then encourages Betty to identify the next area to work on. Betty says she is most concerned with the Self-Care Deficit and the Constipation. The nurse is concerned with the Decisional Conflict about making changes in daily living activities because this is strongly connected to the safety issues. Betty agrees that the safety issues are related, but really wants the other issues dealt with first. Both agree to work on all three areas simultaneously.

The remaining nursing diagnoses, interdisciplinary problems, and problems for referral also will be worked on. For example, the nurse can make the phone calls about the interdisciplinary problem with nutrition and the problem for referral to social services after this visit with Betty and before her next visit. Use the TNT checklist to rate the nurse's thinking while setting priorities.

CLOSING COMMENTS

This chapter has provided an expanded view of how thinking skills, knowledge, and the nursing process are combined, taking into account the patient and the nurse, to work toward great nursing. The *thinking* and *doing* in Betty's case study illustrate how the nurse moves from preencounter thinking to working with Betty in setting priorities for her care. The TNT checklist has provided some structure to follow the thinking as it occurs. The next chapters continue to track the nurse's thinking as plans of care are designed for the major conclusions of assessment.

THINKING LOG #13 ▶

Part of being a caring nurse is thinking about how you would feel and what you would want if you were a patient. It is easy to distance oneself from patients and become impersonal. Put yourself in Betty's situation. What would you think about the nursing process being used if it were used with you? Write a short paragraph describing your thoughts and feelings.

References

Erikson, E. (1963). *Childhood and society* (2nd ed.). New York: WW Norton.
North American Nursing Diagnosis Association. (1996). *NANDA nursing diagnoses: Definitions and classifications, 1997–1998.* Philadelphia: Author.

14

Designing, Doing, and Determining Quality of Care for Actual Problems With Multiple Related Factors

�֍ Learning Outcomes

After reading and doing the activities in this chapter you will be able to:

Explain approaches to caring for a patient with nursing diagnoses categorized as actual problems.

Discuss the importance of identifying all related factors for designing and doing care and determining quality of care.

Critique a poorly developed plan for selected actual problems with multiple related factors, and create a better plan.

It is now time to complete the phases of the nursing process for Betty. Assessment and the early stages of planning with Betty were covered in Chapter 13. To finish the process, designing, doing, and determining quality of care must be completed. As discussed in Chapter 9, "designing" refers to planning care *with* and *for* the patient. "Doing" refers to the implementation phase of care. "Determining quality" focuses on evaluation of the care. These three phases of the nursing process, which are constantly intertwined with assessment, must be accepted as tightly interwoven and approached as a collective set of activities.

This chapter explores care as it is planned, implemented, and evaluated for nursing diagnoses that are actual problems for Betty. Actual problems are those for which the defining characteristics of the problems (signs and symptoms) exist. Betty's potential (Risk for ...) problems, wellness nursing diagnoses, interdisciplinary problems, and problems for referral are discussed in later chapters.

All five of Betty's actual problems have multiple related factors, each of which must be addressed in the overall plan for great nursing care to occur. The role of related factors is highlighted in this chapter to show how critical they are to individualized, thorough nursing care.

The number of factors contributing to problems varies from patient to patient. It often is easy to identify the most obvious related factor, stop at that point, and miss others. Because Betty's case has so many interrelated issues, her problems are complex, with many related factors. Studying her case provides a good example of the value of addressing *all* related factors.

For language clarification, remember that the terms "etiologies," "related factors," and "contributing factors" mean the same thing. Throughout this chapter, "related factors" is used most often.

Although all five of Betty's actual problems are discussed, only two are examined in detail. For those two, care plans of poor quality are presented for study. One of those plans is transformed to a better plan to illustrate the qualitative differences between poor and good plans.

There are two reasons for examining plans of poor and better quality. First, seeing what something should not be is a good way to learn what it should be. Think about that for a minute. Human nature seems to make it easier to critique something someone else did inadequately than to create something from scratch by oneself. Many people can offer suggestions or fix something that doesn't "look right" more easily than they can put words on a blank sheet of paper. Critiquing something that is done poorly is frequently less anxiety-producing than attempting to create a high-quality product from one's own resources.

The second reason involves trying to understand qualitative differences. One way to understand something is to describe what it is not. This works especially well for abstract ideas related to quality. Suppose, in planning to hire a nurse–manager, one tried to describe ideal characteristics. A first response might be, "We want someone who really works well with people." To clarify the abstract notion of working well with people, a common response would be to describe what is not wanted. "Someone who doesn't push her views over everyone else's" or "Someone who doesn't get upset easily" might be given as descriptions. Describing what one does not want is a common method of communicating what one does want. Therefore, studying some lesser-quality (but not unusual) care plans provides a safe, low-anxiety learning opportunity that builds on human nature.

REVIEW OF BETTY'S ACTUAL PROBLEMS

In Chapter 13, a list of the conclusions of assessment made from analyzing the data in Betty's situation was presented. Several nursing diagnoses were made, which included five actual problems that fall within the domain of independent nursing practice:

Self-Care Deficits
Impaired Home Maintenance Management
Diversional Activity Deficit

Decisional Conflict

Constipation

Each of these problems has several factors contributing to it. The formal diagnostic statements included all the related factors. The next few pages explore those statements and the thinking involved in planning care for the problems. The first two nursing diagnostic statements are:

Bathing and Grooming Self-Care Deficits related to weakness, shortness of breath, and unstable movement, 2° amyotrophic lateral sclerosis (ALS), and no safety bars in bathroom

and

Impaired Home Maintenance Management related to weakness and unsteady gait, 2° ALS, and two-floor apartment living arrangement

Both are challenging problems. Because the related factors are similar, the thinking that goes into planning care for one of these problems can be applied to the other. The reason these problems are so challenging is that the related factors are brought on by the ALS, which will get progressively worse. Setting up outcomes that focus on regaining function is unrealistic. If the weakness, shortness of breath, unstable movements, and unsteady gait cannot be reversed, one might well question whether anything can be done about these related factors.

A shift of thinking is needed—away from regaining function toward compensating for those deteriorating areas. Compensation calls for using the patient's strengths to overcome the deficits. Remember, Betty said she was logical and a good problem solver. A creative nurse will get her engaged in considering safe, energy-saving ways to manage some of her own care and decrease the clutter in her house.

The third diagnosis is

Diversional Activity Deficit related to difficulty reading, confinement to apartment, recently quitting job, and limited energy 2° ALS

This is a highly personal issue. Not everybody likes to watch TV, tie fishing flies, or play card games. Finding pleasurable diversional activities is important to emotional health. When usual activities are impossible, however, finding comparably rewarding ones calls for creativity and individualized interventions on the nurse's part.

The fourth diagnosis is

Decisional Conflict about making changes in daily living activities and home environment to maintain safety related to changes being symbolic of decreased independence, reluctance to burden friends at holiday time, and limited finances to purchase support bars for bathroom

This is a complex problem. Because Betty is having trouble deciding to make changes, she is adding to her safety risks. A first impulse in planning care for this problem might be to say sternly to Betty, "You've just got to make these decisions because it is a matter of safety."

⤴ACTION LEARNING #71: Thoughts on Being Directive With Betty About Her Decisional Conflict

Think about the approach to dealing with Betty's decisional conflict (that is, sternly saying "You've just got to make those decisions because it is a matter of safety.") described in the preceding paragraph. Answer these questions:

1. What are the advantages and disadvantages of this approach, the purpose of which is to promote patient safety?

2. Does this approach promote safety?

3. How does this approach reflect the nurse's knowledge and thinking about the intellectual and emotional components of behavior change?

4. How does this approach reflect planning *with* the patient?

5. What are some likely outcomes of this approach?

THINK ABOUT THIS ■ This approach might work; it could intimidate Betty into cooperation, which would result in safety being maintained, but at what cost? Decision making is an emotional and intellectual activity that is very personal. Simply knowing that something should be done is not enough. If you do not believe that, think about the health behaviors you know you should be practicing—exercising, dieting, quitting smoking, relaxing, and others. If you know you should exercise daily, why do you not just make up your mind and do it? Well, there are many reasons that are personal to you. Someone saying, "You've just got to exercise" is not going to make a big difference, is it? Remember this when you work *with* patients. This diagnosis is explored further, with poor and better care plans, later in this chapter.

The last nursing diagnosis concerns the actual problem of constipation. It also has multiple related factors.

Constipation related to inadequate fluid intake, side effects of medications, and decreased mobility 2° ALS

This diagnosis entails somewhat less complexity than the emotion-laden decisional conflict, but care for this problem must take into account other factors, such as the patient's swallowing problems and the progressive nature of her mobility deficits. This diagnosis also is examined further, with a written care plan, later in this chapter.

Before moving to the written care plans, notice again that each of the actual problems has many related factors. The significance of related factors and their role in achieving great nursing care cannot be treated lightly.

THE ROLE OF RELATED FACTORS AND THEIR SIGNIFICANCE TO CARE

Identifying all of the factors contributing to each actual problem is very likely one of the least well done parts of the nursing process. Yet it is one of the most valuable parts of designing individualized care. Find the item on the Tracking Nursing Thinking (TNT) checklist (Appendix D) that addresses related factors.

Often nurses will correctly identify a problem but list only the medical diagnosis as a contributor to the problem. Betty's case illustrates how easily this can be done. Almost all of Betty's problems can be traced back to her ALS. It would be easy to say she has Constipation related to ALS, Self-Care Deficits related to ALS, Diversional Activity Deficits related to ALS, Impaired Home Maintenance Management related to ALS, and a Decisional Conflict related to ALS. Except for the Decisional Conflict, which seems to be pushing the issue a bit far, all of the problems are present because she has ALS. Any nurse recording nursing diagnoses in this short manner would be correct; however, such diagnoses would be hard to plan care for. Essentially, the ALS is a "done deal"—nothing can undo it—and the nurse therefore would have nothing to work with in planning care.

That is not to say that ALS is not a contributing factor to those problems. Indeed, it is important to know that ALS is a related factor. If Betty had self-care deficits because of a stroke, very different approaches could be taken. People who suffer strokes can regain some of their function; many return almost to prestroke function. Amyotrophic lateral sclerosis is, however, progressive; it gets worse instead of better. Care can focus only on compensating for the decreased function, not on regaining lost function.

The medical diagnosis may be listed as a related factor by itself or it may be linked to the functional changes caused by it. In Betty's case, the term "secondary to" (2°) is added to make clear which functional areas are linked to the medical problem.

By itself, however, the medical diagnosis as a related factor is limiting. It is much more helpful to stretch one's thinking to the next level and ask what functional issues are contributing to the problem. Those functional issues, although traceable to the medical problem, often are areas for which care can be planned. Knowing, for example, that Betty's difficulty with home maintenance is related to her living in a two-floor apartment, that she has trouble going up and down stairs, and that she has weakness and an unsteady gait secondary to ALS, allows the nurse to focus on helping Betty move her center of living to one floor and find ways to compensate for her weakness. ALS by itself would not provide that direction.

Delineating more specific related factors allows the nurse and patient to develop individualized outcomes and corresponding nursing interventions. In Betty's case, nursing interventions might include, among other things, getting her a long-handled duster, putting a bin by the stairs where she could place things that needed to go upstairs, and getting devices to help her grip more easily.

Such nursing interventions are much more individualized than they would be if the only identified related factor were the ALS. Individualization of care, therefore, depends almost completely on a well identified list of related factors that goes beyond the obvious one, which is usually the medical problem.

Hindrances to Thinking Beyond the Medical Diagnosis as the Only Related Factor

Several obstacles limit the nurse in identifying all of the appropriate related factors. The primary cause is forgetting to engage all five thinking modes. Stopping the search for related factors once the medical diagnosis is listed is symptomatic of a nurse's use of just the HABIT mode; it can become a habit to link everything to the medical problem.

A second cause is the nurse's limited understanding of the domain of independent nursing practice. If only the medical diagnosis is listed as a related factor for a nursing diagnosis, it implies that nursing care is needed only to care for the complications of the medical diagnosis. A problem identified in this way actually becomes an interdisciplinary problem, and not a nursing diagnosis.

The third obstacle, one that takes a lot of time and energy to overcome, is limited experience and knowledge. Limits in experience and knowledge hinder the nurse from conducting more extensive data analysis, including:

- Looking for relationships among data and data clusters that point to related factors
- Accepting the fact that problems rarely have only one related factor
- Thinking ahead to planning
- Considering the big picture of the patient's situation as planning commences

The final obstacle that plagues even expert nurses is time. Thinking requires time. For beginning nurses, who may not be totally convinced that they need to find all the related factors, the additional time it takes becomes a concern. Hopefully, the value of taking the time is becoming apparent.

Recognizing When Related Factors Have Been Missed

Often it is not until a plan is being developed that less-obvious related factors are found. Sometimes additional factors become apparent as a plan is being implemented; perhaps something is not working or something seems to be missing. An evaluation that reveals unmet goals also may be the point of realization. Suppose, for example, that while implementing Betty's care plan for Impaired Home Maintenance Management, the nurse found that Betty had always pampered and picked up after her son, who had a habit of leaving piles of stuff by the front door, rarely hung up his clothes, and left a trail of food wrappers and dirty dishes everywhere. The nurse might not have seen this behavior if the home visits occurred while the son was at school. Betty's son's behavior and her past habits would be additional factors contributing to her inability to maintain her home. A plan that did not address these factors would fall short of the goal of a less cluttered, clean environment. Weeks might go by with Betty using her new techniques to no avail before that additional factor emerged.

Another clue that related factors have been missed is difficulty in planning care. The nurse looks at the problem and the related factors and feels stumped as to what can be done. The usual methods of linking the patient outcomes to the related factors just do not work, as might be the case when only the medical diagnosis is identified as a contributor. When that happens, and there seems to be no logical flow in "reversing" the related factor to find outcomes, the nurse should question the diagnostic statement. If the problem is one for which the nurse feels something can be done, but the outcomes are not being achieved, there is a high probability that the related factors are not well defined. It is then time to look back to the existing data or collect more data to find all the factors contributing to the problem.

Still another clue to inadequate identification of related factors emerges when the nursing diagnosis for one patient looks just like those for other patients. Related factors are very individual. Although nursing diagnosis texts list many possible related factors for each nursing diagnosis, most patients will have specific factors not found in other patient situations or in books. In Betty's case, although weakness and unsteadiness are common to many patients with ALS who have self-care deficits, the fact that she has no safety bars in her bathroom is unique to her living situation.

Uniqueness of Related Factors to Patients

Very few, if any, patients have exactly the same response to anything, because everyone has unique resources and deficits. It is easy to lose sight of this while caring for several patients who do share many similarities. For an example, consider caring for several patients with Alzheimer's disease. Some nursing homes have units specially planned for these patients because they have many common problems. These patients lose part of their memory and often act in ways that are baffling to their families and care providers. There is no treatment for this disease, but these patients require extensive nursing care. Commonly, these patients wander, forget who they are and where they are, eat inedible things, get upset easily, and exhibit a host of other behavioral responses.

While planning care for these patients, it is easy to identify the related factor for most of their problems as confusion secondary to Alzheimer's disease. However, there also are unique factors that contribute to each person's responses. A man who was a soldier might get more confused around loud noises; a woman who was a piano teacher might be calmed when she hears music and more confused in a completely quiet environment. The challenge to nurses is to go beyond the obvious confusion factor to other, less obvious related factors. Often, the less obvious factors are keys to effective interventions.

There is no magic number of related factors that one can expect to find for each problem. There may well be only one, but in most cases there are several. There also are cases in which the related factors are unknown. For example, "Anxiety related to unknown causes" might be a diagnosis for a person who has a vague feeling of dread but who cannot figure out why that feeling is there. When the related factor is unknown, the nurse initially aims the care toward helping the patient identify the possible factors contributing to the problem. The desired outcome of care would be for the patient to try to identify the causes of the anxiety. If that proved impossible, the next best plan would be to deal with the signs and symptoms of the anxiety.

A nurse also may have a hunch about related factors yet not feel a high degree of certainty about them. Rather than leave those less-certain factors out of the diagnostic statement, it is best for the nurse to add the word "possible" in front of those factors. An example of a nursing diagnosis written in that format is "Functional Incontinence related to immobility and possible reluctance to ask for help." In a case like this, the nurse might suspect the patient is not asking for help, but may not know for certain that this is happening. Having that possible related factor is important for providing thorough care; leaving it off until the nurse is certain of the factor would delay necessary interventions focused on the patient asking for help. Including "possible" related factors is an excellent example of the nurse's thinking-in-process about the patient's problem. Find the item(s) on the TNT checklist that address "Thinking toward planning ... "

DESIGNING CARE WITH BETTY FOR HER ACTUAL PROBLEMS

Each of Betty's actual problems has been discussed briefly. Now it is time to look at two of these in greater detail. First, the Decisional Conflict will be explored. Two plans of care are presented. The first is one completed by Sue Swift, a fast-moving nurse whose major priority is efficiency. Her plans focus on the immediately recognized, usual interventions. Even though she has the benefit of a well-worded, thorough diagnostic statement to start her plan, she develops a poor plan. Another nurse, Thelma Thoreau, expands that plan into a more individualized, complete approach that addresses all the components of the problem and its related factors. Following the plan for Betty's Decisional Conflict is a plan for Betty's Constipation, also completed by Sue. You will be asked to take on Thelma's role and transform that plan into a better one.

Sue's Care Plan for Decisional Conflict

Look at Sue's Care Plan #1. Before reading Thelma's Care Plan, do Action Learning #72.

▼ **Sue's Care Plan #1**

Nursing Diagnosis:
  Decisional Conflict about making changes in daily living activities and home environment to maintain safety, related to changes being symbolic of decreased independence, reluctance to burden friends to help during holiday time, and limited financial resources to purchase support bars for bathroom.

Goal:
  By the end of 1 month, the patient will have made the right decision to make changes in her daily activities and home environment.

continued

▼ **Sue's Care Plan #1 continued**

OUTCOMES	NURSING INTERVENTIONS	RATIONALE
Patient will:		
1. Identify three problem-solving techniques.	1a. Ask pt. what she knows about problem-solving techniques b. Teach her about problem solving c. Ask her to list three techniques	Determining what a pt. knows before teaching something new saves time
2. Select a technique she likes.	2. Explain which technique would be best in her situation and encourage her to use it	Helping pt. pick options increases chances of success
3. Learn how to use technique with decision conflict.	3a. Help her use technique with the changes she needs to make b. Correct errors in her use and support her	Correcting errors increases chances of success
4. Make good decisions.	4a. Talk to her friends and tell them she really needs them to help because she is having trouble asking b. Check out other community resources for financial assistance c. Monitor patient's follow-through on decisions	Using all available resources increases chances of success

⊃Action Learning #72: Critique of Sue's Plan

Carefully analyze Sue's plan, write down what areas are poorly developed, and explain why you think they are less than ideal. Use the TNT checklist to help your critique.

THINK ABOUT THIS ■ Compare what you wrote with these observations:

Sue's care plan follows an appropriate format. It has a goal, outcomes, and nursing interventions. The goal is client centered and has a time frame. The goal comes close to flowing from the problem statement by addressing "decision making." The outcomes, nursing interventions, and rationales are numbered sequentially.

This critique, however, exhausts the positive comments. Unfortunately, there are more problems with Sue's plan than there are positive aspects. First, the goal is quite value laden. The "right" decision implies there is only one "correct" choice. A month as a time frame is probably too long, considering the safety ramifications of this problem.

The outcomes should flow from the goal and relate back to the related factors. In Sue's plan, the outcomes are not focused on the related factors. There is no outcome that focuses directly on the symbolism of changes, reluctance to burden friends, or finding resources. Sue's outcomes focus on Betty learning problem-solving techniques, which are intellectual processes, but they are devoid of reference to the emotional issues in this conflict. The first two outcomes are measurable and specific, but the last two are vague and not measurable. Outcome #3 uses the verb "learn" as a behavioral outcome. Although this term is often used, it is not measurable. Can one see learning? Not really; one can see the consequences of learning, such as passing a test, demonstrating something, or applying knowledge. If one is aiming for "learning" a technique, then an outcome such as applying the technique to the decision conflict would be measurable. The fourth outcome has that vague, value-laden "good," which is like "right." What is "good?" The desired decision would need to be spelled out (eg, "will decide to ask for help").

On the whole, the outcomes fall short because they are not individualized to Betty. The factors contributing to her conflict are not used as guides for the desired outcomes. They superimpose an intellectual fix onto an emotional conflict, which could seem to the patient to be a devaluation of her emotional concerns.

The nursing interventions, on face value, fit with the outcomes, but there is very little that is individual to Betty's situation. The interventions are vague. "Teach her about problem solving" does not give much guidance or reflect much thought. Even if problem-solving teaching were what Betty needed, she would not get much with those general guidelines. How should those be taught?

Which techniques would be best in Betty's situation? Why teach her three techniques; why not two or four or one?

The nursing interventions that accompany outcome #2 do nothing to help Betty *select* a technique. The nurse is only advocating telling Betty which is best. If a nurse truly wants a patient to choose, then care should be directed to helping the patient make the choice, not to directing the choice.

The nursing interventions for outcome #3 are so vague they are hardly worth writing down. "Help" is a catch-all word. The type of help needs to be specified. "Correcting errors" implies, again, that there is a right and wrong way to use a technique. It is a fluff-type of nursing action with very little depth to it.

The interventions for the fourth outcome simply do not fit with that outcome. If the nurse wanted the patient to make the decisions, why would the nurse make the decisions for her? That is what is recorded in 4a and 4b, under "Nursing Interventions." These last interventions could be seen as the nurse's true intent—to do this *for* the patient. It is akin to saying, "Here is what should be done; I'll just do it." It takes away the patient's participation in care.

Thelma's Care Plan for Betty's Decisional Conflict

Thelma's plan of care shows thought that went back to the nursing diagnosis itself. There is a clear focus on the emotional aspects of this problem, and there are no attempts to devalue Betty or her dilemma.

The selection of Decisional Conflict as a valid nursing diagnosis was based on several factors. First, there is clear evidence that Betty is having a decisional conflict. The definition of Decisional Conflict fits with her situation, as do the defining characteristics and the related factors as found in a nursing diagnosis textbook.

Second, the decisional conflict is prohibiting her from restructuring her lifestyle and environment to maintain an acceptable level of safety. Without these changes, she is very likely to fall and experience unnecessary pain and discomfort from bruises or, worse, broken bones. This could increase her immobility, which would increase her risk for infections, especially respiratory infections. This could very likely accelerate her death.

In thinking through these issues, Thelma considered changing the nursing diagnosis instead of planning care for that specific problem. Looking at the big picture, it was obvious that one of Betty's major problems was "Risk for Injury." Because this was already a diagnosis, Thelma thought at first that it would save time simply to add "Decisional Conflict" as an additional related factor to that conclusion. The resulting diagnosis would then read:

> Risk for Injury related to unsteady gait, weakness, living in a two-floor apartment, spending much time alone, history of falls, slippery kitchen floor, clutter on floors, patient's usual pattern of wearing socks rather than shoes at home, and **decisional conflict about making changes in daily living activities and safety of home environment**

Although there is nothing wrong with this approach (it's one Sue would be apt to take), Thelma did not believe it would be the best way to handle the situation, for two reasons. First, it would make the care plan for " Risk for Injury ... " very long and cumbersome. Second, this approach would not highlight or recognize as clearly the strong emotional impact of these changes for Betty.

By developing a separate plan, Thelma was able to channel more of Betty's energy into examining the underlying issues and how they related to Betty's goals for dealing with her illness. This could, of course, be done in the "Risk for Injury ... "

▼ **Thelma's Care Plan**

Nursing Diagnosis: Decisional Conflict about making changes in daily living activities and home environment to maintain safety, related to changes being symbolic of decreased independence, reluctance to burden friends during holiday time, and limited finances to purchase safety bars.

Goal: By the end of 1 week, the patient will have made appropriate decisions to maintain safety in daily living activities and home environment.

OUTCOMES	NURSING INTERVENTIONS	RATIONALE
1. Share thoughts and feelings about changing her mind frequently, making changes that symbolize decreased independence, and her personal goals for dealing with her illness.	1a. Assist pt. to elaborate on her feelings about issues identified in objective #1 b. Actively listen, support, and comfort in decision making c. Discuss alternative ways to interpret change, eg, "change is reflection of strength and healthy problem solving"; encourage pt. to look at problem solving in different ways	1. Behavior change most sucessful if both cognitive and affective components are addressed Redefining the problem helps pt. explore new alternatives that may increase probability of change
2. List changes in daily living and home environment that will maintain safety.	2a. Help pt. identify most important changes to focus on first b. Explore with pt. current and new resources to help with changes, eg, other friends, church members, groups that assist the disabled	2. Clarification of pt.'s priorities helps nurse and pt. focus energy most effectively Use of outside resources increases probability of change
3. Describe consequences of making and not making changes regarding her goal/s for dealing with her illness.	3. Ask pt. to identify the pros and cons of making and not making changes, and impact on her goals	3. Helping pt. think ahead to outcomes of decisions helps pt. to select best decision
4. Agree to ask for help in 3 days for moving furniture, adding safety bars.	4a. Role-play with pt. to practice asking for help b. Contact alternative resources for moving and purchase of safety bars c. Assist pt. in setting date for taking action d. Monitor plan and modify as needed	4. Role-play, identifying additional resources and establishing set date increases probability of action occurring Ongoing evaluation increases probability of successful behavior change and maintaining patient safety

plan as well, but it was more likely to be slighted in that plan because the plan had become so lengthy.

Once the thinking about the diagnosis itself was accomplished, Thelma used the related factors to direct the expected outcomes for Betty's plan of care. Because of the complexity of the related factors, there are several outcomes that address each factor. With emotional issues, in particular, it often is necessary to break down how each factor is addressed into measurable increments of change. Betty needs to process these changes; quick-fix outcomes as seen in Sue's plan are unrealistic for an emotional issue with several related factors.

The "how-tos" are clearly spelled out in the nursing interventions. Specifics, such as having Betty identify what is most important, give direct guidance to any nurse who might need to follow through with this plan. There are many references to helping Betty deal with her feelings. Ultimately, it is a plan that helps Betty work through this problem, rather than one in which the nurse will take care of the problem.

Now that Thelma's plan has been analyzed, check the TNT checklist again, as you did for your analysis of Sue's plan. Look at how much better Thelma's work is in comparison. For a second chance at analysis, consider another of Sue's plans.

▼ Sue's Care Plan #2

Nursing Diagnosis:
   Constipation related to inadequate fluid intake, side effects of medications, and decreased mobility 2° ALS.

Goal: By the end of 1 week, the patient will have no constipation.

OUTCOMES	NURSING INTERVENTIONS	RATIONALE
Patient will:		
1. Increase fluid intake immediately.	1a. Teach patient about relationship between fluid intake and constipation b. Tell patient to drink things like coffee and prune juice that promote intestinal motility	1a. Fluid intake less than 1000 mL per day will lead to constipation b. Common sense
2. Change medications to ones without constipation side effects during next visit to MD.	2a. Tell patient to talk over medications with doctor and ask for changes to other medications	2a. Side effects of ferrous sulfate, baclofen, and nortriptyline = constipation
3. Continue to take Metamucil and Correctol daily.	3a. Let patient know that these may be necessary, considering the nature of her illness	3a. Limitations of activity will cause constipation

Sue's Plan for Constipation

Look at Sue's plan for Betty's constipation problem. Again, she has taken a quick-fix approach. Unlike the decisional conflict problem, constipation may seem like one that could be dealt with simply. There are few emotional issues to take into account. However, other complex aspects of Betty's situation must be kept in mind in dealing with this physiologic problem. Remember earlier discussions of how no problem can be viewed in isolation from the other problems and the big picture of the patient's situation.

⊃Action Learning #73: Becoming Thelma

Now it is your turn to try your hand at being Thelma. Analyze Sue's care plan and transform it into a plan that addresses the problem and all the related factors, taking into account the big picture of Betty's situation. Here is a hint: remember that Betty has trouble swallowing. Thin liquids are more apt to be aspirated into her lungs than are thick liquids. Remember, outcomes should be measurable and specific. Nursing interventions should be specific enough to allow another nurse to use the plan and continue interventions. Look at the resources you have to help you with this task. If you have the NIC and NOC books, you can find suggestions for outcomes and interventions by cross-referencing them with this nursing diagnosis. If you have a care plan guide book, you may find sample plans to help you get started.

Use the TNT checklist to help you check your work. Share your plan with a classmate. Note where your plans differ, and discuss how you each came to the conclusions you used in planning. So that you have plenty of room to write, think, revise, and rewrite, you may want to do this exercise on a separate sheet of paper.

THINK ABOUT THIS ■ How did it go? Are you a better care planner than Sue? Was your plan similar to or different from that of your classmate? How did the big picture guide your planning? What is the most useful thing you learned from this activity that will help you the next time you write a plan for a patient's constipation?

DOING AND DETERMINING QUALITY OF CARE WITH BETTY

Most of the exploration of Betty's actual problems has focused on the designing of care, or care planning. As everyone knows, that is only part of the picture of the nursing process. Because this is a book, however, the implementation of care can only be discussed, not actually carried out. Because the care, as designed, cannot be implemented, it cannot be evaluated. Therefore, anything said about implementation and evaluation is conjecture only. Nevertheless, it is important to think about how Thelma's plans would be implemented and evaluated.

If the plan was developed *with* Betty, rather than *for* Betty, chances are that some of the implementing, or "doing" of the care, would have started as the plan was being developed. Betty would have started thinking about and sharing her ideas about the decisional conflict and, therefore, would already have started to meet some of the outcomes. As the plan was implemented, the nurse and Betty would start to evaluate the outcomes by comparing Betty's progress with the preset outcomes.

A most important thing to keep in mind is that implementing and evaluating must be considered during the planning phase. A well-designed plan of care will take into account the realities of doing the plan. It will allow for ease of evaluation; for example, the outcomes will be specific and measurable. Also, remember that implementing and evaluating may reveal new data that were not addressed in the original plan. In particular, additional factors contributing to the problems may emerge.

Thelma's plan for Betty's decisional conflict had a goal that was to be met in 1 week. If Thelma visited Betty daily, they might work on the decisional conflict plan a little each day. Thelma very likely would evaluate the plan as the week progressed and make changes as needed. Look at Thelma's SOAP note to see what may have occurred. (If you need to review the basics of the SOAP form of documentation, review Chapter 11.) Notice how the changes in the plan are based on the new data that were found when Thelma implemented the plan. The new data are documented in the "S" and "O" parts of the note. The "O" also includes the report of what the nurse did. Thelma specified which outcomes had been met and which were not yet met in the "A" part. Remember, the "A" is the conclusion part of the SOAP note. The conclusions of evaluation focus on how the patient is progressing, as measured against the preset goals and outcomes. In the "P" part of her note, Thelma referred to the plan's changes.

Here is Thelma's SOAP note:

12/20/98 3 PM Problem: Decisional Conflict
S: "It has been helpful to talk about this. I know I just need to get this
done, but I really cannot ask anyone to help me until after the holi-

days. Could you check with the Independent Living Center (ILC) about putting in the safety bars in January?"

O: ILC offered as resource for installing bars without expense to patient. Lengthy discussions with patient about need to make decisions as soon as possible.

A: Goal partially met. Outcomes 1, 2, and 3 met. Objective 4 unmet due to patient's insistence on waiting until after the holidays.

P: Time frame changed to 4 weeks for goal. Outcome 4 time frame mid-January. Role playing will be done at that time. Will contact ILC in early January.—T. Thoreau, S.N.

Thelma's note documents what was done in relation to the problem of Decisional Conflict, and how the patient is progressing toward the goal and outcomes on the plan. The implementation and evaluation of care and Thelma's thinking are evident. Look at the TNT checklist and check which of the areas under "Conclusions of Evaluation" are completed well, as evidenced by Thelma's note.

CLOSING COMMENTS

The process a nurse would use to plan care for two of Betty's five actual problem nursing diagnoses has been described. It is important to remember that this represents only part of the process. A full regimen of nursing care for Betty would include plans relative to the other three problems as well.

Betty's case illustrates the complexity of designing great nursing care. From Sue's care plans, one can see that quick-fix approaches compromise patient individuality and safety. Thelma's plan, although it required more time to develop, reflects the type of individualized care that most people would want for themselves and their loved ones.

Taking the time and energy to discover all the possible related factors for each actual problem is worthwhile in terms of the guidance that related factors provide during care planning. Thinking through the complexities of each patient's unique situation and looking for the less-obvious relationships among data provide the nurse with a means to find those related factors.

Once the problems and all the related factors are identified, individualized care can be designed if the nurse is continually aware of the big picture of the patient's situation. Thinking about how each patient response affects others and thinking ahead to implementing and evaluating care gives the nurse the tools to design great nursing.

Implementation and evaluation complete the cycle of the nursing process. Evaluation "returns" to assessment as the nurse collects more information to see how the patient is progressing.

THINKING LOG #14 ➤

Compare your thinking style with Sue's and Thelma's. Which nurse do you think you will be more like? Knowing how you think, what areas of designing care for actual problems will come easily to you? What areas will be most difficult? Hopefully, Thelma will be your ideal. Develop some memory aids for yourself so that you can think in the manner that Thelma does.

15

Designing, Doing, and Determining Quality of Care for Potential (Risk) Problems

✳ *Learning Outcomes*

After reading and doing the activities in this chapter you will be able to:

Explain approaches to caring for a patient with nursing diagnoses categorized as potential (risk) problems.

Describe the differences in thinking, structuring, and planning when working with actual problems and risk problems.

Critique and improve a poorly developed plan for a selected risk problem.

In this chapter, as in the last one, Betty's case is used to illustrate how great nursing is planned, implemented, and evaluated. Whereas the last chapter focused on actual problems, this chapter focuses on the problems for which Betty is at risk. After discussion of several important issues that differentiate actual problems from risk problems, one of Sue's plans for a potential problem is presented. A critique of her plan and a revised plan illustrate differences in quality of planning. An additional plan of Sue's is presented for your critique and revision.

At several points in this chapter, the reader is reminded of other chapters in which particular concepts were first discussed or discussed in greater depth. Use your KNOWING HOW YOU THINK mode to determine how you want to use these reminders. Some like to go back immediately and check the material. Others find this too disruptive to their continuity of thinking, and choose to ignore the cross-referencing for the time being. They would rather do the cross-referencing later, when they reread. Use whichever system works best for you.

DEFINING POTENTIAL (RISK) PROBLEMS

Terminology Clarification

As was mentioned in earlier chapters, synonymous terms are used in the nursing literature to describe problems for which patients are at risk, including "risk problems," "high risk problems" and "potential problems." The North American Nursing Diagnosis Association (NANDA) moved from using "potential" to "high risk" in 1992. Later, the "high" was dropped so that "risk for" is currently the terminology used in the NANDA Taxonomy (NANDA, 1996). Recently published nursing diagnosis books use the later terminology; earlier books use the term "potential" or "high risk."

The change from "potential" to "risk for" helps clear some of the confusion that can arise in distinguishing between the terms and among types of nursing diagnostic statements. For example, "possible" and "potential" are two terms that are sometimes confused. "Possible" problems are hunches, or problems that the nurse thinks exist but for which there is insufficient data to say for certain. With potential—or risk—problems, the data exist, but they are risk factors for a problem that could occur, not data that support an existing problem.

Another clarification of terms is the distinction between risk factors for illness-related responses and risk factors for wellness responses, in which there is potential for change to a higher level of wellness. The terminology recommended by NANDA for wellness nursing diagnoses is "Potential for enhanced"—for example, "Potential for enhanced parenting."

A brief review of Chapters 6 and 8, which describe the conclusions nurses make after analyzing data, including conclusions about potential problems, might be helpful before continuing with this chapter.

Differences Between Actual Problems and Potential (Risk) Problems

Because actual problems exist, the focus of care is to diminish or remove them. Potential problems do not exist, so the focus of care is health promotion or illness prevention, which makes up a big part of a nurse's job. These activities are not simple, however. Identifying problems that are likely to occur and planning care to prevent those problems require a well-functioning thinking cap and a sound knowledge base.

Some of the differences between actual problems and risk problems were discussed in Chapters 6 and 8. Three of those differences are reviewed and expanded on in this chapter: thinking differences, structural differences, and planning differences.

Thinking Differences

The biggest differences between diagnosing actual and potential problems lie in the thinking skills used and the amount of knowledge and experience needed for the thinking. Actual problems are easier to diagnose because they are more easily supported by patient data. Potential problems are a bit trickier. One has to "know" from books and from experience which conditions are likely to contribute to certain problems. The nurse must use INQUIRY to see that A + B + C, especially when D is present, will very likely lead to problem #1.

To illustrate this formula, consider a familiar nursing diagnosis, "Risk for Impaired Skin Integrity," which is a potential problem that many patients have. In any given patient situation the nurse especially needs to know, among other things, the following about skin:

> Skin is the body's main defense against infection and must be maintained intact.
> The skin does its job best when it is clean, dry, and has good circulation.
> Breaks in the skin disrupt the normal functioning of the skin and allow organisms to enter the body.
> Organisms grow well in warm, wet, dark places.
> Urine is irritating if left in contact with the skin for long periods of time (incontinent patients experience this).
> Sitting for long periods of time cuts off circulation to the parts of the body that are being sat on.
> Skin that is overly dry and thin or fragile is more easily broken down than skin that is normally moist and healthy.
> Good skin turgor means the skin will "bounce back" after it is moved or pressed.
> Sitting for long periods of time in one place creates warm, moist, dark places on the perineum and the buttocks.

This list could be much longer, but the point is that a nurse must have at least this level of knowledge and experience to anticipate potential problems with skin integrity. Along with this knowledge, the nurse uses INQUIRY to see the relationships between these facts and the individual patient situation, and then comes to the conclusion that a patient is or is not at risk for impaired skin integrity.

⊃Action Learning #74: What Is the Risk?

Look at the following three situations and determine whether the patient in each situation is at risk, and if so, for what. Explain your thinking to a classmate and indicate what knowledge was needed to make your decision.

1. Tommy has just started to crawl. His parents are collectors of blown glass art pieces and like to display them on the floor-to-ceiling shelves and the coffee table in the living room. The art work is very colorful.
   Is Tommy at risk?
   If yes, for what?
   Knowledge needed?

2. Mr. West has just read a new food fad book and is trying to convince you that nature's wonder food is bananas. He has decided to eat nothing but bananas for the next 2 weeks to cleanse his body of all the toxins it has built up over the years.

> *Is Mr. West at risk?*
> *If yes, for what?*
> *Knowledge needed?*

3. Ms. North has just lost her husband. She is new to the city and has no close friends. She just started a new job and says she just wants to bury herself in her work and get on with life.

> *Is Ms. North at risk?*
> *If yes, for what?*
> *Knowledge needed?*

THINK ABOUT THIS ■ How did you come to your conclusions? Which pieces of your thinking fit with TOTAL RECALL? Which fit with INQUIRY?

Structural Differences

EXISTENCE OF THE PROBLEM

An actual problem exists when the patient data "paint a picture" of that problem. A potential problem exists when the problem is "likely to occur" if something isn't done; data that support the related factors are found, but the actual problem does not exist.

TERMINOLOGY

For actual problems, the nurse simply states the nature of the problem (patient response). Examples include "Self-Care Deficit," "Impaired Gas Exchange," and "Parental Role Conflict." For potential problems, the problem label is preceded by the words, "Risk for." Examples are "Risk for Self-Care Deficit," "Risk for Impaired Gas Exchange," and "Risk for Parental Role Conflict."

EXISTENCE OF DEFINING CHARACTERISTICS TO SUPPORT THE PROBLEM

Defining characteristics *must* exist to support the problem if it is to be labeled an *actual* problem. Defining characteristics *do not exist* for potential problems. If the defining characteristics existed, there wouldn't be a potential problem anymore; there would be an actual problem.

DATA TO SUPPORT THE RELATED FACTORS

Data to support the related factors almost always exist for actual problems. Sometimes an actual problem can exist and the causes are "unknown," but there is no denying that the problem exists. A common example is, "Anxiety related to unknown causes." With a potential problem, however, there must always be data to support the related factors, or there wouldn't be a potential problem.

One might wonder how many related factors need to exist before the nurse diagnoses a potential problem. The answer comes with experience. In some cases, one factor is enough to alert the nurse; in other cases, several factors must exist before the nurse's antennae go up. This is another one of those probability issues. After nurses have taken care of several people with similar circumstances, they are able to make those judgments with a higher probability of accuracy. Think of this situation: An alien from another planet is driving a car. The car stops running when the gas gauge moves from "F" to "E." The first time this happens, the alien might not see the connection; however, after it happens a second or third time, she would say, "Oh, when that little thing moves toward `E,' the car is likely to stop; I'd better do something before that happens." She has learned from experience that there is a potential problem. She also could have read about this situation in a manual for operating a car to obtain some "knowledge."

Planning Differences

FOCUS OF THE PATIENT GOAL

When dealing with an actual problem, it obviously makes sense to try to remove or alleviate the problem. Basically, nursing is focused on *restoring* the patient to the optimum level of health, and that means diminishing or eliminating the problem. (An aside: It is important to note here that there are situations in which the patient has an actual problem but it is not feasible to restore health or eliminate the problem because the patient has a chronic or acute deteriorating condition. In these cases, maintenance and comfort are appropriate goals. For a patient who has total incontinence because of irreversibly damaged nerves, for example, a goal of continence is not realistic. A goal of comfort without constant wetness is the only option.)

The focus of the goal when dealing with a potential problem is different. Because the problem doesn't exist (yet), there are two basic approaches to planning care. One approach is to try to keep the patient at his or her existing level of health (*maintain*) and not let things get worse. Maintenance goals are often written in the negative form. The identified problem for which the patient is at risk will not occur; for example, "the patient will have no skin breakdown" if he is at risk for skin impairment. The other option is to help put the patient at even less risk (*promote* to a higher status of health). Here are two examples that show the difference between maintenance and promotion:

Maintaining status: A patient who has had a stroke can easily get contractures (shortening of ligaments and tendons so that a part of the body stays in a permanently flexed position). A typical nursing diagnosis is "Risk for contractures related to paralysis and lack of active movement." The goal for this patient would be to **maintain** full range of motion. Stated another way, it could be, "The patient will not develop contractures."

Promoting higher status: A patient who has diabetes, but who does not follow his diet carefully and who does not take insulin as directed, can have problems such as hypoglycemic or hyperglycemic reactions (blood sugar levels that are too low or too high), circulatory problems, infections, and many others. A typical nursing diagnosis is "Risk for hyperglycemic or hypoglycemic reactions related to nonadherence to diabetic diet and insulin schedule." The goal for this patient is to **promote** a higher level of care. Often the word "promote" is not actually used. Rather, the specific action that indicates health promotion is used; in this case that might be, "Patient will adhere to diet and insulin regimen."

Table 6-1 in Chapter 6 summarizes the differences between actual and potential problems. You may want to return to that chapter for a review.

INTERFACE OF POTENTIAL PROBLEMS DIAGNOSED BY NURSES, MEDICAL PROBLEMS DIAGNOSED BY PHYSICIANS, AND PROBLEMS DIAGNOSED BY OTHER PROVIDERS

At times, diagnosing potential problems gets into the fuzzy realm of what is a nursing diagnosis, what is a medical diagnosis, and what is a diagnosis made by another health care provider. Recall earlier discussions of the conclusions nurses reach from analyzing data—patients' strengths and health concerns—with the health concerns being nursing diagnoses, interdisciplinary problems, and problems for referral.

Usually, the distinctions among the three different types of health concerns in the domain of nursing are easy to see. If a patient has severe chest pain, obviously a nurse would refer that person to a physician. It is fairly easy to see that a person who has hypertension and who needs counseling on diet and lifestyle changes has interdisciplinary problems. If a patient who has trouble getting to the bathroom because of mobility deficits is incontinent, a clear nursing diagnosis conclusion can be made (Functional Incontinence related to mobility deficits). Or if a family is adjusting well to the new baby and wants to continue, the wellness diagnosis is Potential for enhanced family growth. Other times, however, the distinction is not so clear. Subtle differences must be distinguished.

In the realm of nursing diagnoses, nurses focus on patients' response patterns, not on diseases. The actual problems that nurses are licensed to treat and are capable of treating independently are human responses. When it comes to diagnosing and treating areas of risk, however, nurses go beyond the confines of responses to include risks for diseases as well. Diagnosing *actual* pathologic conditions (illness or disease) is the domain of physicians. But diagnosing the *risk* for a disease is within the realm of nursing because nurses can intervene to prevent a disease from occurring.

For an illustration of the difference between diagnosing an actual disease and diagnosing the risk for a disease, look at these examples:

> Mrs. Grey has an indwelling urinary catheter and she does not drink very much. Mr. Brown, the nurse, knows that most people who have indwelling catheters get urinary tract infections, especially those who do not drink lots of fluids. Although the nurse would not diagnose an actual urinary tract infection, the nurse would diagnose the patient's high risk for a urinary tract infection and work with Mrs. Grey to increase her fluid intake to prevent the infection from occurring. If Mr. Brown suspected the patient had a medical problem, because of blood in the urine and an elevated temperature, he would refer the patient to a physician to diagnose that problem.

> Ms. French, the school nurse, talks with a group of adolescents about their sexual practices. She finds that very few of the sexually active youths use condoms. She concludes that they are at high risk for pregnancy and contracting AIDS or other sexually transmitted diseases. She diagnoses the risk, although she would not diagnose the diseases themselves. Her interventions include helping the adolescents change their behaviors to decrease their risk.

This review and enhancement of previous information on potential problems is presented to help the reader see how the nurse came to the conclusions about Betty's risk problems and how care was planned, implemented, and evaluated for those risk areas.

DESIGNING CARE WITH BETTY FOR HER POTENTIAL PROBLEMS

In Chapter 13, these three nursing diagnoses of potential problems were made based on the data in Betty's case:

> Risk for Injury related to unsteady gait, weakness, living in two-floor apartment, spending much time alone, history of a fall, slippery kitchen floor, clutter on floors, and patient's usual pattern of wearing socks at home.
> Risk for Infection (especially respiratory and urinary) related to weakness of muscles of respiratory system, decreased mobility, swallowing difficulty 2° amyotrophic lateral sclerosis (ALS), insuffi-

cient fluid intake, environmental irritants during cold weather, and exposure to many people bringing in food.

Risk for Aspiration related to swallowing difficulties due to weakened muscles 2° ALS.

At first glance, these diagnoses seem very long-winded. That is often the nature of "risk" nursing diagnoses for patients who have many factors contributing to one area of risk. Betty, like many patients with chronic illnesses, has many risk factors that must be addressed. Some nurses shorten the diagnostic statement by indicating the risk factors just once (such as on the care plan), and then recording only the area of risk (eg, injury, infection, aspiration) for future documentation (such as SOAP notes). This practice would seem logical for the first two diagnoses described here.

How the ``Risk" Nursing Diagnoses Fit Into the Big Picture of Betty's Care: The Nurse's Thinking

One could ask why the nurse decided on these three areas of risk. Here is some of the nurse's thinking that took place as the areas of risk were considered relative to the big picture of Betty's care:

Is there a need to address the risk of infection and the risk for aspiration separately? Yes, the two are closely related because aspiration ultimately can lead to pneumonia, which is an infection, but aspiration also can be immediately life threatening because Betty could completely occlude her trachea and not be able to breathe. If the aspiration risk is addressed only in terms of the infection, a plan of action for an aspiration emergency might not be addressed.

Are these potential problems more of a priority than the actual problems? Yes, although they are not life threatening yet, they are potentially more life threatening than the Constipation, Self-Care Deficit, Diversional Activity Deficit, and Impaired Home Maintenance Management, which have been identified as actual problems. The Decisional Conflict actual problem is closely related to the Risk for Injury, so it is of equal priority to the potential problems. Injury, infection, and aspiration could each result in early death; therefore, it is a high priority to intervene to prevent these things from occurring.

How do these "risk" diagnoses overlap with the other health concerns? Risk for Injury is closely related to Betty's decisional conflict. If she can make decisions to move her bed downstairs, she will eliminate some risks for injury. The plan of care for the decisional conflict should be referred to in the plan for decreasing the risks for injury. The risks for aspiration and infection are related to the interdisciplinary nutrition problem. Interventions by the dietitian and speech therapist could decrease Betty's risk for aspiration and therefore decrease her risk for infection. As plans are developed for the aspiration and infection risks, the interdisciplinary plan should be addressed simultaneously.

How well did the nurse do toward achieving the items on the Tracking Nursing Thinking (TNT; see Appendix D) checklist, under the category "Consider the `big picture' when finalizing all conclusions of assessment?"

Sue's Plan for Betty's Risk for Aspiration

Once again, Sue's nursing care plan provides food for thought. With her usual speed she developed a plan for Betty's "Risk for Aspiration" nursing diagnosis. Read Sue's Care Plan #1 and think about how it could be better.

Sue's goal is that the patient will have no episodes of aspiration. This is the easy way out—to say that the problem for which Betty is at risk will not occur. In Betty's case, however, this goal, although ideal, is not realistic. Despite all that Betty or her nurse might do, Betty still could have an episode of aspiration. Sue should be focusing on decreasing the risks for aspiration. In other words, she should be promoting a higher level of functioning (decreasing the risk) rather than just maintaining present functioning.

Sue, then, merely repeats the goal as an outcome. There is very little that can be measured in terms of patient outcomes based on that goal. This outcome only offers two options, either there is *no* aspiration or there is aspiration. There is no in-

---

▼ Sue's Care Plan #1

Nursing Diagnosis: Risk for Aspiration related to swallowing difficulties due to weakened muscles 2° ALS

Goal: Patient will have no episodes of aspiration

OUTCOMES	NURSING INTERVENTIONS	RATIONALE
1. No aspiration.	**a.** Make sure patient knows about dangers of aspiration	Aspiration can occur when muscles in mouth and throat are weakened
	b. Teach patient and son the Heimlich maneuver	Everyone should know this emergency procedure
	c. Make sure patient sits upright when eating	Gravity helps food and liquids go down
	d. Tell patient not to drink thin liquids	Thin liquids can be aspirated more easily when muscles of swallowing are weakened

between option for the reality of Betty's situation. The related factor of the nursing diagnosis is not addressed in the outcome. The swallowing difficulties are what put Betty at risk. Outcomes that provide criteria to measure the status of the swallowing difficulties are needed; otherwise there is no way to determine whether any change in the risk factors has occurred.

The nursing interventions, in Sue's usual form, are very short and provide very little detail for any other nurse who might need to follow this plan with Betty. The first intervention (a) is important, but if implemented as stated, it could scare the patient into not eating. Betty is already nutritionally compromised, so it would not be clinically sound to act in any way that would make one problem worse while trying to correct another problem.

The second intervention (b) is a good idea, but there is not enough detail about the best method for teaching the patient. Because of the age of Betty's son and the fact that Betty could be alone when she aspirated food or fluid, individualized approaches to teaching should be spelled out in greater detail, especially considering Betty's decreased mobility.

The third intervention (c) is not realistic. Sue could not "make sure patient sits upright when eating" because Betty lives at home and does not have a nurse present at all times. The nursing intervention must focus on how the patient can manage at home. Betty needs to understand how sitting upright is relevant to decreasing her risk of aspiration so that she can adapt her life at home to doing just that. Sue's nursing interventions do not suggest ways for nurses to help her do that.

The fourth intervention (d) is dangerous because of Betty's existing low level of fluid intake. Merely telling Betty not to drink thin liquids would make the fluid intake problem worse, and would be counterproductive to the plans to alleviate Betty's risk for infection and her constipation problem (see Chapter 14).

Each rationale in Sue's plan is related to its corresponding nursing intervention. The list of rationales, however, is incomplete because Sue's planned nursing interventions are incomplete. If she studied any references on the care of patients who are at risk for aspiration, she would have found that there are much better rationales for much better nursing interventions.

Thelma's Plan for Betty's Risk for Aspiration

Thelma's plan is much more comprehensive and reflects much more study of the principles of care for patients at risk for aspiration. She clearly had the big picture of Betty's case in mind as she developed this individualized, clinically sound plan. As you examine Thelma's plan, compare her work with the items on the TNT checklist.

The goal of Thelma's plan is realistic. It does not indicate that Betty will not aspirate, as Sue's plan did. Considering the nature of Betty's illness, it would be impossible to ensure that Betty never has an episode of aspiration. Thelma focuses on decreasing Betty's risk by promoting a higher level of functioning. She also focuses on Betty's need to have an emergency plan for an aspiration episode.

▼ **Thelma's Care Plan**

Nursing Diagnosis: Risk for Aspiration related to swallowing difficulties due to weakened muscles 2° ALS.

Goal: Within 2 weeks, patient will decrease risk of aspiration and have plan for dealing with aspiration emergency, as evidenced by:

OUTCOMES	NURSING INTERVENTIONS	RATIONALE
1. Describing the mechanisms of swallowing and how her muscle weakness puts her at risk (week 1).	1a. Explain to Betty how swallowing muscles work to prevent food from going into trachea b. Use pictures to show her the anatomic landmarks that are relevant to swallowing c. Reinforce Betty's present understanding of need to chew longer and eat slowly	1a. An increased level of knowledge will allow patient to understand the risks b. Multisensory learn- will enhance understanding of abstract information c. Building on present knowledge and strengths will enhance learning
2. Agreeing to eat and drink only while sitting upright with head tilted slightly forward (week 1).	2a. Determine Betty's usual position for eating b. Using pictures, show Betty how the position of the body and head helps food move into the esophagus, not the airway	2a. Eating is often associated with other behaviors that are unique to each person b. The upright position keeps the tongue forward and allows food to be better formed into a bolus; tilting the head back opens the airway
3. Describing the best foods and fluid consistency to prevent aspiration (week 1).	3a. Assess Betty's food likes and dislikes and help her plan how to adapt these to a mechanical soft consistency b. Help Betty plan for moving to pureed foods as muscles weaken further c. Reinforce need to eat foods that are not too hot d. Encourage Betty to maintain a fluid intake of at least 2000 mL per day	3a. Adapting patient's favorite foods to therapeutic diet will increase compliance with dietary changes b. Pureed foods are less apt to be aspirated c. Hot foods can cause a gasp reaction, which could trigger aspiration d. Fluid intake is vital to maintaining circulation and kidney function, and to preventing infection

Continued

▼ **Thelma's Care Plan** *continued*

OUTCOMES	NURSING INTERVENTIONS	RATIONALE
	e. Suggest drinks that are of nectar consistency by adding thickening agent (eg, gelatin) to favorite juices and eating foods high in fluids, such as custards, creamed cereals, creamed soups, and milk shakes	**e.** Thin liquids may be aspirated more easily than thick liquids; thick liquids allow patient more time to swallow, giving weakened muscles a better chance to work fully
	f. Incorporate all diet changes into written list for neighbors who bring food	**f.** People who prepare foods need guidelines; otherwise patient has to adapt foods
	g. Coordinate actions with interdisciplinary plan with dietitian and speech therapist	**g.** Coordinated interventions provide for better continuity of care.
4. Developing a plan for managing an aspiration emergency (week 2).	**4a.** Teach Betty and her son how the Heimlich maneuver is done, using a stuffed shirt and pants "dummy" for practice Help Betty find furniture of correct height to use to push against if she should choke while alone	**4a.** Actual practice with the technique will allow for better learning and will allow nurse to correct imperfections in technique
	b. Provide a written set of directions to post in the house as reminders	**b.** Written reminders will allow others to be prepared for an emergency and will reinforce teaching
	c. Encourage Betty to eat alone as little as possible; suggest that she eat high-risk favorite foods only when someone is present	**c.** It is much more likely that effective removal of aspirated food can be accomplished by others than by patient herself

For more details on swallowing disorders, see Emick-Herring, B., & Wood, P. (1990). A team approach to neurologically based swallowing disorders. *Rehabilitation Nursing,* *15*(3), 126–132.

The outcomes on Thelma's plan are specific and measurable. When the time comes for evaluation, Thelma will have clear outcomes developed to compare with Betty's future behaviors to determine change. The outcomes also focus on controlling the factors contributing to the risk (the swallowing difficulties). By aiming for control of the related factors, Thelma will decrease Betty's risk, which is the goal. In acknowledging that full control is impossible, Thelma's outcome of Betty having an emergency plan is realistic.

Thelma's planned nursing interventions are specific enough that any nurse could continue the plan in Thelma's absence. Rather than just making comments like "teach the patient ... ," Thelma records teaching strategies. She advocates using pictures and indicates how to make a dummy for Heimlich maneuver practice.

Thelma's interventions are individualized for Betty. They focus on assessing Betty's usual patterns so that necessary changes can be incorporated into the patient's individualized habits and tastes. There is a clear orientation of the interventions to a home care situation. Whereas Sue wrote "make sure patient sits upright while eating," Thelma addressed her interventions to an adaptation of Betty's usual position for eating; she helped Betty come to the conclusion that sitting upright was best. Thelma's individualized plan also addressed Betty's strengths. Betty already knew that she needed to chew longer and eat slowly. By reinforcing that behavior, Thelma was acknowledging Betty's strength and using it to overcome a potential problem.

All of Thelma's nursing interventions are clinically sound. There are no interventions that would be harmful to other areas of Betty's health. Clearly, Thelma kept the big picture of Betty's situation in mind and did some research on swallowing problems and risks of aspiration. She adapted what she found to Betty's individual situation without compromising the soundness of the proposed interventions.

The rationales listed give additional testimony to Thelma's focus on clinically sound nursing interventions. Each rationale is clearly linked to a nursing intervention, and no intervention is left without a rationale to explain it. Thelma even added a note about a good reference on the subject of swallowing difficulties. Other nurses could check that reference if they wanted more details on this clinical problem.

Did Thelma miss any of the items on the TNT checklist?

Sue's Plan for Betty's Risk for Infection

Are you ready to critique Sue's second plan? She approached Betty's risk for infection in much the same way that she approached the aspiration risk. Again, you get to critique the plan and make it better. It is time to readjust your thinking cap and take on Thelma's role.

▼ **Sue's Care Plan #2**

Nursing Diagnosis: Risk for Infection (especially respiratory and urinary) related to weakness of muscles of respiratory system, decreased mobility, swallowing difficulty 2° ALS, insufficient fluid intake, environmental irritants during cold weather, and exposure to many people bringing in food.

Goal: Patient will have no infections, as evidenced by:

OUTCOMES	NURSING INTERVENTIONS	RATIONALE
1. Having a regular exercise program.	1a. Teach patient how she can get regular exercise b. Explain the value of exercise to prevention of infection	Increased mobility decreases risk of infection by improving circulation and respiratory function
2. Following recommendations of dietitian and speech therapist for swallowing problems.	2. Coordinate plan with other providers	
3. Increasing her fluid intake.	3a. Let patient know she should have about 2000 mL of fluid each day b. Remind patient to avoid too many thin liquids	2000 mL per day recommended for optimal fluid intake Thin liquids increase swallowing risks
4. Avoiding contact with too many people.	4a. Explain to patient how increased contact increases her exposure to germs	The more people, the more chances of infection

⊃ACTION LEARNING #75: Becoming Thelma Again

In the last chapter, you had an opportunity to try your hand at improving Sue's plan for Betty's constipation problem. Now you can do the same for Betty's risk for infection. Examine Sue's plan; find some books that address risks for infection, think about the big picture of Betty's case, and develop a plan as you think Thelma would. Use the planning part of the TNT checklist to check your work. Share your plan with a classmate and compare your approaches. As you did with Action Learning #73 in Chapter 14, you may want to use a larger sheet of paper so that you can "think" on paper as you develop your plan.

> **THINK ABOUT THIS** ■ How has your thinking evolved? Did this exercise go faster than the one in the last chapter, when you first took on Thelma's role? Chances are it still took you a long time to develop a great plan. Planning great nursing care takes time, especially for beginners, but each plan you develop gets easier. Through practice, you start to home in on the important issues more quickly.

DOING AND DETERMINING QUALITY OF CARE WITH BETTY FOR HER RISKS

Consider now how Thelma would implement and evaluate care for Betty. (Continue to track her activities on the TNT checklist.) Thelma's plan for the aspiration risk will be discussed to show how this is done. Although only one plan is discussed in this section, remember that Thelma would be implementing and evaluating all parts of Betty's care, including care for the actual problems discussed in Chapter 14 and the wellness, interdisciplinary, and referred concerns discussed in Chapter 16. She would use the same process for each part of the plan.

To implement the plan for the aspiration risk, Thelma would set up a visit with Betty. First, because she probably wrote much of the plan after her last visit with Betty, she would share all elements of the plan and ask Betty what she would like added to it. Thelma would want to find out from Betty the best times to focus on the aspiration issues. At the specified time, Thelma would begin the implementation with data collection. There are several places on the plan where interventions indicate a need to assess Betty's usual patterns—including positions for eating and Betty's food likes and dislikes. Getting Betty's personal perspective early on would allow Thelma to incorporate more personalized information into the other interventions.

Because much of the plan involves teaching, Thelma would stop periodically to see whether Betty was clear about the topics being discussed. She would ask Betty to explain what she had learned. Doing this would allow Thelma and Betty to evaluate the care because Betty's answers would indicate whether the outcomes were being met.

Thelma and Betty set a 2-week time frame for meeting the goal of this plan. The first three outcomes have 1-week time frames. Thelma and Betty, therefore, would aim to meet the first three outcomes during the first visit and would set up a second visit to focus on the fourth outcome. Such a time frame and plan would make sense, considering that Betty is being seen at home and that her son needs to be involved in the last part of the plan, which focuses on outcome number four.

Thelma therefore would bring to the first visit her teaching materials for outcomes one through three. If Betty didn't have any other pressing needs, Thelma would implement all the interventions for the first three outcomes and adapt those interventions to whatever came up during the session with Betty.

At the end of the first visit, Betty and Thelma could evaluate the first three outcomes. Using an evaluation SOAP note format (review Chapter 11 for discussion of SOAP notes), here is what an evaluation of the care at the end of week 1 might look like:

> 12/14/98 3 PM Problem: Risk for Aspiration
>
> S: "It really helps to see the pictures of my muscles involved in swallowing. I know how easy it is to choke now. I will definitely sit up whenever I eat. I've already started to see how much easier it is to swallow thicker liquids, but I never thought about using gelatin to thicken things like juice. My son should be here in the evening next Tuesday so we can practice the Heimlich maneuver. I will remember all of this much better if I can have everything in writing."
>
> O: Patient participated actively in all parts of interventions and picked up information quickly.
>
> A: Outcomes 1–3 met. Interventions effective. Goal of decreased risk being met.
>
> P: Next visit Tuesday, 12/21/98. Focus on outcome #4; son will be present. Bring written information to leave with patient. Review areas covered this week and reinforce with written materials.—T. Thoreau, S.N.

This note shows how Thelma reviewed the patient's response to the interventions by recording selected quotations from Thelma as subjective data. Thelma also recorded objective data—her observations of Betty's response. Under the "A," Thelma recorded her conclusion, which related to how the outcomes and goals were being met. Under the "P" section, Thelma recorded any plans for the future. She could have written the additional information on the plan itself and stated, "See changes in plan."

This example of evaluation shows the nursing process cycle and how nursing care is constantly adapted according to the patient's changing responses. It also shows that the nurse is thinking about the patient's progress in this area of risk.

How effective was Thelma's care according to the TNT checklist? Did you see any areas that needed improvement?

CLOSING COMMENTS

This chapter has reviewed some of the issues surrounding nursing diagnoses of patients' health concerns that involve areas of risk. By applying this knowledge to a complex patient situation, one can appreciate the importance of defining the conclusion (nursing diagnosis) accurately, viewing that conclusion as part of the big picture of the patient's situation, and planning sound care for the patient. The cycle of the nursing process continues as the nurse evaluates and revises care after it is implemented.

Although Betty's case is more complex than the case studies presented earlier in this book, the same nurse thinking processes apply. As patient complexity increases, there are more pieces of information to add to the thinking, but the thinking itself is not new.

Thinking Log #15 ➤

Continue to play Thelma's role and develop a plan for the nursing diagnosis "Risk for Injury ... ." As you develop the plan, track your thinking according to the T.H.I.N.K. modes (**T**otal Recall, **H**abits, **I**nquiry, **N**ew Ideas and Creativity, and **K**nowing How You Think). If you do not have time to develop a new plan, go back to the plan you created in Action Learning #75 for the "Risk for Infection" diagnosis, and track your thinking through that process.

References

North American Nursing Diagnosis Association (1996). *Nursing diagnoses: Definitions and classification 1997–1998*. Philadelphia: Author.

16

Designing, Doing, and Determining Quality of Care for Wellness Diagnoses, Interdisciplinary Problems, and Problems for Referral

❋ *Learning Outcomes*

After reading and doing the activities in this chapter you will be able to:

Explain approaches to care for wellness diagnoses, interdisciplinary problems, and problems for referral.

Examine the differences, similarities, and overlap among all the major conclusions of assessment: strengths, actual problems/wellness diagnoses, potential problems, interdisciplinary problems, and problems for referral.

Wellness diagnoses, interdisciplinary problems, and problems for referral are the focus of this final discussion on planning, implementing, and evaluating care for all the conclusions of assessment. That these are discussed last in no way implies that they are of less importance. Great nursing means that nurses have identified all relevant conclusions of assessment and have acted on all aspects of a patient's health care responses.

This chapter focuses on brief descriptions of wellness diagnoses, interdisciplinary problems, and problems for referral as well as the thinking behind planning, implementing, and evaluating such conclusions in Betty's case. By this time it should be self-evident that all five modes of thinking are needed to address all conclusions of assessment.

WELLNESS DIAGNOSES

Wellness diagnoses have been the focus of much debate within the nursing profession during the last decade. One point of view is that wellness issues are simply strengths. People taking this stand note that the word "diagnosis" implies a problem; wellness issues, therefore, do not fit well within the existing taxonomy. It appears that most nurses on this side of the fence work primarily in acute care settings.

Another point of view is that wellness diagnoses are very appropriate nursing diagnoses because the basic foundation of nursing is health promotion and illness prevention. Many proponents of the wellness diagnoses work in community health, maternal–child, or well child nursing settings.

This debate has been addressed in several NANDA conferences. Ongoing debate has focused on the taxonomy itself. Some nurse scholars propose a companion wellness taxonomy to parallel the current taxonomy. Another proposed approach is to consider one taxonomy with different axes for incorporating wellness diagnoses as options for any area of care.

This debate will probably continue, but meanwhile, NANDA has added wellness diagnoses to the existing taxonomy. In the proceedings of the ninth NANDA conference (Carroll-Johnson, 1991), the following guidelines for review of wellness nursing diagnoses were established:

> A wellness nursing diagnosis is a clinical judgment about an individual, family, or community in transition from a specific level of wellness to a higher level of wellness.
> 1. Label: The term "Potential for Enhanced" will be the designated qualifier. Enhanced is defined as made greater, to increase in quality, or more desired. Wellness diagnoses will be one-part statements.
> 2. Definition: The definition of the label provides a clear, precise description. The definition delineates its meaning and helps differentiate this diagnosis from all others.
> 3. Literature/Clinical Validation: A narrative review of literature is required to support the rationale for the diagnosis. A sample one-part wellness nursing diagnostic statement with related outcome criteria and nursing-prescribed interventions must accompany the submission. (pp. 375–376)

Designing Care With Betty for Her Wellness Diagnosis

Although Betty has several areas that might be considered wellness diagnoses, there was one area that particularly lent itself to a wellness diagnosis—her acceptance of and planning for her death. A search of the NANDA taxonomy did not reveal an appropriate diagnostic label for Betty's situation. Therefore, the nurse and

Betty created a diagnosis to fit the situation, "Potential for Enhanced Effective Preparation for Death."

If the nurse considers this a useful diagnosis, and it can be supported with literature and clinical validation, he or she might submit it to NANDA to review for inclusion in the taxonomy at a future date. Right now, however, the nurse's primary concern is helping Betty to continue to prepare effectively for her death. The accompanying care plan was developed.

The goal of this plan is to maintain the healthy attitudes and behaviors that Betty is already demonstrating. The outcomes also reflect a continuation of specific attitudes and behaviors. The nursing interventions include monitoring and adjust-

---

▼ Care Plan for Betty's Wellness Diagnosis

Nursing Diagnosis: Potential for Enhanced Effective Preparation for Death

Goal: Betty will maintain attitudes and behaviors that promote effective preparation for death

OUTCOMES	NURSING INTERVENTIONS	RATIONALE
1. Continue to share thoughts and feelings with nurse and significant others.	1a. Maintain therapeutic relationship by active listening and support b. Monitor for any decrease in her sharing	1. Maintaining and monitoring nurse–pt. relationship increases opportunities for caring
2. Continue to follow through on decisions regarding legal, financial, and child care issues.	2a. Discuss status of decisions, what is finalized, what is in progress b. Provide assistance in further problem solving and decision making as needed	2. Support and assistance increases effective problem solving
3. Continue to meet with pastor on weekly basis.	3. Monitor frequency of contact with pastor and pt.'s responses to those meetings; suggest increase or decrease as needed	3. Monitoring effectiveness of resources promotes effective use
4. Continue to modify living arrangements to maintain safety and minimal stress.	4. Monitor impact of declining functions and modification of lifestyle on effective coping with impending death	4. Because increase stressors can diminish coping skills, additional help may be needed soon
5. Identify changing needs as death approaches.	5. Assess for changing needs and add additional resources to plan of care when required, eg, hospice care, increased frequency of home care, respiratory equipment, and the like	5. As functioning declines additional resources can support coping skills

ing as needed, especially as Betty's physical condition worsens. The emotional stress from declining functional abilities can decrease energy for dealing with the emotional aspects of impending death.

Doing and Determining Quality of Care With Betty for Her Wellness Diagnosis

At this point in Betty's care, this plan is working very well. The nurse includes time to address Betty's preparation for death during each visit. An evaluation SOAP note after one visit might look like this:

> 12/14/98 3 PM Diagnosis: Potential for Enhanced Effective Preparation for Death
>
> S: "I really enjoy the visits from the pastor, he is a very caring person. I know he is busy but I wouldn't mind seeing him more often, I'm just afraid to bother him."
>
> O: Patient's voice tone and body language relaxed and peaceful when discussing conversations with pastor. Receptive to gentle encouragement to ask pastor for additional visits.
>
> A: Outcome #3 met, interventions effective, goal of maintaining effective preparation for death being met.
>
> P: Next visit 12/21/98. Follow up to see whether pastor was asked and whether he can increase his visits. Continue to monitor her need and family's need in this area. Continue to monitor Outcomes 1, 2, 4, and 5.

This note shows how the nurse documented implementation and evaluation of care. Betty's progress is tracked clearly by using the plan's outcomes as the standards for desired behaviors.

INTERDISCIPLINARY PROBLEMS

Before examining interdisciplinary problems specifically, it is helpful to review briefly the concept of collaboration. Collaboration is best described as cooperation and working together. It does not mean that one person supervises, directs, or manages other people. Such activities are called supervising, directing/delegating, or managing.

Collaboration means that people with different areas of expertise are working as equals to define issues, design solutions, and achieve high-quality outcomes. In a sense, all conclusions made about a patient's situation are collaborative because the nurse collaborates with the patient; however, collaboration with patients is a given in great nursing care. The term "interdisciplinary problem" is applied to issues that require collaboration between nurses and other health care disciplines.

In health care, as in other arenas, collaboration among professionals occurs along a continuum. The continuum refers to the back-and-forth flow of accountability and responsibility for different aspects of a patient's care. All health care providers are considered equal partners in the team providing care, but there are times when one partner's expertise has a predominant influence on the design of specific aspects of care. For example, Mr. Jidou, age 83 years, is experiencing severe pain in his knees from degenerative joint disease. He is being seen in a primary care clinic on an outpatient basis. His health care team includes the physician, the home care nurse, and the physical therapist. Both the physician and the nurse know that Mr. Jidou needs exercises, but the physical therapist is the primary designer of the details for this aspect of care. The physical therapist will design the type and frequency of exercises needed for achieving the physician's order of "Nonweight-bearing exercises to the lower extremities," and the nurse will work with the patient and family to find the best ways for the patient to do the exercises at home.

A nursing conclusion in Mr. Jidou's case, categorized as an interdisciplinary problem, would be written as, "Pain in both knees related to chronic degenerative joint disease." With a more complete data base there would likely be additional related factors that would help to individualize care better. Additional data might include information such as Mr. Jidou's inability to tolerate most over-the-counter medications for reducing pain, or a chronic respiratory condition that limits his activity tolerance for nonweight-bearing strengthening exercises.

Another way of writing interdisciplinary problems is in the format of "Risk for . . . ." Consider an example of a patient who is admitted to an alcohol rehabilitation unit. The first priorities for care include life-threatening and safety issues, and are matters of collaboration between the nurse and the physician. The major life-threatening and safety issues in alcohol rehabilitation are related to the signs and symptoms of withdrawal of the toxic chemical ethyl alcohol from all body systems, especially the cardiovascular system. A typical interdisciplinary problem at this point of treatment is, "Risk for complications of alcohol withdrawal." The related factors will vary depending on the patient. An example of a related factor for this diagnosis might be, "related to detoxification after 20 years of daily alcohol intake averaging 1 pint/day."

Relationships exist among the type of health care setting, the nature of the patient's health concerns, and the number of interdisciplinary problems that are identified as nursing conclusions. In most inpatient settings where patients experience acute levels of health problems, more nursing conclusions are in the realm of interdependent practice (interdisciplinary problems). In outpatient settings, home care, or wellness care settings, more nursing conclusions are in the realm of independent nursing care (nursing diagnoses). These generalities are by no means always the case, however.

Designing Care With Betty for Her Interdisciplinary Problem

Five nursing conclusions made in Betty's case were classified as actual problems, the care of which could be provided in the independent realm of nursing. Another nursing conclusion is in the realm of interdependent nursing practice. This conclusion required collaboration with other health care providers: "Altered Nutrition and Fluid Intake related to impaired swallowing and meal preparation by neighbors." To design effective care in this area, the nurse enlists the expertise of a dietitian and a speech therapist to define the issues accurately, design treatment plans, and evaluate outcomes.

This interdisciplinary problem is closely related to the Risk for Aspiration diagnosis addressed in Chapter 15. Because the risk for aspiration pointed to a need for immediate action, the nurse will have started the interventions on that plan already. One of the interventions on that plan was to coordinate those actions with recommendations on this interdisciplinary plan.

Because collaboration can take more time when the patient is at home, the nurse could not wait and address the risk for aspiration and the nutrition and fluid intake problem together as one issue. If Betty had been hospitalized, the nurse would have had quick access to the speech therapist and the dietitian and, therefore, could have combined the risk diagnosis and the interdisciplinary problems into one plan. Further along in Betty's care, however, the two plans very likely might become one interdisciplinary plan.

The first part of the *preliminary* care plan for "Altered Nutrition . . . " is presented in the Preliminary Care Plan for Betty's Interdisciplinary Problem. This plan illustrates the first steps in incorporating the collaboration aspect. The actual interdisciplinary plan cannot be completed until after the collaboration occurs with the other health care professionals.

Notice that the goal of this plan is focused on improving a condition that is not currently acute but probably will be if left untreated. The time frame of 1 month probably is realistic, depending on how quickly the nutritionist and speech therapist can make recommendations.

The outcomes are patient centered, measurable, and flow from the related factors. They focus on the patient, describing her understanding of the seriousness of the problem, her willingness to participate in the evaluations, and her compliance with the recommendations. The last outcome brings the focus back to the need to share information with the neighbors who prepare her meals by addressing the second related factor for this interdisciplinary problem.

The nursing interventions are nurse centered, realistic, and clearly flow from their respective patient outcomes. The interventions (as well as the outcomes and rationales) specifically related to collaboration with other health care providers are in **boldface**. The speech therapist will assess and diagnose the degree of swallowing difficulty, and make suggestions for swallowing techniques and the types of foods and liquids that are least likely to stimulate choking. The nutritionist will assess and diagnose the current nutritional state, and make suggestions regarding how to maintain adequate intake of food and fluids without increasing the risk of aspiration. If all works well, the dietitian and the speech therapist will collaborate in their final recommendations and a revised care plan will be designed. An interdisciplinary care plan has many of the same characteristics that a nursing care plan has but includes the special recommendations of all the collaborators, including the patient.

▼ **Preliminary Care Plan for Betty's Interdisciplinary Problem**

INTERDISCIPLINARY PROBLEM:

Altered Nutrition and Fluid Intake related to impaired swallowing and meal preparation by neighbors

Goal: Within 1 month, Betty will have attained adequate nutrition and hydration

OUTCOMES	NURSING INTERVENTIONS	RATIONALE
1. Describe significance of impaired swallowing to maintain adequate food and fluid intake.	1a. Ask Betty to describe her understanding of the problem and assess her awareness of the importance of dealing with it b. Explain as needed the purpose of collaboration with speech therapist and dietitian	1. Patients who understand the reason for change are more cooperative in seeking change
2. **Participate in evaluation of swallowing status and nutritional and fluid intake.**	2. **Collaborate with MD, speech therapist, and dietitian, and help Betty set up appointments for evaluation**	2. **Effective referrals include getting patient to proper providers**
3. **Follow up on recommendations of speech therapist and dietitian.**	3a. **Discuss recommendations with Betty and ask her to explain them and share how she feels about them** b. **Assess how well she can follow recommendations at home** c. **Consult with dietitian and speech therapist to modify plans as needed to fit best her individual needs**	3. **Effective referrals include evaluation of the results**
4. Share needs for specific food requirements with neighbors.	4a. Discuss how she will share needs with neighbors, role-play as needed b. Develop a written list that can be given to neighbors for reference	4. Helping patients adapt recommendations to their specific needs improves quality of care

Doing and Determining Quality of Care
With Betty for Her Interdisciplinary Problem

As it so happens, we know what occurred in this situation. One of the recommendations of the dietitian was the following outcome, "Increase fluid intake to eight glasses of thickened fluid a day." This recommendation did not work well for Betty. It increased her need to urinate to the point of diminishing any activities outside the home. Diminished ability to be far from a toilet created increased problems related to Diversional Activity Deficit. This recommendation also caused nausea and occasional gagging. The nausea was unpleasant, but the gagging was dangerous for Betty.

After the nurse begins to implement care directed toward this outcome, an evaluation SOAP note might look like this.

> 12/17/98 10 AM Interdisciplinary Problem: Altered Nutrition and
>   Fluid Intake
> S: "The nutritionist and the speech therapist both said to add the
>   thickening agent to fluid and drink eight glasses a day. I have been
>   trying, but I have to go to the bathroom so much I can't leave the
>   house, and I added the thickener to water and it made me sick to
>   my stomach. I'm gagging at times."
> O: Dietitian contacted by nurse and recommendations changed to
>   drinking three glasses of thickened apple juice and three glasses of
>   apricot nectar. Betty agreed to try this change.
> A: Outcome #3 partially met. Modifications above made. Goal of at-
>   taining adequate nutrition being achieved.
> P: Call Betty tomorrow and assess for decreased frequency of urina-
>   tion and decrease in or absence of nausea. Follow up on Betty's in-
>   teraction with neighbors, outcome #4.—G. Rubenfeld, R.N.

Both the speech therapist and the nutritionist will continue to see Betty for modifications as her chronic terminal illness progresses. It is important for the nurse to maintain contact with all health care providers involved in the patient's care. This task is somewhat easier in an acute care setting, where all the providers usually are in the same organization. But in other settings, such as clinics and homes, it becomes particularly important for the nurse to assume the role of case manager–coordinator. This role provides for increased continuity and completeness of care.

PROBLEMS FOR REFERRAL

The nurse's skill in effectively identifying and referring problems depends directly on three factors: accepting that nursing cannot be all things to all people; the nurse's knowledge about the domains of other health care disciplines; and the nurse's degree of experience. Beginning nursing students generally make fewer referrals than do experienced nurses, but this is not always the case.

Accepting the Limitations of the Nursing Profession and Oneself

The first factor that influences the nurse's skill in identifying problems for referral and making effective referrals requires some additional thinking. From the beginning of nursing school, nurses are taught how to assess, plan, implement, and evaluate care for nursing problems. At some point, nurses also must learn about the limitations of their profession. Nurses cannot do everything for everybody. There are situations in which patients' problems and concerns do not fit at all within the domain of nursing. It is the responsibility of the nurse to recognize this and properly refer the patient to providers who can meet those needs. This is part of the nurse's professional responsibility.

Nurses may make referrals to other nurses as well as to nonnurse providers. For example, it is perfectly appropriate for a nurse who has worked for 20 years in obstetrics to say that he or she is not qualified or comfortable caring for gerontologic patients. It is, however, that nurse's responsibility to assist the patient or family in finding the proper resource to deal with the problems related to gerontologic concerns. Those other resources very likely may be gerontologic nurses or other specialists in gerontology.

Accepting one's own limitations goes beyond accepting a lack of knowledge and experience in another area of care. Sometimes a nurse's values and beliefs are in conflict with an area of patient need. Deciding when one's values and beliefs are hindrances to care is not an easy judgment. There are professional and ethical issues to consider as well. Nurses, for example, cannot simply refuse to care for people they do not like; however, when nurses honestly believe that their values and beliefs could interfere with the quality of their care in any given situation, they should refer patients to other providers, whether they be nurses or other health care workers.

⊃Action Learning #76: Identifying Problems for Referral

As a beginning nurse, examine the following situations and think about your knowledge, experience, values, and beliefs. Which would you consider problems for referral and which would you deal with yourself or collaboratively? Why? Share your reasoning with a classmate.

Peter is experiencing all the signs and symptoms of diabetes—frequent urination and excessive thirst and hunger. He has a strong family history of diabetes. He asks you for help.

Alicia is 13 years old and tells you she needs an abortion and wants you to help her in finding out how to get one.

Fred is complaining of bad stomach aches after 2 weeks of eating only chili dogs and French fries. He is asking for help in getting rid of the stomach aches.

Bill has been gaining weight and is asking you for help in finding a weight management program that he can live with. He is feeling very stressed because his companion, John, just moved out and John did all the cooking.

THINK ABOUT THIS ■ What criteria did you use to determine whether you could deal with the patient's requests or whether you needed to make a referral? How did your values and beliefs about each situation influence your decisions? Except for the first situation with Peter, all of the situations could appropriately be handled by experienced nurses. It would not, however, be inappropriate for even experienced nurses to make referrals if they believed their values and beliefs about abortion or homosexuality would interfere with the objectivity of their thinking or their judgments about care.

Knowledge

Knowledge about the domains of other health care disciplines is initially obtained through nursing education programs, reading, attending conferences, and so forth. The more the nurse knows about the other health professions, the more likely patient problems for referral will be recognized and appropriately referred. Most nursing programs include a large amount of information in the biomedical field.

This knowledge, plus the close collaboration between nurses and physicians, makes referrals to the physician fairly easy to identify. It takes more effort on the part of the nurse to learn about the kinds of care other health care professionals can provide, and to learn how to make those referrals.

⊃ACTION LEARNING #77: Increasing Your Knowledge for Referring Problems

Select a health care profession other than nursing or medicine. Find someone who works in that profession and ask that person the following questions. Share your findings with a classmate. (This Action Learning exercise will be helpful for interdisciplinary problems as well.)

1. What is your primary responsibility in patient care?

2. What kinds of things should I be looking for in terms of patient behaviors, signs or symptoms, and the like, to make appropriate referrals to you?

3. What is the most effective way to make sure you and the patient get connected?

THINK ABOUT THIS ■ What was your most interesting finding? What is the best way for you to store this information in your long-term memory for future use?

Experience

Experience is a great teacher. The more the nurse works directly with other providers, the clearer the understanding of their roles and responsibilities will be. Probably one of the best role models for knowledge and experience about health care services, patient resources, and how to make referrals is a community health nurse. A major responsibility of all community health nurses is to know who in the community can do what for whom, and how to get patients effectively connected with the resources they need.

Display 16-1 lists some basic guidelines for making effective referrals. These guidelines are broad enough to be used in many settings. Additional specific guidelines usually are found in the policy and procedure manuals of each health care setting.

Designing, Doing, and Determining Quality of Care With Betty for Her Problem for Referral

The area of finances frequently presents problems that require a referral. Even community health nurses, who directly assist patients with examining the impact of finances on their overall health and living situation, usually make referrals to other organizations to work on the details. Such organizations include the Department of Social Services, Credit Counseling Services, emergency rent payment groups, and the like.

The nurse worked with Betty to define the issues with regard to finances. This frequently is a very difficult subject for the patient and the nurse to discuss. Many people are taught from a very early age that it is inappropriate to discuss one's financial status with anyone but a personal banker. Discussing a person's financial

---

DISPLAY 16–1.   Basic Guidelines for Making Referrals

GUIDELINES	QUESTIONS TO BE ANSWERED
Collaborate with patient	What specifically is needed? How soon is it needed? How does the patient think the need could best be met?
Identify available resources	Which providers/resources focus specifically on this patient's needs? What is the cost? Does the patient go to them or will they come to the patient? Does the patient meet the criteria for obtaining help from this resource?
Assist patient in making contact	How is contact made: by phone, letter of referral, in person? Can the patient complete forms? Does patient have transportation, baby sitting, and so forth, to keep appointment?
Determine quality of results	Did patient get connected? Was need met? How does patient feel about the resource? Are modifications in plan needed?

situation is sometimes more difficult than talking about elimination or sexuality. The nurse approached this delicate topic by saying,

> "Betty, many people have a lot of difficulty sharing information about their financial situation. These are very private matters. It is important, however, for us to discuss this because it significantly affects you and your sons' future lifestyle. I am not an expert in financial matters but I can begin to help you find resources as they are needed.
>
> "The other reason to discuss this is to make you aware of resources that you are entitled to and eligible for as a hardworking taxpayer of many years.
>
> "Tell me how you feel about talking about your financial situation and what I can do to make it easier. I should remind you at this point that all of this information, as well as all other information about you and your family, is strictly confidential."

Once the discussion began, it became clear that Betty had had no income since her retirement, which had been necessary for medical reasons. The nurse knew from experience that Betty was probably eligible for disability income through Social Security and contacted the Social Security Office. Because of Betty's difficulty in talking for any length of time on the phone, the nurse contacted the agency directly. In other circumstances, the nurse would have helped the patient to make the contact and learn how to negotiate the system. Negotiating the health care delivery system to obtain the needed resources is a skill that is invaluable to all patients.

The appointment was set up, transportation was arranged, and Betty kept the appointment. She was, however, disappointed. Because she had a small certificate of deposit in a local bank, she was not eligible to receive her disability benefits at that time. A plan was developed for her to use up the funds, after which she would be eligible to reapply in 3 months. In the meantime, the nurse worked with other agencies to be sure that Betty received home care services and additional food until she could receive her benefits. Luckily, she did not have to worry about paying rent and utilities because her former employer was providing that.

CONCLUDING COMMENTS ON DESIGNING, DOING, AND DETERMINING QUALITY OF CARE FOR WELLNESS DIAGNOSES, INTERDISCIPLINARY PROBLEMS, AND PROBLEMS FOR REFERRAL

Providing care for these last three conclusions of assessment requires the use of all five modes of thinking—just as much as addressing actual and potential problems did. Wellness diagnoses require more NEW IDEAS AND CREATIVITY, simply because there currently are fewer options in this area of the NANDA taxonomy. Interdisciplinary problems and problems for referral also require extra knowledge to be identified effectively. Skill in identifying these last three conclusions of assessment significantly enhances the delivery of comprehensive, great nursing care.

SUMMARY OF CHAPTERS 13 THROUGH 16

The last four chapters were meant to show how thinking and the nursing process are applied in a complex patient situation. Although no written description can ever capture the full scope of any real-life situation, we hope that the reader has been able to appreciate how the nurse's thinking was used to coordinate the many aspects of care.

Betty's case required that the nurse collect and analyze a large amount of data and make many conclusions. Many conclusions about Betty's strengths were addressed in care plans as a means to help her deal with her health concerns. The conclusions about Betty's health concerns touched on all categories—nursing diagnoses of wellness issues, actual problems, and potential problems; interdisciplinary problems; and problems for referral.

While these examples from Betty's case are fresh in the reader's mind, it may be helpful to review the differences and similarities among all the major conclusions of assessment. As was pointed out in earlier chapters, nursing is like life in general: things don't always fit into nice, neat boxes or categories. There are always gray areas and fuzzy edges. Keeping the gray areas and fuzzy edges in mind, examine Table 16-1, which gives the characteristics of each of the major conclusions of assessment. Remember, there are always exceptions to any rules, but these distinctions work for most situations.

⊃Action Learning #78: Distinguishing the Category of the Conclusion of Assessment

Examine the conclusions listed below. Select the conclusion category from Table 16-1 that would most likely fit with each conclusion. Explain your reasoning to a classmate. The first conclusion category is provided as an example.

Conclusion Label

1. Unsafe sanitation in day care center
2. High risk for complications of open heart surgery
3. Altered Cardiac Output related to . . .
4. High Risk for Injury to toddler related to unsecured kitchen cabinets containing cleaning fluids
5. Potential for Enhanced individual coping

Conclusion Category

1. Problem for referral

Table 16–1 Overview of the Differences and Similarities Among the Major Conclusions of Assessment

QUESTIONS TO ASK	WELLNESS NURSING DIAGNOSIS	ACTUAL PROBLEM NURSING DIAGNOSIS	POTENTIAL PROBLEM NURSING DIAGNOSIS	INTERDISCIPLINARY PROBLEM	PROBLEM FOR REFERRAL
Who identifies the concern?	Nurse	Nurse	Nurse	Nurse or other provider	Nurse or other provider
Who deals with the concern?	Nurse (independent practice)	Nurse (independent practice)	Nurse (independent practice)	Nurse (interdependent practice) and other provider	Other provider
What knowledge is needed?	Nursing science Sciences Basic studies	Nursing science Sciences Basic studies	Nursing science Sciences Basic studies	Nursing science Sciences Basic studies Domain of other providers	Nursing science Sciences Basic studies Domain of other providers
What minimum work experience is needed?	Average	Average	Better than average	Average	Average
What modes of thinking are needed?	All five modes	All five modes	All five modes	All five modes	All five modes
What does first part of conclusion statement look like?	"Potential for Enhances . . ."	Taxonomy label or other descriptive label	Usually taxonomy label of "Risk for . . ."	Taxonomy label or other descriptive label	Variable
Are related factors included?	NO—N/A	Yes, unless unknown	Yes (mandatory)	Sometimes	N/A
What might complete statement look like?	Potential for Enhanced Family Coping; Growth	Self-Esteem Disturbance r/t knowledge deficit, ineffective coping as new mother, and loss of job	Risk for Impaired Skin Integrity r/t immobility, incontinence and fragile skin	Risk for complications of kidney transplant	Unsafe housing

THINK ABOUT THIS ■ How well did you do? Did you consider #1 a problem for referral? For most beginning nurses it might be, but for an experienced community health nurse it also could be considered a community-focused interdisciplinary problem. This wasn't meant to be a trick question, but was meant to show you that "rules" are not rigid; there are always exceptions.

THINKING LOG #16 ➤

The best way to internalize everything you have been reading and thinking about during the last four chapters is to continue to put your learning to work. Select a patient you previously cared for, or one you are currently caring for, and find your care plans. Using the Tracking Nursing Thinking checklist as a guide, think back over your care in that situation, and rate your thinking. Plan whether or how you will do things differently in the future.

If you haven't begun to collect your care plans already, start now. Create your own Care Plan Portfolio, and include this one in it. Your portfolio will be a valuable resource for many years to come.

Reference

Carroll-Johnson, R.M. (Ed.). (1991). *Classification of nursing diagnoses: Proceedings of the ninth conference.* Philadelphia: J.B. Lippincott.

17

Thinking Into the Future: From Linear Equation to a Paradigm of Great Nursing and Beyond

✳ *Learning Outcomes*

After reading and doing the activities in this chapter you will be able to:

Discuss your learning and thinking as it has evolved from the beginning chapters through the last chapter.

Design and explain a visual illustration of the relationships among all the components of great nursing.

Embrace the future of *your* professional nursing practice.

This final chapter is an overview of where you started, where you are, and where you are going as you continue your journey in nursing. The journey has just begun.

WHERE YOU STARTED

The first three chapters of this text introduced the basic concepts of *thinking*, *doing*, and *the nursing process*. The second and third sections of the text, Chapters 4 through 12, explored the details of the nursing process and the importance of effective verbal and written communication. The fourth section, Chapters 13 through 16, examined thinking, doing, and the nursing process in the context of a more complex patient situation. You have come a long way.

Knowing the five modes of thinking is the foundation for critical thinking and sound clinical judgment. Clearly understanding the multiple roles of direct and indirect care activities helps define the domain of what nurses do, and appreciating the intertwining of thinking and doing with the nursing process is necessary to move beyond the role of beginner (Fig. 17-1).

In Chapter 3, a linear equation for great nursing was examined. It looked like this:

FIGURE 17–1   Thinking into the future.

$$\text{Patient} + \text{You} + \frac{\text{Thinking}}{\text{Skills}} + \text{Knowledge} + \frac{\text{Nursing}}{\text{Process}} = \text{Great Nursing}$$

At that point in time this basic equation was sufficient, but by now readers who have expanded their thinking are questioning the simplicity of this linear equation. It is time to examine where your thinking is now, after reading, rereading, and doing the many Action Learning exercises and Thinking Logs throughout all of the chapters. It is time to reexamine the equation with your ever-growing thinking skills.

WHERE YOU ARE

The basic components of the equation are still appropriate; however, their definitions need expanding. The simple addition of each component to the others does not do justice to the dynamic relationship among the components and the resulting great nursing.

Appreciating the phrase "The whole is greater than the sum of the parts" is critical to this discussion. Consider as an example the now famous cake that has served to illustrate several issues. The ingredients of the cake are the parts of the whole. The cake itself, the finished product, is the whole. How different are the separate parts from the whole? The cake is a tasty result of the appropriate amounts of each ingredient, blended in the proper sequence, and then baked at the appropriate temperature for the optimum length of time. The cake is a new and unique whole that cannot simply be separated back into its original parts.

Likewise, the simple equation of the five components, added to each other to achieve great nursing, does not fully represent the whole of great nursing as you are now visualizing it.

The next few pages contain a brief overview of each of the components of the Great Nursing Equation. As you read, think about, ask questions about, and find answers for each component. At the end of this overview you will find the last Action Learning Activity for this book. This last activity asks you to create a new version of the old linear equation.

Thinking Skills

By now you have gained new insight into your thinking skills as well as how to nurture and develop their growth. Reflect back, using your KNOWING HOW YOU THINK mode, to appreciate fully some of the changes in your thinking. You have every reason to be proud of your accomplishments thus far.

It is the growing level of comfort and ease in using all five modes of thinking skills that is of particular importance at this point. The key modes of thinking that were introduced in Chapter 1 (TOTAL RECALL, HABITS, INQUIRY, NEW IDEAS AND CREATIVITY, and KNOWING HOW YOU THINK) have been identified consistently throughout this text.

Now, to broaden your perspective on thinking, consider these thinking skills as more than separate entities. Picture these five modes as working in harmony with each other all at the same time. Compare the modes of thinking with the strings on a guitar. Each mode, like each string, has its own special purpose, but when all the strings are used together to play a piece of music, the result is much nicer than if just one or two strings were played alone. The same idea applies to the use of the thinking modes. The more they are used in harmony with each other, the better the result.

Also consider the fact that the five modes of thinking are integral parts of the patient as well as of the nurse. Thinking skills are developed over time and can be enhanced for both nurse and patient. One of the major roles of nursing is to help patients learn how to help themselves. Guiding and enhancing patients' understanding of their own thinking and problem-solving skills is one of the major goals of nursing care.

KNOWING HOW YOU THINK is the key mode for nurturing the growth of all thinking modes for both the nurse and the patient. Some refer to this mode as "reflective thinking." Reflective thinking has been studied for over a decade. Even popular literature considers reflective thinking to be the common denominator among the world's great thinkers (Begley, 1993).

Knowledge

There is never an end to the learning of knowledge. What is learned today may be different tomorrow, or maybe even in a few minutes. Great nursing is impossible if nurses stop learning.

Knowledge was first discussed in Chapter 2, when the *doing* part of nursing was explored. If nurses do not understand the many direct and indirect aspects of nursing care, great nursing is impossible.

Nurses also must know about the activities of other health professionals to effectively identify, collaborate on, and refer health concerns. Most of the knowledge required of nurses, aside from nursing knowledge, is in the biomedical field. Although many expert nurses are sophisticated enough in their knowledge base to determine medical diagnoses, it *is **not** within the legal realm of nursing practice to make medical diagnoses*.

The purpose of having strong knowledge in the biomedical field is not to make medical diagnoses but to supplement nursing practice. For example, a patient with all the signs and symptoms of diabetes can be identified by the nurse and referred to the physician for an official diagnosis. The nurse then diagnoses the many possible and probable nursing needs of the patient, who must manage the activities of daily living affected by the disease. The nurse and patient determine how the diabetes is affecting sleep patterns, activity patterns, eating patterns, skin care, and so forth. All of these effects of the disease become the human responses for which nurses are responsible as they diagnose and design care in collaboration with patients.

The sources of knowledge are ever-expanding. Lectures, workshops, books, journals, computer searches, other health professionals, patients, significant others, and experience are only some of the many sources of information.

The strong connections between knowledge and thinking become obvious as the nurse looks for the many possible and probable relationships among the multiple content areas: the patient's individual responses to the situation at hand; the patient's strengths and resources; what the nurse knows or needs to look up about health and illness; the domain of nursing; and the domain of other health care professionals.

The Nursing Process

Several chapters have addressed the details of the components of the nursing process—assessing, planning, implementing, and evaluating—as well as the big picture of the nursing process components working together. The components of the process each require thinking skills (all five modes) and knowledge to be completely effective. Each of the components also has many subcomponents or subprocesses within the overall process. The components also interact and interrelate constantly, like guitar strings, if they are working well. Thus, the nursing process is a dynamic entity consisting of multiple processes within a larger process, all working in harmony to achieve great nursing care.

A brief review of Chapters 3 through 10 and 13 through 16 will refresh the reader's perspective on the details as well as the whole of the nursing process.

The Patient

This activity book consistently has referred to the "patient" as an individual. It is important to remember, however, that families, groups, and communities also are patients, and have their own unique nursing needs and interventions. After you become skilled in applying the nursing process to individuals, you will need to expand your skills to work with families, groups, and communities.

It also is important to remember that patients have thinking skills, knowledge, and feelings just as nurses have. Patients are unique individuals with unique needs. On top of that, the patient has automatic ownership of the health situation. Great nursing cannot exist if the patient is depersonalized and not recognized as the ultimate controller of his or her health situation.

All of these factors make patients special individuals who deserve thinking nurses—nurses who do not simply dole out standardized, cookbook care.

You—The Nurse

The next component of great nursing is you. You, and every other nurse, are a unique blend of thinking skills, knowledge (including knowledge of the nursing process), and—the most vital part of all—a unique personality. It is your personality that provides the values, the feelings, and the caring. It is your personality that makes your nursing practice unique to you. Without you and your caring, "great nursing" is simply a nice-sounding phrase with a very hollow ring.

Great Nursing

This brings us to the last part of the original equation, great nursing. It continues to be a concept that is not easy to describe precisely and clearly. Great nursing usually is easy to recognize when it is found, but it is elusive to pin down with words. Consider the following comparison of adequate nursing with great nursing to help make the distinction clearer.

> *Adequate nursing care:* Safe care because all parts of the nursing process are used. (Unsafe, poor nursing care is the result of skipping one or more of the parts.) The nurse who provides adequate care mechanically plods through all the components of the nursing process in a series of separate steps that simply follow each other in a linear fashion. The primary thinking modes used are TOTAL RECALL and HABITS.
>
> *Great nursing care:* Safe, efficient, and effective care that results from using the nursing process as the dynamic tool it was designed to be. Assessing, planning, implementing, and evaluating are done by nurses using all modes of thinking. The nursing process becomes embedded into the nurse's thinking process. The nursing process is no longer a separate entity that requires retrieval from a textbook or even from conscious memory, during each patient encounter. Care is focused on the patient as a unique individual. When nursing is great, it is a caring art as well as a sophisticated science.

Great nursing is not an elusive ideal that can only be written about by nursing scholars. Great nursing is practiced hourly, by nurses in all health care settings, including homes, long-term care facilities, schools, clinics, intensive care units, urgent care clinics, and hospitals, to name only a few. Great nursing will be practiced by *you* as you incorporate the components of the equation into your practice.

This brings us to the last Action Learning: Your Paradigm of Great Nursing. A paradigm is a model (usually seen as a large, important model) that illustrates how two or more ideas are related and what that relationship produces. You could also think of a paradigm as a sophisticated recipe. In addition to including all of the ingredients of the recipe, the paradigm shows how all the ingredients are related and what the final product looks like. One of our students completed this activity by drawing a big pot (the nursing process) filled with all the different ingredients of a stew (different pieces of knowledge), being heated over a fire (thinking), and being mixed, blended, and cooked (by the nurse and the patient) to produce a delicious meal (great nursing). Now it is your turn to engage your thinking cap and create your own unique paradigm. The ideas (concepts) that you need to include in your paradigm are the same concepts used in the original linear equation that is no longer descriptively adequate. Those are: *the patient, you, thinking skills, knowledge, the nursing process, and Great Nursing.*

⊃ACTION LEARNING #79: My Paradigm of Great Nursing

THINK ABOUT THIS ■ What do you think of your creation? How is it similar to and different from those created by your classmates? What parts do you think will change the most by graduation? Are you willing to make the changes at that time and continue to grow toward great nursing? In particular, remember that this is *your* paradigm; it will be similar to others, but no others will have "you" as a critical component.

The preceding review and paradigm development were designed for two reasons. First, they demonstrate how you have grown in your thinking and your ability to see relationships among the components of great nursing. Identifying relationships and examining their values are extremely valuable thinking abilities. Seeing relationships permits you to see the "big picture" of a patient's needs.

The second, and equally important, reason for designing your own paradigm is to help you internalize the concepts of the original equation. To "internalize" means to absorb new information into your existing understanding so that you can use the new information automatically. It is the process of developing HABITS—very useful HABITS. The more thoroughly you incorporate the concepts into your repertoire of thinking and doing, the more likely you will be to use the concepts effectively and efficiently in nursing practice. Concepts that are not internalized can be "parroted" back on an examination, but rarely can be applied to real-world nursing care.

One of the best ways to internalize information is to feel a sense of ownership of the information. The paradigm you have created is yours and yours alone; you own it. It took your thinking, your personality, and your energy to create it. You are more likely to value, remember, and use what is your private property than you are likely to use someone else's diagram memorized from a textbook. Therefore, you were encouraged to create a personal paradigm in the hope that it would mark your entry into a new level of thinking and doing in your journey toward great nursing.

WHERE YOU ARE GOING

Now that you have identified where you are, what about where you are going? The future holds many challenges for nursing and nurses. This next section will very briefly address issues related to nursing in the new millennium. You will be among the first nurses to practice in the 21st century. We cannot predict the future but we can help you think ahead about issues that will definitely have an impact on your critical thinking as a professional nurse. And, we can offer some suggestions on how to nurture your thinking and doing as you prepare to practice nursing in the new century.

Legal Issues

Legal issues are becoming increasingly relevant as we move into the new century. As discussed in Chapter 12, nurses are required to be more accountable for their actions and their care. State Nurse Practice Acts delineate the roles and responsibilities of nurses. These are the standards by which nurses are judged if there is a question of negligence or malpractice. Because Nurse Practice Acts vary from state to state, it is important that all nurses be aware of the specific regulations governing their practice in their state. In addition to Nurse Practice Acts, nurses also are subject to legal decisions based on Standards of Practice as established by the American Nurses Association. Liability insurance for nurses is something that requires some serious thought. Most major nursing textbooks, journals, and local nursing associations are valuable resources for detailed information on these issues, which have been only briefly introduced here. Some valuable legal resources are also listed at the end of Chapter 12.

Ethical Issues

Ethical issues and ethical decision making require skills in all five thinking modes. "Ethics are principles of conduct governing one's relationships with others—basic beliefs about values for right and wrong" (Ellis & Hartley, 1992, p. 158). The American Nurses Association and the International Council of Nurses have both developed Codes of Nursing Ethics. Although the basic principles of ethics have more sophisticated names, they essentially address doing good and not harm; accepting patients' autonomy in making decisions; being fair to all people; being faithful to one's commitments; and being truthful. As the next century arrives, there will be many ethical questions with regard to health care. Who will receive health care and who will not? Will someone receive a bone marrow transplant when there is no insurance to pay for it? Who can get an abortion and who cannot? Should life be prolonged when quality of life is gone? What is quality of life? What or who should be cloned? How far should we go with gene therapy? How can privacy be maintained in this information age? Should insurance companies know a person's genetic pattern? Nurses need to be part of the dialogue about such issues. They will be asked to contribute suggestions for solutions to tough questions.

Economic Issues

Many of the ethical questions also are economic questions. As individuals, families, communities, and nations we have limited health care resources. How should these resources be used? The fact that health care is expensive is not a news flash anymore. Even beginning level students in health care today recognize the term "cost containment." Why this is an issue and the complexity of the issue is addressed in widely diverse places, from basic textbooks to sophisticated specialty journals.

Economic issues have impacts on many aspects of nursing. The most traumatic impacts have involved loss of jobs, retraining, and/or cross-training of nurses. Nurses have been challenged to redesign many traditional methods of delivering nursing care. For example, one health care corporation is designing a 40-bed intensive care unit to care for the entire gamut of acutely ill patients. Nurses working in such an area will need extensive knowledge of all body systems and complex biomedical conditions as well as sophisticated nursing interventions. An era of the generalist-specialist nurse may be one answer to new delivery models. Some change is not so bad because it forces us to examine some long-standing HABITS that may no longer be useful. However, the biggest economic impact has been on patients and the quality of their care. With the "downsizing" of professional nursing staff, many ancillary staff are now performing nursing care. As good as these unprofessional staff members are, they do not have the education, the experience, or the highly developed critical thinking skills of the professional nurse.

Because economic issues have significantly affected quality of care, nurses must be knowledgeable about economics and the language of economics (eg, "product line," "zero-based budget," "proprietary status," and "capitation") in order to have their opinions heard. There are no simple solutions to these economic issues and nurses must use their critical thinking to be active participants in finding ways to achieve both cost containment and quality care. Nurses often align themselves with patient advocacy groups to increase the power of their voices.

Political Issues

Politics is a method of using power and influence to have an impact on decision making. There is a saying, "It's not what you know but who you know that counts." This is only partly true in nursing because what you know is very important, especially as it relates to patient care. But, there are times when "who you know" also affects patient care. If you were coordinating health care in a homeless shelter and you had 20 very hungry families because the food for the day didn't arrive, you would probably start thinking about WHO you knew who could help supply food. If you knew the owner of a local restaurant, you might call her for an emergency donation of food. You would be using political (who you know) power.

You also have a responsibility as a thinking citizen and a thinking nurse to be aware of health care issues that are being discussed and decided at your local, state/provincial, and national governmental levels. You have influence as an individual, but you can have even more impact as a group through professional nursing organizations. The voices of nurses must be heard at all levels of decision making (local, state/provincial, national, and international) if we are to have health care policies that are fair and just for all people.

Knowledge and Technology Issues

It does not take a rocket scientist to figure out that today's knowledge and technology will look like stone-age vintage in the next few years. Anyone who has used or bought a computer (such as an author!) will tell you that the one used today will be obsolete tomorrow. The phenomenal access to knowledge that is afforded by today's technology is mind-boggling. Learning how to keep up with that knowledge can be an insurmountable chore. The most that nurses (and most mortals) can hope for is to keep up with the number of "doors" that open to allow access of knowledge. The knowledge itself is useless if you cannot access it. Thus, nurses will need to be computer literate along with their other skills. They will need to know how to gain access through data bases, web sites, and good old books and journals. There is no question that computers will be a given in health care. Their presence will allow for faster access to all kinds of information.

Nurses must also be aware of what Drucker (1998) calls "The Next Information Revolution." This revolution will address the "meaning" and "purpose" of information as opposed to the volume of information or simple access to information. The impact of this revolution will help redefine many institutions in our society, including the health care industry.

HOW WILL CRITICAL THINKING GROW IN NURSING?

In the preceding section many references were made to nurses using their critical thinking skills to deal with the many changes in society and health care. Although it may not surprise readers to find, in a textbook on critical thinking, that critical thinking is touted as an answer to nursing dilemmas, it would be reasonable to question whether we know enough about critical thinking to use it fully.

One might well ask where we stand as a profession relative to our critical thinking. The answer lies partly in nursing research. There are two areas of research that are relevant here; one is research on nursing care itself—the knowledge base of nursing—and the other is research on the critical thinking process.

Nursing Care Research

The body of knowledge in every discipline is expanded and refined through research. For example, biomedical research has provided knowledge about new antibiotics to treat new infections; astronomical research has provided knowledge of how planets and galaxies work; engineering research has provided knowledge about how to build safer buildings in earthquake zones. Nursing has done the same. Professional nursing's founder, Florence Nightingale, is still respected for her pioneering work as a researcher, which involved collecting and analyzing data that helped the care situation for soldiers during the Crimean War. Her work began the process of using research to validate and support nursing practice with an empirical body of knowledge.

It was not until recently, however, that nursing research and the use of research findings to guide practice (research utilization) became widespread. Today, nursing has a formal division in the National Institutes of Health within the federal government to provide grants to fund nursing research. It was this kind of funding that supported the recent major research projects on Nursing Outcomes Classification (NOC) and Nursing Interventions Classification (NIC).

Even with the growing body of nursing knowledge from research, there are still many nursing practices that are based on tradition. You can recognize this basis for care when you hear statements such as, "It has always been done like this." Still other nursing interventions were borrowed from other disciplines (eg, psychology, sociology, and education) because of the overlap in knowledge that nursing shares with those other disciplines. Examples of this overlap include situations in which nurses use principles of family dynamics from sociology to help families use their strengths to cope with an ill member, or occasions when a nurse uses principles of teaching and learning to determine (assess) what a patient already knows about diabetes before teaching that patient about the disease.

In today's world of cost containment and demands for accountability, nurses must go beyond doing things based only on tradition or borrowed knowledge, to a research-based practice that can validate the importance of what nurses do. Although most people intuitively believe that nursing makes a difference in health care, the time has come for nurses to back up that belief with hard evidence. Such evidence is obtained through research. Through research testing, some nursing interventions have been refined, some have been discarded, and some have remained the same. The NIC research is an excellent example of this process of identifying and fine-tuning what nurses do. The NOC research is providing a better understanding of what patients should be doing if nursing interventions are working.

It is your job, as a nursing student now and as a professional nurse later, to use all your T.H.I.N.K. modes when you are practicing nursing. It is the responsibility of each nurse to question rationales such as "This is what we have always done." Nurses in all specialty areas and in all kinds of positions need to wonder about things they see daily. They need to wonder, for example, why a large majority of mental health patients have hypothyroidism. They need to ask, for example, what nurses are doing to make a difference in the lives of patients with chronic diseases such as hypertension and how such efforts might be improved.

As a professional nurse it is also your job to be aware of and familiar with the different types of nursing research, how to find research, how to read and understand research, and how to implement nursing research findings. Baccalaureate programs in nursing usually include a course on nursing research and/or integrate nursing research throughout the program of study. Knowledge gained from such a course is another one of the many aspects of education that enhances critical thinking abilities.

Critical Thinking Research

In the past few years the number of journal articles on critical thinking in nursing has exploded. Some of these articles have been reports of research studies, but more of them have been reports of various strategies to teach and learn critical thinking. A few have presented models of critical thinking in nursing.

Critical thinking research is still in its infancy partly because of the challenge of measuring critical thinking (Rane-Szostak & Robertson, 1996). Before a phenomenon can be measured fully it must be defined explicitly. Thus far in nursing, definitions of critical thinking often are those borrowed from other fields and adapted to nursing (Videbeck, 1997a). New models of critical thinking in nursing are focused on teaching and learning (Videbeck, 1997b; Whiteside, 1997).

For a quick review, readers can study the reference list at the end of this chapter and the additional bibliography at the end of the book. Many of the cited research articles measure critical thinking in students (eg, Behrens, 1996; Brooks & Shepherd, 1992; Graham, 1995; Perciful & Nester, 1996; Saucier, 1995; Sedlak, 1997; Wong, Kember, Chung, & Yan, 1995). The measure of critical thinking that is used most often is the "Watson-Glaser Critical Thinking Appraisal" (Watson & Glaser, 1964), which is not nursing-specific.

Reports of teaching and learning strategies that are used to promote critical thinking make up the largest segment of current literature in nursing critical thinking. These strategies include *debate* (Garrett, Schoener & Hood, 1996), *concept or mind mapping* (Roberts, Sucher, Perrin & Rodriguez, 1995; Rooda, 1994), *use of case studies* (Neill, Lachat & Taylor-Panek, 1997; Vanetzian & Corrigan, 1996), *use of mnemonics* (Beitz, 1977), *use of journals and journaling* (Brown & Sorrell, 1993; Degazon & Lunney, 1995; Heinrich, 1992; Patton, Woods, Agarenzo, Brubaker, Metcalf & Sherrer, 1997), *gaming* (Kuhn, 1995), *use of learning circles* (Heibert, 1996), *"Think Aloud" seminars* (Lee & Ryan-Wenger, 1997), *strategies for large classroom learning* (Elliot, 1996), *computerized programs* (Lange, et al.,

1977), and *reflective learning* (Baker, 1996; Carkhuff, 1996; Lauterbach & Becker, 1996; Wong, Kember, Chung & Yan, 1995). Some authors report more generally on teaching critical thinking throughout a program (Alexander & Giguere, 1996; Beeken, Dale, Enos & Yarbrough, 1997; Chubinski, 1996; Dexter et al., 1997; Facione & Facione, 1996; O'Sullivan, Blevins-Stephens, Smith & Vaughan-Wrobel, 1997). Some focus on specific practice areas, such as critical care (Bucknall & Thomas, 1997; Whiteside, 1997).

As the reader can see from these examples alone, there are many ideas on critical thinking out there in the literature. Still in its infancy is the whole issue of just what critical thinking in nursing is all about. One idea is that critical thinking is the same in every discipline. Another is that the overall process may be the same but that the tasks are discipline specific. Yet another is that critical thinking in nursing is different from critical thinking in other fields.

The authors of this book, as mentioned in Chapter 1, have, during the past few years, conducted a study to arrive at a consensus definition of critical thinking in nursing. An international panel of nurses were asked to describe the (cognitive) skills and habits of the mind (affective dispositions or inclinations) that are characteristic of critical thinking in nursing. Using a research method that allows for a qualitative analysis of data (The Delphi Method), the authors have, through five rounds of mailed questions and answers, teased out the essence of critical thinking in nursing and have arrived at the consensus statement found in Chapter 1 and repeated here. Approximately 80 nurses were involved in at least some rounds of this study and approximately 55 responded to most or all rounds. Those nurses were from eight countries and 25 U.S. states.

> Critical thinking in nursing is an essential component of professional accountability and quality nursing care. Critical thinkers in nursing exhibit these habits of the mind: confidence, contextual perspective, creativity, flexibility, inquisitiveness, intellectual integrity, intuition, open-mindedness, perseverance, and reflection. Critical thinkers in nursing practice the cognitive skills of analyzing, applying standards, discriminating, information seeking, logical reasoning, predicting and transforming knowledge. (Scheffer & Rubenfeld, 1999, in press)

The Delphi Method, which was used to arrive at this statement, has been used many times in nursing and in other fields. For example, the group that eventually became NANDA used it to initially identify nursing diagnoses. It also was the process used by the American Philosophical Association (APA) to collect information from a multidisciplinary group and arrive at their consensus statement on critical thinking (Facione, 1990). That statement is as follows:

> We understand critical thinking to be purposeful, self-regulatory judgment which results in interpretation, analysis, evaluation, and inference as well as explanation of the evidential, conceptual, methodological, criteriological, or contextual considerations upon which that judgment is

based.... Critical thinking is a pervasive and self-rectifying human phenomenon. The ideal critical thinker is habitually inquisitive, well-informed, trustful of reason, open-minded, flexible, fair-minded in evaluation, honest in facing personal biases, prudent in making judgments, willing to reconsider, clear about issues, orderly in complex matters, diligent in seeking relevant information, reasonable in the selection of criteria, focused in inquiry, and persistent in seeking results which are as precise as the subject and the circumstances of inquiry permit.

Many nurses in the Scheffer and Rubenfeld study indicated that they were familiar with the APA critical thinking statement and may have been influenced by it and/or by other definitions. However, although there obviously are similar themes in the two statements, there also are differences. It may be that there are some unique features of critical thinking in nursing.

As other descriptions of critical thinking in nursing become available for critical review, the debate over the uniqueness of nurse critical thinking may become answerable. We strongly recommend that readers continually engage their critical thinking as they study research reports on critical thinking. We are making significant progress but we are by no means at the end of the journey toward understanding critical thinking in nursing and other disciplines.

CONTINUING THE JOURNEY

So, what can you do to continue to nurture your thinking and doing as you move toward your professional career? The answers to that question could fill another complete book with several volumes. In the interest of time, here are some simplified versions of the answers.

- Prepare yourself for the reality of the kind of nursing you will find in the real world. You may want to work or volunteer in a hospital or other health care setting while you are in school. Remember to keep your thinking cap on as you view the real world; compare it with the ideal that you learned in school. Don't give up your ideals when the world is not ideal.
- Consider the vast array of career options available to you. Remember, despite the fluctuating job market, there is always a job for a nurse, especially a nurse who can visualize nursing outside traditional settings. You can design your own position using your critical thinking skills.
- Develop networks with colleagues and professional organizations. Critical thinking is easiest when it is done with other critical thinkers.
- Explore graduate education, certification, and interdisciplinary degrees. If you don't choose to participate in a formal program, teach yourself. Don't stop learning.
- Make your voice heard where health care policies and health care decisions are being made.

- Continue to use all five modes of critical thinking and don't allow yourself to get too comfortable with the HABIT mode.
- Take care of yourself physically, emotionally, and spiritually. Remember, thinking is not just dependent on your brain. (Read the story below.)

A colleague once shared with me a valuable rule. I was a graduate student in psychiatric nursing. My clinical assignment included co-leading a therapy group at a crisis intervention clinic. My co-leader, who had been practicing therapy for several years, asked me, "What is the number one rule of therapy?" Being an ever-conscientious student, my thoughts raced for an answer. Was he asking about assessing for suicidal intentions? Should I say something about helping the patient to get in touch with feelings? Or maybe he was asking about one of the theoretical frameworks, such as Carl Rogers's "unconditional positive regard." Finally I just admitted I didn't know.

He then, very seriously, told me this: "The number one rule of therapy is survival of the therapist. The rationale for that rule being you can't help anyone else if you don't take care of yourself."

I have always remembered those words. I find they apply to many aspects of nursing and life. One of the most common problems of those of us who want to help others is that we give and give and give and forget that we have to replenish our physical, emotional, and spiritual resources continually or the "well runs dry." When our well runs dry we are diagnosed with "burnout." One danger of burnout is that, for survival, the nurse uses merely HABIT thinking.

To coin a cliché, there are no crystal balls to help predict where you or health care may be going. Change, however, is guaranteed, and the best you can do is be prepared for it as you continue your journey into the future. As you prepare, consider incorporating these three basic principles to navigate successfully the troughs and waves (and maybe even tidal waves) as they come:

- Nurture and value your thinking in all five modes: TOTAL RECALL, HABITS, INQUIRY, NEW IDEAS AND CREATIVITY, and especially KNOWING HOW YOU THINK.
- Acknowledge the patient as a unique individual with strengths and health concerns *and* as the person who has the final word in determining his or her own health care.
- Know that great nursing is an achievable goal if you believe in and internalize your own paradigm.

The future of the nursing profession and patient care is in your hands, your heart, and your head. As you continue your journey we wish you great health and GREAT THINKING.

References

Alexander, M.K. & Giguere, B. (1996). Critical thinking in clinical learning: A holistic perspective. *Holistic Nursing Practice, 10* (93), 15–22.

Baker, C.R. (1996). Reflective learning: A teaching strategy for critical thinking. *Journal of Nursing Education, 35* (1), 19–22.

Beeken, J.E., Dale, M.L., Enos, M.F., Yarbrough, S. (1997). Teaching critical thinking skills to undergraduate nursing students. *Nurse Educator, 22* (3), 37–39.

Begley, S. (1993, June 28). The puzzle of genius: Where do great minds come from? And why are there no Einsteins, Freuds or Picassos today? *Newsweek*, 46–50.

Behrens, P.J. (1996). The Watson-Glaser critical thinking appraisal and academic performance of diploma school students. *Journal of Nursing Education, 35*, 34–36.

Beitz, J.M. (1997). Unleashing the power of memory: The mighty mnemonic. *Nurse Educator, 22* (2), 25–29.

Brooks, K. & Shepherd, J.M. (1992). Professionalism versus general critical thinking abilities of senior nursing students in four types of nursing curricula. *Journal of Professional Nursing, 8* (2), 87–95.

Brown, H.N. & Sorrell, J.M. (1993). Use of clinical journals to enhance critical thinking. *Nurse Educator, 18* (5), 16–19.

Bucknall, T. & Thomas, S. (1997). Nurses' reflections on problems associated with decision-making in critical care settings. *Journal of Advanced Nursing, 25*, 229–237.

Carkhuff, M.H. (1996). Reflective learning: Work groups as learning groups. *Journal of Continuing Education in Nursing, 27* (5), 209–214.

Chubinski, S. (1996). Creative critical-thinking strategies. *Nurse Educator, 21* (6), 23–27.

Degazon, C.E. & Lunney, M. (1995). Clinical journal: A tool to foster critical thinking for advanced levels of competence. *Clinical Nurse Specialist, 9* (5), 270–274.

Dexter, P., Applegate, M., Backer, J., Claytor, K., Keffer, J., Norton, B. & Ross, B. (1997). A proposed framework for teaching and evaluating critical thinking in nursing. *Journal of Professional Nursing, 13* (3), 160–167.

Drucker, P.F. (1998). The next information revolution. *Forbes ASAP,* August 24, 47–58.

Elliot, D. (1996). Promoting critical thinking in the classroom. *Nurse Educator, 21* (2), 49–52.

Ellis, J.R. & Hartley, C.L. (1992). *Nursing in today's world* (4th ed.). Philadelphia: J.B. Lippincott.

Facione, P. (1990) *Critical thinking: A statement of expert consensus for purposes of educational assessment and instruction*. Millbrae, CA: The California Academic Press.

Facione, N.C. & Facione, P.A. (1996). Externalizing the critical thinking in knowledge development and clinical judgment. *Nursing Outlook, 44* (3), 129–136.

Garrett, M., Schoener, L. & Hood, L. (1996). Debate: A teaching strategy to improve verbal communication and critical-thinking skills. *Nurse Educator, 21* (4), 37–40.

Graham, M.E. (1995). The relationship between critical thinking and how time is structured in the clinical setting for students in a baccalaureate nursing program. *ABNF Journal, 6* (6), 149–157.

Heinrich, K.T. (1992). The intimate dialogue: Journal writing by students. *Nurse Educator, 17* (6), 17–21.

Hiebert, J.L. (1996). Learning circles: A strategy for clinical practicum. *Nurse Educator, 21* (3), 37–42.

Jacobs, P.M., Ott, B., Sullivan, B., Ulrich, Y. & Short, L. (1997). An approach to defining and operationalizing critical thinking. *Journal of Nursing Education, 36* (1), 19–22.

Kuhn, M.A. (1995). Gaming: A technique that adds spice to learning? *Journal of Continuing Education in Nursing, 26* (1), 35–39.

Lange, L.L., Haak, S.W., Lincoln, M.J., Thompson, C.B., Turner, C.W., Weir, C., Foerster, V., Nilasena, D., & Reeves, R. (1997). Use of Iliad to improve diagnostic performance of nurse practitioner students. *Journal of Nursing Education, 36* (1), 36–45.

Lauterbach, S.S. & Becker, P.H. (1996). Caring for self: Becoming a self-reflective nurse. *Holistic Nursing Practice, 10* (2), 57–68.

Lee, J.E.M. & Ryan-Wenger, N. (1997). The "Think Aloud" seminar for teaching clinical reasoning: A case study of a child with pharyngitis. *Journal of Pediatric Health Care, 11* (3), 101–110.

Neill, K.M., Lachat, M.F. & Taylor-Panek, S. (1997). Enhancing critical thinking with case studies and nursing process. *Nurse Educator, 22* (2), 30–32.

O'Sullivan, P.S., Blevins-Stephens, W.L., Smith, F.M. & Vaughan-Wrobel, B. (1997). Addressing the national league for nursing critical thinking outcome. *Nurse Educator, 22* (1), 23–29.

Patton, J.G., Woods, S.J., Agarenzo, T., Brubaker, C., Metcalf, T. & Sherrer, L. (1997). Enhancing the clinical practicum experience through journal writing. *Journal of Nursing Education, 36* (5), 238–240.

Perciful, E.G. & Nester, P.A. (1996). The effect of an innovative clinical teaching method on nursing students' knowledge and critical thinking skills. *Journal of Nursing Education, 35* (1), 23–28.

Rane-Szostak, D. & Robertson, J. F. (1996). Issues in measuring critical thinking: Meeting the challenge. *Journal of Nursing Education, 35* (1), 5–11.

Roberts, C.M., Sucher, K., Perrin, D.G, & Rodriguez, S. (1995). Concept mapping: An effective instructional strategy for diet therapy. *Journal of the American Dietetic Association, 95* (8), 908–911.

Rooda, L.A. (1994). Effects of mind mapping on student achievement in a nursing research course. *Nurse Educator, 19*(6), 25–27.

Sedlak, C.A. (1997). Critical thinking of beginning baccalaureate nursing students during the first clinical nursing course. *Journal of Nursing Education, 36* (1), 11–18.

Saucier, B.L. (1995). Critical thinking skills of baccalaureate nursing students. *Journal of Professional Nursing, 11*, 351–357.

Vanetzian, E. & Corrigan, B. (1996). "Prep" for class and class activity key to critical thinking. *Nurse Educator, 21* (2), 45–48.

Videbeck, S.L. (1997a). Critical thinking: Prevailing practice in baccalaureate schools of nursing. *Journal of Nursing Education, 36* (1), 5–10.

Videbeck, S.L. (1997b). Critical thinking: A model. *Journal of Nursing Education, 36* (1), 23–28.

Watson, G. & Galser, E. (1964). *Critical thinking appraisal manual.* New York: Harcourt, Brace & World.

Whiteside, C. (1997). A model for teaching critical thinking in the clinical setting. *Dimensions of Critical Care Nursing, 16* (3), 152–162.

Wong, F.K.Y., Kember, D., Chung, L.Y.F. & Yan L. (1995). Assessing the level of student reflection from reflective journals. *Journal of Advanced Nursing, 22*, 48–52.

Appendix A
NURSING DIAGNOSES, NORTH AMERICAN NURSING DIAGNOSIS ASSOCIATION, 1997–1998, WITH UPDATES FOR 1999-2000

Pattern 1: Exchanging

1.1.2.1	Altered Nutrition: More than Body Requirements
1.1.2.2	Altered Nutrition: Less than Body Requirements
1.1.2.3	Altered Nutrition: Risk for More Than Body Requirements
1.2.1.1	Risk for Infection
1.2.2.1	Risk for Altered Body Temperature
1.2.2.2	Hypothermia
1.2.2.3	Hyperthermia
1.2.2.4	Ineffective Thermoregulation
1.2.3.1	Dysreflexia
1.2.3.2	Risk for Autonomic Dysreflexia
1.3.1.1	Constipation
1.3.1.1.1	Perceived Constipation
1.3.1.2	Diarrhea
1.3.1.3	Bowel Incontinence
1.3.1.4	Risk for Constipation
1.3.2	Altered Urinary Elimination
1.3.2.1.1	Stress Incontinence
1.3.2.1.2	Reflex Urinary Incontinence
1.3.2.1.3	Urge Incontinence
1.3.2.1.4	Functional Urinary Incontinence
1.3.2.1.5	Total Incontinence
1.3.2.1.6	Risk for Urinary Urge Incontinence
1.3.2.2	Urinary Retention
1.4.1.1	Altered (Specify Type) Tissue Perfusion (Renal, cerebral, cardiopulmonary, gastrointestinal, peripheral)
1.4.1.2	Risk for Fluid Volume Imbalance
1.4.1.2.1	Fluid Volume Excess
1.4.1.2.2.1	Fluid Volume Deficit
1.4.1.2.2.2	Risk for Fluid Volume Deficit
1.4.2.1	Decreased Cardiac Output
1.5.1.1	Impaired Gas Exchange
1.5.1.2	Ineffective Airway Clearance
1.5.1.3	Ineffective Breathing Pattern
1.5.1.3.1	Inability to Sustain Spontaneous Ventilation
1.5.1.3.2	Dysfunctional Ventilatory Weaning Response (DVWR)
1.6.1	Risk for Injury
1.6.1.1	Risk for Suffocation
1.6.1.2	Risk for Poisoning

1.6.1.3	Risk for Trauma
1.6.1.4	Risk for Aspiration
1.6.1.5	Risk for Disuse Syndrome
1.6.1.6	Latex Allergy
1.6.1.7	Risk for Latex Allergy
1.6.2	Altered Protection
1.6.2.1	Impaired Tissue Integrity
1.6.2.1.1	Altered Oral Mucous Membrane
1.6.2.1.2.1	Impaired Skin Integrity
1.6.2.1.2.2	Risk for Impaired Skin Integrity
1.6.2.1.3	Altered Dentition
1.7.1	Decreased Adaptive Capacity: Intracranial
1.8	Energy Field Disturbance

Pattern 2: Communicating

2.1.1.1	Impaired Verbal Communication

Pattern 3: Relating

3.1.1	Impaired Social Interaction
3.1.2	Social Isolation
3.1.3	Risk for Loneliness
3.2.1	Altered Role Performance
3.2.1.1.1	Altered Parenting
3.2.1.1.2	Risk for Altered Parenting
3.2.1.1.2.1	Risk for Altered Parent/Infant/Child Attachment
3.2.1.2.1	Sexual Dysfunction
3.2.2	Altered Family Processes
3.2.2.1	Caregiver Role Strain
3.2.2.2	Risk for Caregiver Role Strain
3.2.2.3.1	Altered Family Process: Alcoholism
3.2.3.1	Parental Role Conflict
3.3	Altered Sexuality Patterns

Pattern 4: Valuing

4.1.1	Spiritual Distress (Distress of the Human Spirit)
4.1.2	Risk for Spiritual Distress
4.2	Potential for Enhanced Spiritual Well-Being

Pattern 5: Choosing

5.1.1.1	Ineffective Individual Coping
5.1.1.1.1	Impaired Adjustment
5.1.1.1.2	Defensive Coping
5.1.1.1.3	Ineffective Denial
5.1.2.1.1	Ineffective Family Coping: Disabling
5.1.2.1.2	Ineffective Family Coping: Compromised

5.1.2.2	Family Coping: Potential for Growth
5.1.3.1	Potential for Enhanced Community Coping
5.1.3.2	Ineffective Community Coping
5.2.1	Ineffective Management of Therapeutic Regimen (Individuals)
5.2.1.1	Noncompliance (Specify)
5.2.2	Ineffective Management of Therapeutic Regimen: Families
5.2.3	Ineffective Management of Therapeutic Regimen: Community
5.2.4	Effective Management of Therapeutic Regimen: Individual
5.3.1.1	Decisional Conflict (Specify)
5.4	Health Seeking Behaviors (Specify)

Pattern 6: Moving

6.1.1.1	Impaired Physical Mobility
6.1.1.1.1	Risk for Peripheral Neurovascular Dysfunction
6.1.1.1.2	Risk for Perioperative Positioning Injury
6.1.1.1.3	Impaired Walking
6.1.1.1.4	Impaired Wheelchair Mobility
6.1.1.1.5	Impaired Wheelchair Transfer Ability
6.1.1.1.6	Impaired Bed Mobility
6.1.1.2	Activity Intolerance
6.1.1.2.1	Fatigue
6.1.1.3	Risk for Activity Intolerance
6.2.1	Sleep Pattern Disturbance
6.2.1.1	Sleep Deprivation
6.3.1.1	Diversional Activity Deficit
6.4.1.1	Impaired Home Maintenance Management
6.4.2	Altered Health Maintenance
6.4.2.1	Delayed Surgical Recovery
6.4.2.2	Adult Failure to Thrive
6.5.1	Feeding Self Care Deficit
6.5.1.1	Impaired Swallowing
6.5.1.2	Ineffective Breastfeeding
6.5.1.2.1	Interrupted Breastfeeding
6.5.1.3	Effective Breastfeeding
6.5.1.4	Ineffective Infant Feeding Pattern
6.5.2	Bathing/Hygiene Self Care Deficit
6.5.3	Dressing/Grooming Self Care Deficit
6.5.4	Toileting Self Care Deficit
6.6	Altered Growth and Development
6.6.1	Risk for Altered Development
6.6.2	Risk for Altered Growth
6.7	Relocation Stress Syndrome
6.8.1	Risk for Disorganized Infant Behavior
6.8.2	Disorganized Infant Behavior
6.8.3	Potential for Enhanced Organized Infant Behavior

Pattern 7: Perceiving

7.1.1	Body Image Disturbance
7.1.2	Self Esteem Disturbance
7.1.2.1	Chronic Low Self Esteem
7.1.2.2	Situational Low Self Esteem
7.1.3	Personal Identity Disturbance
7.2	Sensory/Perceptual Alterations (Specify) (Visual, Auditory, Kinesthetic, Gustatory, Tactile, Olfactory)
7.2.1.1	Unilateral Neglect
7.3.1	Hopelessness
7.3.2	Powerlessness

Pattern 8: Knowing

8.1.1	Knowledge Deficit (Specify)
8.2.1	Impaired Environmental Interpretation Syndrome
8.2.2	Acute Confusion
8.2.3	Chronic Confusion
8.3	Altered Thought Processes
8.3.1	Impaired Memory

Pattern 9: Feeling

9.1.1	Pain
9.1.1.1	Chronic Pain
9.1.2	Nausea
9.2.1.1	Dysfunctional Grieving
9.2.1.2	Anticipatory Grieving
9.2.1.3	Chronic Sorrow
9.2.2	Risk for Violence: Self-Directed or Directed at Others
9.2.2.1	Risk for Self-Mutilation
9.2.3	Post-Trauma Syndrome
9.2.3.1	Rape-Trauma Syndrome
9.2.3.1.1	Rape-Trauma Syndrome: Compound Reaction
9.2.3.1.2	Rape-Trauma Syndrome: Silent Reaction
9.2.4	Risk for Post-Trauma Syndrome
9.3.1	Anxiety
9.3.1.1	Death Anxiety
9.3.2	Fear

(North American Nursing Diagnosis Association. [1998]. *NANDA nursing diagnoses: Definitions and classification 1999–2000*. Philadelphia: NANDA.)

Appendix B

NURSING INTERVENTIONS CLASSIFICATION (NIC) TAXONOMY

Overview of the NIC Taxonomy

On the following pages, the interventions in NIC are organized in a three-level taxonomy. At the top, most abstract level are six *domains* (numbered 1 to 6). Each domain includes *classes* (assigned alphabetical letters) or groups of related interventions (each with a unique code of four numbers) that are at the third level of the taxonomy. Only intervention label names are used in the taxonomy. Refer to the alphabetical listing for the definition and activities for each intervention.

The taxonomy clusters related interventions for ease of use. Nurses in any specialty should remember that they will need to use the whole taxonomy with a particular patient, not just interventions from one class or domain. The taxonomy is theory neutral; the interventions can be used with any nursing theory and in any of the various nursing and health care delivery systems. The interventions can also be used with various diagnostic classifications, including NANDA, ICD, DSM, and Omaha.

Each of the interventions has been assigned a unique number to facilitate computerization. If one wishes to identify the class and domain in which the intervention is included, then one would use six digits (e.g., 1A-0140 = Body Mechanics Promotion located in the Activity and Exercise Management class in the Physiological: Basic domain). Activities are not coded in this book, but if one wishes to assign codes, then each intervention's activities can be numbered using two spaces after a decimal (e.g., 1A-0140.01). Some interventions have been included in two classes but are coded according to the primary class. We have attempted to keep cross-referencing to a minimum. Interventions are listed in another class only if they were judged to be sufficiently related to the interventions in that class. No intervention is listed in more than two classes. Each class has been assigned 300 codes, which have been distributed across existing interventions, leaving space for future additions. Interventions that are more concrete (i.e., those with colons in the title) have been coded at the fourth digit (e.g., Exercise Therapy: Ambulation is coded 0221). Occasionally, an intervention is located in only one class but has a code that is assigned to another class (e.g., Nutritional Counseling is located in class D Nutrition Support but is coded 5246 to indicate that it is a counseling intervention). In the current version of the taxonomy, the interventions are numbered in progressive order and listed alphabetically, but, in the future when additional interventions are added, the order will be more difficult to maintain. Only the class of Elimination Management is not in alphabetical order because interventions related to the bowel and bladder have been grouped separately within the class. The last two classes in the domain Health System have been assigned small numerical letters (Health System Management is "a" and Information Management is "b"). These classes contain many of the indirect care interventions (those that would be included in overhead costs rather than directly billed), and this coding of the class represents a convenient way to assist users in identifying them.

NIC Taxonomy

	DOMAIN 1	DOMAIN 2	DOMAIN 3
Level 1 Domains	**1. Physiological: Basic** Care that supports physical functioning	**2. Physiological: Complex** Care that supports homeostatic regulation	**3. Behavioral** Care that supports psychosocial functioning and facilitates life-style changes
Level 2 Classes	*A Activity and Exercise Management:* Interventions to organize or assist with physical activity and energy conservation and expenditure *B Elimination Management:* Interventions to establish and maintain regular bowel and urinary elimination patterns and manage complications due to altered patterns *C Immobility Management:* Interventions to manage restricted body movement and the sequelae *D Nutrition Support:* Interventions to modify or maintain nutritional status *E Physical Comfort Promotion:* Interventions to promote comfort using physical techniques *F Self-Care Facilitation:* Interventions to provide or assist with routine activities of daily living	*G Electrolyte and Acid-Base Management:* Interventions to regulate electrolyte/acid base balance and prevent complications *H Drug Management:* Interventions to facilitate desired effects of pharmacological agents *I Neurologic Management:* Interventions to optimize neurologic functions *J Perioperative Care:* Interventions to provide care before, during, and immediately after surgery *K Respiratory Management:* Interventions to promote airway patency and gas exchange *L Skin/Wound Management:* Interventions to maintain or restore tissue integrity *M Thermoregulation:* Interventions to maintain body temperature within a normal range *N Tissue Perfusion Management:* Interventions to optimize circulation of blood and fluids to the tissue	*O Behavior Therapy:* Interventions to reinforce or promote desirable behaviors or alter undesirable behaviors *P Cognitive Therapy:* Interventions to reinforce or promote desirable cognitive functioning or alter undesirable cognitive functioning *Q Communication Enhancement:* Interventions to facilitate delivering and receiving verbal and nonverbal messages *R Coping Assistance:* Interventions to assist another to build on own strengths, to adapt to a change in function, or to achieve a higher level of function *S Patient Education:* Interventions to facilitate learning *T Psychological Comfort Promotion:* Interventions to promote comfort using psychological techniques

DOMAIN 4	DOMAIN 5	DOMAIN 6
4. Safety Care that supports protection against harm	**5. Family** Care that supports the family unit	**6. Health System** Care that supports effective use of the health care delivery system
U *Crisis Management:* Interventions to provide immediate short-term help in both psychological and physiological crises V *Risk Management:* Interventions to initiate risk-reduction activities and continue monitoring risks over time	W *Childbearing Care:* Interventions to assist in understanding and coping with the psychological and physiological changes during the childbearing period X *Lifespan Care:* Interventions to facilitate family unit functioning and promote the health and welfare of family members throughout the lifespan	Y *Health System Mediation:* Interventions to facilitate the interface between patient/family and the health care system a *Health System Management:* Interventions to provide and enhance support services for the delivery of care b *Information Management:* Interventions to facilitate communication among health care providers

Level 1 Domains	**1. PHYSIOLOGICAL: BASIC** **Care That Supports Physical Functioning**		
Level 2 Classes	**A Activity and Exercise Management** Interventions to organize or assist with physical activity and energy conservation and expenditure	**B Elimination Management** Interventions to establish and maintain regular bowel and urinary elimination patterns and manage complications due to altered patterns	**C Immobility Management** Interventions to manage restricted body movement and the sequelae
Level 3 Interventions	0140 Body Mechanics Promotion 0180 Energy Management 0200 Exercise Promotion 0202 Exercise Promotion: Stretching 0221 Exercise Therapy: Ambulation 0222 Exercise Therapy: Balance 0224 Exercise Therapy: Joint Mobility 0226 Exercise Therapy: Muscle Control 5612 Teaching: Prescribed Activity/Exercise **S***	0410 Bowel Incontinence Care 0412 Bowel Incontinence Care: Encopresis **X** 0420 Bowel Irrigation 0430 Bowel Management 0440 Bowel Training 0450 Constipation/Impaction Management 0460 Diarrhea Management 0470 Flatulence Reduction 0480 Ostomy Care **L** 0490 Rectal Prolapse Management 0550 Bladder Irrigation 0560 Pelvic Floor Exercise 1876 Tube Care: Urinary 0570 Urinary Bladder Training 0580 Urinary Catheterization 0582 Urinary Catheterization: Intermittent 0590 Urinary Elimination Management 0600 Urinary Habit Training 0610 Urinary Incontinence Care 0612 Urinary Incontinence Care: Enuresis **X** 0620 Urinary Retention Care 1804 Self-Care Assistance: Toileting **F**	0740 Bed Rest Care 0762 Cast Care: Maintenance 0764 Cast Care: Wet 6580 Physical Restraint **V** 0840 Positioning 0846 Positioning: Wheelchair 0910 Splinting 0940 Traction/Immobilization Care 0960 Transport
	0100 to 0399	**0400 to 0699**	**0700 to 0999**

*Letter indicates another class where the intervention is also included.

D	**Nutrition Support** Interventions to modify or maintain nutritional status	**E**	**Physical Comfort Promotion** Interventions to promote comfort using physical techniques	**F**	**Self-Care Facilitation** Interventions to provide or assist with routine activities of daily living
1020	Diet Staging	1320	Acupressure	1610	Bathing
1030	Eating Disorders Management	1340	Cutaneous Stimulation	1620	Contact Lens Care
		6482	Environmental Management: Comfort	1630	Dressing
1050	Feeding **F**			1640	Ear Care
1056	Enteral Tube Feeding	1380	Heat/Cold Application	1650	Eye Care
1080	Gastrointestinal Intubation	1400	Pain Management	1050	Feeding **D**
		1460	Progressive Muscle Relaxation	1660	Foot Care
1100	Nutrition Management			1670	Hair Care
1120	Nutrition Therapy	1480	Simple Massage	1680	Nail Care
5246	Nutritional Counseling	5465	Therapeutic Touch	1710	Oral Health Maintenance
1160	Nutritional Monitoring	1540	Transcutaneous Electrical Nerve Stimulation (TENS)		
1803	Self-Care Assistance: Feeding **F**			1720	Oral Health Promotion
1860	Swallowing Therapy **F**			1730	Oral Health Restoration
5614	Teaching: Prescribed Diet **S**			1750	Perineal Care
				1770	Postmortem Care
1200	Total Parenteral Nutrition (TPN) Administration **G**			1780	Prosthesis Care
				1800	Self-Care Assistance
1874	Tube Care: Gastrointestinal			1801	Self-Care Assistance: Bathing/Hygiene
1240	Weight Gain Assistance			1802	Self-Care Assistance: Dressing/Grooming
1260	Weight Management			1803	Self-Care Assistance: Feeding **D**
1280	Weight Reduction Assistance			1804	Self-Care Assistance: Toileting **B**
				1850	Sleep Enhancement
				1860	Swallowing Therapy **D**
				1870	Tube Care

1000 to 1299	**1300 to 1599**	**1600 to 1899**

Level 1 Domains	**2. PHYSIOLOGICAL: COMPLEX** **Care That Supports Homeostatic Regulation**		

Level 2 Classes	**G**	**Electrolyte and Acid-Base Management** Interventions to regulate electrolyte/acid base balance and prevent complications	**H**	**Drug Management** Interventions to facilitate desired effects of pharmacological agents

Level 3 Interventions				
	1910	Acid-Base Management	2210	Analgesic Administration
	1911	Acid-Base Management: Metabolic Acidosis	2214	Analgesic Administration: Intraspinal
	1912	Acid-Base Management: Metabolic Alkalosis	2840	Anesthesia Administration **J**
	1913	Acid-Base Management: Respiratory Acidosis **K***	2240	Chemotherapy Management **S**
			2260	Conscious Sedation
	1914	Acid-Base Management: Respiratory Alkalosis **K**	2300	Medication Administration
			2301	Medication Administration: Enteral
	1920	Acid-Base Monitoring	2302	Medication Administration: Interpleural
	2000	Electrolyte Management		
	2001	Electrolyte Management: Hypercalcemia	2303	Medication Administration: Intraosseous
	2002	Electrolyte Management: Hyperkalemia	2304	Medication Administration: Oral
	2003	Electrolyte Management: Hypermagnesemia	2305	Medication Administration: Parenteral
	2004	Electrolyte Management: Hypernatremia	2306	Medication Administration: Topical
	2005	Electrolyte Management: Hyperphosphatemia	2307	Medication Administration: Ventricular Reservoir
	2006	Electrolyte Management: Hypocalcemia	2380	Medication Management
			2390	Medication Prescribing
	2007	Electrolyte Management: Hypokalemia	2400	Patient-Controlled Analgesia (PCA) Assistance
	2008	Electrolyte Management: Hypomagnesemia	5616	Teaching: Prescribed Medication **S**
	2009	Electrolyte Management: Hyponatremia	2440	Venous Access devices (VAD) Maintenance **N**
	2010	Electrolyte Management: Hypophosphatemia		
	2020	Electrolyte Monitoring		
	2080	Fluid/Electrolyte Management **N**		
	2100	Hemodialysis Therapy		
	2120	Hyperglycemia Management		
	2130	Hypoglycemia Management		
	2150	Peritoneal Dialysis Therapy		
	4232	Phlebotomy: Arterial Blood Sample **N**		
	1200	Total Parenteral Nutrition (TPN) Administration **D**		
	1900 to 2199		**2200 to 2499**	

*Letter indicates another class where the intervention is also included.

I **Neurologic Management** Interventions to optimize neurologic function	**J** **Perioperative Care** Interventions to provide care before, during, and immediately after surgery

2540	Cerebral Edema Management	2840	Anesthesia Administration **H**
2550	Cerebral Perfusion Promotion	2860	Autotransfusion **N**
2560	Dysreflexia Management	6545	Infection Control: Intraoperative
2590	Intracranial Pressure (ICP) Monitoring	0842	Positioning: Intraoperative
2620	Neurologic Monitoring	2870	Postanesthesia Care
2660	Peripheral Sensation Management	2880	Preoperative Coordination **Y**
0844	Positioning: Neurologic	2900	Surgical Assistance
2680	Seizure Management **V**	2920	Surgical Precautions **V**
2690	Seizure Precautions	2930	Surgical Preparation
2720	Subarachnoid Hemorrhage Precautions	5610	Teaching: Preoperative **S**
1878	Tube Care: Ventriculostomy/Lumbar Drain	3902	Temperature Regulation: Intraoperative **M**
2760	Unilateral Neglect Management		

2500 to 2799 | **2800 to 3099**

Level 1 Domains	**2. PHYSIOLOGICAL: COMPLEX** **Care That Supports Homeostatic Regulation—Cont'd**	
Level 2 **Classes**	**K** **Respiratory Management** Interventions to promote airway patency and gas exchange	**L** **Skin/Wound Management** Interventions to maintain or re- store tissue integrity

Level 3
Interventions
	1913 Acid-Base Management: Respi-
	        ratory Acidosis **G**
	1914 Acid-Base Management: Respi-
	        ratory Alkalosis **G**
	3120 Airway Insertion and Stabiliza-
	        tion
	3140 Airway Management
	3160 Airway Suctioning
	3180 Artificial Airway Management
	3200 Aspiration Precautions **V**
	3230 Chest Physiotherapy
	3250 Cough Enhancement
	4106 Embolus Care: Pulmonary **N**
	3270 Endotracheal Extubation
	3300 Mechanical Ventilation
	3310 Mechanical Ventilatory
	        Weaning
	3320 Oxygen Therapy
	3350 Respiratory Monitoring
	1872 Tube Care: Chest
	3390 Ventilation Assistance
		3420 Amputation Care
		3440 Incision Site Care
		3460 Leech Therapy
		0480 Ostomy Care **B**
		3500 Pressure Management
		3520 Pressure Ulcer Care
		3540 Pressure Ulcer Prevention **V**
		3584 Skin Care: Topical Treatments
		3590 Skin Surveillance
		3620 Suturing
		3660 Wound Care
		3662 Wound Care: Closed Drainage
		3680 Wound Irrigation

	3100 to 3399	**3400 to 3699**

*Letter indicates another class where the intervention is also included.

M	**Thermoregulation**	**N**	**Tissue Perfusion Management**
	Interventions to maintain body temperature within a normal range		Interventions to optimize circulation of blood and fluids to the tissue

3740	Fever Treatment	2860	Autotransfusion **J**
3780	Heat Exposure Treatment	4010	Bleeding Precautions
3800	Hypothermia Treatment	4020	Bleeding Reduction
3840	Malignant Hyperthermia Precautions **U**	4021	Bleeding Reduction: Antepartum Uterus **W**
3900	Temperature Regulation	4022	Bleeding Reduction: Gastrointestinal
3902	Temperature Regulation: Intraoperative **J**	4024	Bleeding Reduction: Nasal
		4026	Bleeding Reduction: Postpartum Uterus **W**
		4028	Bleeding Reduction: Wound
		4030	Blood Products Administration
		4040	Cardiac Care
		4044	Cardiac Care: Acute
		4046	Cardiac Care: Rehabilitative
		4050	Cardiac Precautions
		4060	Circulatory Care
		4064	Circulatory Care: Mechanical Assist Device
		4070	Circulatory Precautions
		4090	Dysrhythmia Management
		4104	Embolus Care: Peripheral
		4106	Embolus Care: Pulmonary **K**
		4110	Embolus Precautions
		2080	Fluid/Electrolyte Mangement **G**
		4120	Fluid Management
		4130	Fluid Monitoring
		4140	Fluid Resuscitation
		4150	Hemodynamic Regulation
		4160	Hemorrhage Control
		4170	Hypervolemia Management
		4180	Hypovolemia Management
		4190	Intravenous (IV) Insertion
		4200	Intravenous (IV) Therapy
		4210	Invasive Hemodynamic Monitoring
		4220	Peripherally Inserted Central (PIC) Catheter Care
		4232	Phlebotomy: Arterial Blood Sample **G**
		4234	Phlebotomy: Blood Unit Acquisition
		4238	Phlebotomy: Venous Blood Sample
		4250	Shock Management
		4254	Shock Management: Cardiac
		4256	Shock Management: Vasogenic
		4258	Shock Management: Volume
		4260	Shock Prevention
		2440	Venous Access Devices (VAD) Maintenance **H**

3700 to 3999	**4000 to 4299**

Level 1 Domains	**3. BEHAVIORAL** **Care That Supports Psychosocial Functioning and Facilitates Life-style Changes**					
Level 2 Classes	**O**	**Behavior Therapy** Interventions to reinforce or promote desirable behaviors or alter undesirable behaviors	**P**	**Cognitive Therapy** Interventions to reinforce or promote desirable cognitive functioning or alter undesirable cognitive functioning	**Q**	**Communica-tion Enhance-ment** Interventions to facilitate delivering and receiving verbal and nonverbal messages
Level 3 Interventions	4310 4320 4330 4340 4350 4352 4354 4356 4360 4362 4370 4380 4390 4400 4410 4420 4430 4470 4480 4490 4500 4510 4512 4514 4516	Activity Therapy Animal-Assisted Therapy **Q*** Art Therapy **Q** Assertiveness Training Behavior Management Behavior Management: Overactivity/ Inattention Behavior Management: Self-Harm Behavior Management: Sexual Behavior Modification Behavior Modification: Social Skills Impulse Control Training Limit Setting Milieu Therapy Music Therapy **Q** Mutual Goal Setting Patient Contracting Play Therapy **Q** Self-Modification Assistance Self-Responsibility Facilitation Smoking Cessation Assistance Substance Use Prevention Substance Use Treatment Substance Use Treatment: Alcohol Withdrawal Substance Use Treatment: Drug Withdrawal Substance Use Treatment: Overdose	4640 4680 4700 4720 5520 5540 4760 4820 4860	Anger Control Assistance Bibliotherapy Cognitive Restructuring Cognitive Stimulation Learning Facilitation **S** Learning Readiness Enhancement **S** Memory Training Reality Orientation Reminiscence Therapy	4920 4320 4330 4974 4976 4978 5000 4400 4430 5100	Active Listening Animal-Assisted Therapy **O** Art Therapy **O** Communication Enhancement: Hearing Deficit Communication Enhancement: Speech Deficit Communication Enhancement: Visual Deficit Complex Relationship Building Music Therapy **O** Play Therapy **O** Socialization Enhancement
		4300 to 4599		**4600 to 4899**		**4900 to 5199**

*Letter indicates another class where the intervention is also included.

R	**Coping Assistance** Interventions to assist another to build on own strengths, adapt to a change in function, or to achieve a higher level of function	S	**Patient Education** Interventions to facilitate learning	T	**Psychological Comfort Promotion** Interventions to promote comfort using psychological techniques
5210	Anticipatory Guidance **W**	2240	Chemotherapy Management **H**	5820	Anxiety Reduction
5220	Body Image Enhancement	6784	Family Planning: Contraception **W**	5840	Autogenic Training
5230	Coping Enhancement	5510	Health Education	5860	Biofeedback
5240	Counseling	5520	Learning Facilitation **P**	5880	Calming Technique
5242	Genetic Counseling **W**	5540	Learning Readiness Enhancement **P**	5900	Distraction
5248	Sexual Counseling			5920	Hypnosis
6160	Crisis Intervention **U**	5562	Parent Education: Adolescent **X**	5960	Meditation
5250	Decision-Making Support **Y**	5564	Parent Education: Childbearing Family **W**	6000	Simple Guided Imagery
5260	Dying Care	5566	Parent Education: Childrearing Family **X**	6040	Simple Relaxation Therapy
5270	Emotional Support	5580	Preparatory Sensory Information		
5290	Grief Work Facilitation	5602	Teaching: Disease Process		
5294	Grief Work Facilitation: Perinatal Death **W**	5604	Teaching: Group		
5300	Guilt Work Facilitation	5606	Teaching: Individual		
5310	Hope Instillation	5608	Teaching: Infant Care **W**		
5320	Humor	5610	Teaching: Preoperative **J**		
5330	Mood Management	5612	Teaching: Prescribed Activity/Exercise **A**		
5340	Presence	5614	Teaching: Prescribed Diet **D**		
5360	Recreation Therapy	5616	Teaching: Prescribed Medication **H**		
5370	Role Enhancement **X**	5618	Teaching: Procedure/Treatment		
5380	Security Enhancement	5620	Teaching: Psychomotor Skill		
5390	Self-Awareness Enhancement	5622	Teaching: Safe Sex		
5400	Self-Esteem Enhancement	5624	Teaching: Sexuality		
5420	Spiritual Support				
5430	Support Group				
5440	Support System Enhancement				
5450	Therapy Group				
5460	Touch				
5470	Truth Telling				
5480	Values Clarification				
	5200 to 5499		**5500 to 5799**		**5800 to 6099**

Level 1 Domains	**4. SAFETY** **Care That Supports Protection Against Harm**		
Level 2 Classes	**U**	**Crisis Management** Interventions to provide immediate short-term help in both psychological and physiological crises	**V** **Risk Management** Interventions to initiate risk-reduction activities and continue monitoring risks over time

Level 3 Interventions		
	6140 Code Management 6160 Crisis Intervention **R*** 6200 Emergency Care 6240 First Aid 3840 Malignant Hyperthermia Precautions **M** 6260 Organ Procurement 6300 Rape-Trauma Treatment 6320 Resuscitation 6340 Suicide Prevention **V** 6360 Triage	6400 Abuse Protection 6402 Abuse Protection: Child 6404 Abuse Protection: Elder 6410 Allergy Management 6420 Area Restriction 3200 Aspiration Precautions **K** 6440 Delirium Management 6450 Delusion Management 6460 Dementia Management 6470 Elopement Precautions 6480 Environmental Management 6484 Environmental Management: Community 6486 Environmental Management: Safety 6487 Environmental Management: Violence Prevention 6489 Environmental Management: Worker Safety 6490 Fall Prevention 6500 Fire-Setting Precautions 6510 Hallucination Management 6520 Health Screening 6530 Immunization/Vaccination Administration 6540 Infection Control 6550 Infection Protection 6560 Laser Precautions 6570 Latex Precautions 6580 Physical Restraint **C** 6590 Pneumatic Tourniquet Precautions 3540 Pressure Ulcer Prevention **L** 6600 Radiation Therapy Management 6610 Risk Identification 6630 Seclusion 2680 Seizure Management **I** 6340 Suicide Prevention **U** 2920 Surgical Precautions **J** 6650 Surveillance 6654 Surveillance: Safety 6680 Vital Signs Monitoring
	6100 to 6399	**6400 to 6699**

*Letter indicates another class where the intervention is also included.

Level 1 Domains	**5. FAMILY** Care That Supports the Family Unit			

Level 2 Classes	**W**	**Childbearing Care** Interventions to assist in understanding and coping with the psychological and physiological changes during the childbearing period	**X**	**Lifespan Care** Interventions to facilitate family unit functioning and promote the health and welfare of family members throughout the lifespan
Level 3 Interventions	6700 Amnioinfusion 5210 Anticipatory Guidance **R*** 6710 Attachment Promotion 6720 Birthing 4021 Bleeding Reduction: Antepartum Uterus **N** 4026 Bleeding Reduction: Postpartum Uterus **N** 1052 Bottle Feeding 1054 Breastfeeding Assistance 6750 Cesarean Section Care 6760 Childbirth Preparation 6771 Electronic Fetal Monitoring: Antepartum 6772 Electronic Fetal Monitoring: Intrapartum 6481 Environmental Management: Attachment Process 7104 Family Integrity Promotion: Childbearing Family 6784 Family Planning: Contraception **S** 6786 Family Planning: Infertility 6788 Family Planning: Unplanned Pregnancy 5242 Genetic Counseling **R** 5294 Grief Work Facilitation: Perinatal Death **R** 6800 High-Risk Pregnancy Care 6820 Infant Care 6830 Intrapartal Care 6834 Intrapartal Care: High-Risk Delivery	6840 Kangaroo Care 6850 Labor Induction 6860 Labor Suppression 5244 Lactation Counseling 6870 Lactation Suppression 6880 Newborn Care 6890 Newborn Monitoring 6900 Nonnutritive Sucking 5564 Parent Education: Childbearing Family **S** 6924 Phototherapy: Neonate 6930 Postpartal Care 5247 Preconception Counseling 6950 Pregnancy Termination Care 6960 Prenatal Care 7886 Reproductive Technology Management 6972 Resuscitation: Fetus 6974 Resuscitation: Neonate 6612 Risk Identification: Childbearing Family 6656 Surveillance: Late Pregnancy 5608 Teaching: Infant Care **S** 1875 Tube Care: Umbilical Line 6982 Ultrasonography: Limited Obstetric **6700 to 6999**	0412 Bowel Incontinence Care: Encopresis **B** 7040 Caregiver Support 7050 Developmental Enhancement 7100 Family Integrity Promotion 7110 Family Involvement 7120 Family Mobilization 7130 Family Process Maintenance 7140 Family Support 7150 Family Therapy 7160 Fertility Preservation 7180 Home Maintenance Assistance 7200 Normalization Promotion 5562 Parent Education: Adolescent **S** 5566 Parent Education: Childrearing Family **S** 7260 Respite Care 5370 Role Enhancement **R** 7280 Sibling Support 0612 Urinary Incontinence Care: Enuresis **B** **7000 to 7299**

*Letter indicates another class where the intervention is also included.

Level 1 Domains	**6. HEALTH SYSTEM** **Care That Supports Effective Use of the Health Care Delivery System**				
Level 2 Classes	**Y**	**Health System Mediation** Interventions to facilitate the interface between patient/family and the health care system	**a**	**Health System Management** Interventions to provide and enhance support services for the delivery of care	**b**	**Information Management** Interventions to facilitate communication among health care providers

Level 3 Interventions						
	7310	Admission Care	7610	Bedside Laboratory Testing	7920	Documentation
	7330	Culture Brokerage	7620	Controlled Substance Checking	7960	Health Care Information Exchange
	5250	Decision-Making Support **R***	7640	Critical Path Development	7970	Health Policy Monitoring
	7370	Discharge Planning	7650	Delegation	7980	Incident Reporting
	7400	Health System Guidance	7660	Emergency Cart Checking	8020	Multidisciplinary Care Conference
	7410	Insurance Authorization	7680	Examination Assistance	8060	Order Transcription
	7440	Pass Facilitation	7690	Laboratory Data Interpretation	8100	Referral
	7460	Patient Rights Protection	7700	Peer Review	8120	Research Data Collection
	2880	Preoperative Coordination **J**	7710	Physician Support	8140	Shift Report
	7500	Sustenance Support	7722	Preceptor: Employee	8180	Telephone Consultation
	7560	Visitation Facilitation	7726	Preceptor: Student		
			7760	Product Evaluation		
			7800	Quality Monitoring		
			7820	Specimen Management		
			7830	Staff Supervision		
			7840	Supply Management		
			7880	Technology Management		
	7300 to 7599		**7600 to 7899**		**7900 to 8199**	

*Letter indicates another class where the intervention is also included.

Appendix C
NURSING OUTCOMES CLASSIFICATION (NOC) OUTCOMES AND MEASUREMENT SCALES

The Nursing Outcomes Classification (NOC) was designed specifically for nurses to evaluate the effects of nursing interventions. Patient outcomes are evaluated on a continuum or rating scale to indicate changes in patient conditions. NOC uses 16 different scales (shown in this appendix) that provide a way of measuring not only if an outcome was met but also how well it was met. When the NOC text was printed in 1997, there were 190 outcomes identified, along with definitions, indicators, and measurement scales. The next edition of NOC will reflect refinement of the existing outcomes and additional outcomes identified since the 1997 edition.

This appendix, reprinted with permission, includes all 16 of the NOC measurement scales to show you how different outcomes are placed on different scales. Each of the 16 scales was designed to deal with certain outcomes. For example, Scale #1 addresses the degree to which its 43 outcomes may or may not be compromised, and Scale #3 addresses the degree of the patient's dependency or independency related to its 17 different outcomes.

This appendix was included to help you very briefly see how NOC was designed. To actually use NOC, you will need the text itself.

We strongly believe that NOC, along with the NANDA and NIC classifications, will soon be commonly used in nursing practice, education, and research. NANDA/NIC/NOC provide common languages that delineate nursing care more clearly than has been done in the past.

Measurement Scales Used in NOC

SCALE #		NOC SCALES	
1	Extremely compromised	Substantially compromised	Moderately compromised

		OUTCOMES
Mildly compromised	**Not compromised**	Bowel Elimination
		Cardiac Pump Effectiveness
		Caregiver Emotional Health
		Caregiver Physical Health
		Caregiver Well-Being
		Caregiver-Patient Relationship
		Circulation Status
		Cognitive Ability
		Communication
		Communication: Expressive Ability
		Communication: Receptive Ability
		Electrolyte & Acid/Base Balance
		Endurance
		Fluid Balance
		Hydration
		Immune Status
		Muscle Function
		Neurological Status
		Neurological Status: Autonomic
		Neurological Status: Central Motor Control
		Neurological Status: Consciousness
		Neurological Status: Cranial Sensory/ Motor Function
		Neurological Status: Spinal Sensory/ Motor Function
		Nutritional Status
		Nutritional Status: Energy
		Oral Health
		Quality of Life
		Respiratory Status: Gas Exchange
		Respiratory Status: Ventilation
		Rest
		Sleep
		Spiritual Well-Being
		Thermoregulation
		Thermoregulation: Neonate
		Tissue Integrity: Skin & Mucous Membranes
		Tissue Perfusion: Cardiac
		Tissue Perfusion: Cerebral
		Tissue Perfusion: Peripheral
		Tissue Perfusion: Pulmonary
		Tissue Perfusion: Abdominal Organs
		Urinary Elimination
		Well-Being
		Will to Live

Continued

Measurement Scales Used in NOC–cont'd

SCALE #		NOC SCALES	
2	Extreme deviation from expected range	Substantial deviation from expected range	Moderate deviation from expected range
3	Dependent, does not participate	Requires assistive person & device	Requires assistive person
4	No motion	Limited motion	Moderate motion
5	Not at all	To a slight extent	To a moderate extent
6	Not adequate	Slightly adequate	Moderately adequate

		OUTCOMES
Mild deviation from expected range	**No deviation from expected range**	Growth Nutritional Status: Biochemical Measures Nutritional Status: Body Mass Physical Aging Status Physical Maturation: Female Physical Maturation: Male Vital Signs Status
Independent with assistive device	**Completely independent**	Ambulation: Walking Ambulation: Wheelchair Balance Body Positioning: Self-Initiated Mobility Level Self-Care: Activities of Daily Living (ADL) Self-Care: Bathing Self-Care: Dressing Self-Care: Eating Self-Care: Grooming Self-Care: Hygiene Self-Care: Instrumental Activities of Daily Living (IADL) Self-Care: Non-Parenteral Medication Self-Care: Oral Hygiene Self-Care: Parenteral Medication Self-Care: Toileting Transfer Performance
Substantial motion	**Full motion**	Joint Movement: Active Joint Movement: Passive
To a great extent	**To a very great extent**	Blood Transfusion Reaction Control Dignified Dying Energy Conservation Grief Resolution Immune Hypersensitivity Control
Substantially adequate	**Totally adequate**	Abuse Protection Breastfeeding Establishment: Infant Breastfeeding Establishment: Maternal Breastfeeding Maintenance Breastfeeding Weaning Caregiver Performance: Direct Care Caregiver Performance: Indirect Care Caregiver Endurance Potential Leisure Participation Nutritional Status: Food & Fluid Intake Nutritional Status: Nutrient Intake Parenting Parenting: Social Safety Play Participation

Continued

Measurement Scales Used in NOC—cont'd

SCALE #		NOC SCALES	
6—cont'd			
7	**Over 9**	**7–9**	**4–6**
8	**Extensive**	**Substantial**	**Moderate**
9	**None**	**Limited**	**Moderate**
10	**None**	**Slight**	**Moderate**
11	**Never positive**	**Rarely positive**	**Sometimes positive**

		OUTCOMES
		Role Performance Safety Behavior: Fall Prevention Safety Behavior: Home Physical Environment Safety Behavior: Personal
1–3	**None**	Safety Status: Falls Occurrence
Limited	**None**	Caregiver Stressors Loneliness
Substantial	**Extensive**	Abuse Recovery: Emotional Abuse Recovery: Financial Abuse Recovery: Physical Abuse Recovery: Sexual Acceptance: Health Status Caregiver Adaptation to Patient Institutionalization Caregiver Home Care Readiness Child Adaptation to Hospitalization Comfort Level Hope Knowledge: Breastfeeding Knowledge: Child Safety Knowledge: Diet Knowledge: Disease Process Knowledge: Energy Conservation Knowledge: Health Behaviors Knowledge: Health Resources Knowledge: Infection Control Knowledge: Medication Knowledge: Personal Safety Knowledge: Prescribed Activity Knowledge: Substance Use Control Knowledge: Treatment Procedure(s) Knowledge: Treatment Regimen Psychosocial Adjustment: Life Change Social Interaction Skills Social Involvement Social Support
Substantial	**Complete**	Bone Healing Wound Healing: Primary Intention Wound Healing: Secondary Intention
Often positive	**Consistently positive**	Body Image Self-Esteem

Continued

Measurement Scales Used in NOC—cont'd

SCALE #		NOC SCALES	
12	**Very weak**	**Weak**	**Moderate**
13	**Never demonstrated**	**Rarely demonstrated**	**Sometimes demonstrated**

		OUTCOMES
Strong	**Very strong**	Health Beliefs Health Beliefs: Perceived Ability to Perform Health Beliefs: Perceived Control Health Beliefs: Perceived Resources Health Beliefs: Perceived Threat Health Orientation
Often demonstrated	**Consistently demonstrated**	Abusive Behavior Self-Control Adherence Behavior Aggression Control Anxiety Control Bowel Continence Cognitive Orientation Compliance Behavior Concentration Coping Decision Making Distorted Thought Control Fear Control Health Promoting Behavior Health Seeking Behavior Immunization Behavior Identity Impulse Control Information Processing Memory Mood Equilibrium Pain Control Behavior Parent-Infant Attachment Participation: Health Care Decisions Risk Control Risk Control: Alcohol Use Risk Control: Drug Use Risk Control: Immunization Risk Control: Sexually Transmitted Diseases (STD) Risk Control: Tobacco Use Risk Control: Unintended Pregnancy Risk Detection Self-Mutilation Restraint Suicide Self-Restraint Symptom Control Behavior Treatment Behavior: Illness or Injury Urinary Continence

Continued

Measurement Scales Used in NOC—cont'd

SCALE #		NOC SCALES	
14	Severe	Substantial	Moderate
15	No evidence	Limited evidence	Moderate evidence
16	Extreme delay from expected range	Substantial delay from expected range	Moderate delay from expected range

		OUTCOMES

Slight	**None**	Caregiver Lifestyle: Disruption
		Immobility Consequences:
		    Physiological
		Immobility Consequences:
		    Psycho-Cognitive
		Infection Status
		Pain Level
		Pain: Disruptive Effects
		Safety Status: Physical Injury
		Substance Addiction Consequences
		Symptom Severity

Substantial evidence	**Extensive evidence**	Abuse Cessation Neglect Cessation

**Mild delay from
expected range**
	**No delay from
	expected range**
		Child Development: 2 Months
		Child Development: 4 Months
		Child Development: 6 Months
		Child Development: 12 Months
		Child Development: 2 Years
		Child Development: 3 Years
		Child Development: 4 Years
		Child Development: 5 Years
		Child Development: Middle Childhood
		    (6–11 Years)
		Child Development: Adolescence
		    (12–17 Years)

(Johnson, M., & Maas, M. [1997]. *Iowa Outcomes Project: Nursing Outcomes Classification [NOC]*. St. Louis: Mosby, pp. 52–61.)

TRACKING NURSING THINKING (TNTA) CHECKLIST: GUIDELINES FOR USE

Purposes of the Tool
1. Guidance while preparing a student care plan to make sure all aspects of thinking and doing are included.
2. Self-evaluation to determine if one's care plan has included all the key elements.
3. Peer or instructor evaluation of plans to provide either initial evaluation or validation of the care planner's self-evaluation.

How to Use
1. Make a photocopy of the tool for each plan to be evaluated.
2. Compare the items listed on the far left with any evidence on the written care plan that indicates the item has occurred.
3. Use the "self ranking" scale at the top of each page to judge how well each item was achieved. If there is no evidence indicate a "0" or "N/A" for "not applicable."
4. Add any additional supporting comments or ideas for improvement in the column on the far right.
5. At the end of each of the three sections, in the areas provided, briefly discuss the care planner's overall ability in thinking and doing.
6. Write a summary of additional comments or suggestions for growth in the final section.

Optional Uses for Tracking Nursing Thinking
1. Assign numerical value to each of the items and tally the scores for each. Some items can have more weight than others, for example, "Are outcomes client centered?" might be weighted at 1 point, and "Provide rationale for all nursing actions" might be weighted at 2 points. The number of points would then be multiplied by the self-ranking number for a total score for that particular item.
2. Develop a grading scale based on the scores.
3. Keep a notebook of all the checklists completed over the semester or course to document and acknowledge growth and improvement.

TRACKING NURSING THINKING (TNTa) CHECKLIST

Student _____ Patient Initials _____ Date _____

What is the concern? (Conclusions of Assessment)	Self Ranking	Supporting Comments/Plans For Improvement
Did I …	0…No 1…Good 2…Better 3…Best	
Develop a therapeutic relationship		
Collect objective, subjective data and necessary inferences?		
Know population norms for comparison? (knowledge)		
Compare data to population norms?		
Compare data to individual norms?		
Use branching questions?		
Use D.E.T.A.I.L. questions?		
Develop hunches?		
Identify data gaps?		
Use directed data collection to fill gaps?		
Cluster data effectively?		
Select the best clusters?		
Select the best labels for the clusters?		
Identify all conclusions of assessment (strengths, nursing diagnoses, interdisciplinary problems and problems for referral)?		
Develop conclusions that reflect strong content knowledge?		
Consider alternative conclusions, differential diagnoses?		
Use proper nursing diagnosis format?		
Support all conclusions with data?		
Support all related factors with data?		
Identify all related factors for all nursing diagnoses?		
Think toward planning when finalizing all conclusions?		
Place self in patient's shoes?		
Consider the "big picture" when finalizing all conclusions of assessment?		
Clearly document all data and conclusions of assessment?		

MY OVERALL ABILITY IN THINKING AND DOING DURING ASSESSMENT IS:

TRACKING NURSING THINKING (TNTa) Checklist p. 2 Student_____Date_____		
How can the concern be altered by nursing care? (Conclusions of Planning and Implementation)	**Self Ranking**	**Supporting Comments/Plans for Improvement**
Did I...	0=No 1=Good 2=Better 3=Best	
Make the patient a partner in planning?		
Use the patient's strengths in planning?		
Use the best resources to design care?		
Set priorities based on the guidelines, and the "big picture"?		
Considered life threatening issues?		
Considered safety issues?		
Considered the patient's priorities?		
Considered the nurse's priorities?		
Establish goals that:		
Match with the conclusions?		
Are client-centered?		
Have a realistic time frame?		
Are indicators of direction to move?		
Establish outcomes that:		
Fit with their respective goals?		
Are client-centered?		
Are measurable?		
Include specific criteria?		
Address all behaviors, cognitive, affective, psychomotor, and changes in patient conditions beyond the patient's control?		
Develop nursing interventions that:		
Fit with each outcomes?		
Are nurse-centered?		
Give clear directions?		
Are realistic?		
Are clinically supported by sound rationale?		
Provide rationale for all nursing interventions?		
Identify sources of rationale?		
Design care for all nursing diagnoses, interdisciplinary problems and problems for referral?		
Design care that used effective time and resource management?		
Use standardized care plans as a trigger to thinking and individualized care?		
Clearly document the nursing care plan?		
Implement care safely?		
Implement care efficiently?		
MY OVERALL ABILITY IN THINKING AND DOING DURING PLANNING AND IMPLEMENTATION IS:		

TRACKING NURSING THINKING (TNTa) Checklist p. 3 Student_____Date_____		
Did the plan work? **(Conclusions of Evaluation)**	**Self Ranking**	**Supporting Comments/Plans for Improvement**
Did I...	0=No 1=Good 2=Better 3=Best	
Establish appropriate outcome criteria during the planning?		
Ask patient to assist in the evaluation process?		
Determine patient's progress toward outcomes and goals?		
Clearly document patient's progress toward outcomes and goals?		
Determine degree of patient's achievement of all goals and outcomes?		
Clearly document patient's achievements toward all goals and outcomes?		
Determine if the patient's concerns/problems were resolved?		
Clearly document the status of concerns/problems?		
Modify the plan of care periodically to adapt to the patient's changing needs?		
Clearly document modifications in plan?		
Backtrack through the nursing process to find areas of breakdown in thinking if there were any?		

MY OVERALL ABILITY IN THINKING AND DOING DURING EVALUATION IS:

ADDITIONAL COMMENTS/SUGGESTIONS FOR GROWTH:

Appendix E

TRACKING NURSING THINKING (TNTb) GUIDELINES AND CHECKLIST (STREAMLINED FOR ASSESSMENT AND PLANNING ONLY)

Purpose of the Tool

1. Provide a streamlined tool for student and faculty to make sure key areas of thinking have been done for assessment and planning only.
2. Provide systematic way to evaluate plans and rate them.

How to Use

1. Make a photocopy of the tool for each plan to be evaluated
2. Compare the items listed on the far left with any evidence on the written care plan that indicates the item has occurred.
3. Use the "self ranking" scale at the top of each page to judge how well each item was achieved. If there is no evidence, indicate a "0" or "N/A" for "not applicable."
4. Add any additional supporting comments or ideas for improvement in the column on the far right.
5. At the end of each checklist, briefly discuss the care planner's overall ability in thinking and doing.
6. Write a summary of additional comments or suggestions for growth in the final section.

Optional Uses for the TNTb

1. Develop a grading scale based on the scores.
2. Keep a notebook of all the checklists completed over the semester or course to document and acknowledge growth and improvement.
3. This checklist can be used with any form of nursing care plan, traditional column format, concept map format, or others.

Tracking Nursing Thinking (TNTb) Checklist
(Streamlined for Assessment and Planning)

Student _____ Patient Initials _____ Date _____

Categories	Self/Instructor's Rating 0 = No 1 = Needs much improvement 2 = Needs some improvement 3 = Good 4 = Best	Supporting Comments
Relevant data identified		
Referenced norms (knowledge base and source)		
Initial data clusters made		
Clusters labeled (hunches)		
Data gaps identified		
Conclusions of Assessment: Strengths identified		
Nursing diagnoses: Proper format		
Data to support label (def. characteristics)		
All related factors identified		
Interdisciplinary problems labelled		
Data to support label		
Problems for referral identified		
Conclusions of Planning: Priorities set appropriately		
Goal statement: Time frame identified		
Addresses diagnostic label		
Patient centered		
Patient outcomes: Measurable statements		
Patient centered		
All related factors addressed		
Nursing interventions: Nurse centered		
Fit with outcomes		
Individualized to patient		
Clear, specific directions		
Rationale for nursing interventions Specific to each intervention		
Source identified		

Overall use of the five T.H.I.N.K. modes:

T.   (Total Recall)
H.   (Habits)
I.   (Inquiry)
N.   (New Ideas and Creativity)
K.   (Knowing How You Think)

Appendix 7

THINKING WORKSHEET FOR TRACKING NURSING THINKING (TNTB) CHECKLIST

Directions

Read the Case Study provided by your instructor.

Use the categories identified below as a guide to your thinking. (You may want to simply use the categories on another sheet of paper to allow more room to write.)

After completing the worksheet, review the first half of the Tracking Nursing Thinking (TNTb) Checklist.

Be sure you can rate yourself in each of the categories through "Priorities Set Appropriately."

Develop your nursing care plan for the priority nursing diagnosis in whatever format your instructor requests.

After completing the care plan, review the second half of the TNTb Checklist and rate yourself in each of the categories.

Student _____ Date _____

Relevant Data	Why? Compared to What Norms? (Include reference)

Initial Data Clusters	Cluster Label (Hunch)	Data Gaps

Conclusions of Assessment:
   Strengths:

Nursing Diagnoses:	Data to Support

Interdisciplinary Problems:	Data to Support

   Problems for Referral:

Priority Nursing Diagnosis: (Include diagnostic label with *all* related factors)

Rationale for Choosing Priority Nursing Diagnosis:

Defining Characteristics for Diagnostic Label	Data to Support Related Factor

Appendix G
MIND MAP FOR CLINICAL SITUATION

Mind maps, also called concept maps, are ways to show one's thinking processes. They allow for the presentation of not only data but also the linkages among those data. They are individual processes that are most helpful when they are not highly structured by someone other than the person doing the map. Each person's mind works in a different way; a map allows for expression of that unique process. The map presented here is adapted from one done by a student over 2 weeks of clinical work with a patient who had suffered a brain injury (TBI). The student was told to start with whatever issues struck her as important and to record her mind's patterns as she studied information relative to this patient's condition and made plans for the next week's work with this patient. Another person in the same situation might have produced a map very different from this one.

The value of mapping is that it allows one's mind to move in a natural flow. There are no constraints such as forms, columns, wording, specific requirements, etc. The energy that a person might put into making things fit within an assigned format can be used to explore details that he or she sees as relevant. Mapping promotes Inquiry thinking, in particular because the questions asked along the way are as important as the end results of that questioning.

Some people use a variety of colors when mapping so that types of information can be coded. Others use shapes or graphics to code things. Most people start their maps in the middle of a piece of paper so that they have room to record their mind's movements in any direction. Some start with a large piece of paper, and others add paper around the edges of the first one as needed.

Mind maps work best for people who are non-linear thinkers, those who feel restricted by forms or columns. They are difficult for people who feel a need to have "order" in their work. (Maps can seem very disorderly.) They are helpful learning experiences for dualistic thinkers who try to be more relativistic because it helps them to address multiple connections among information.

(Evaluation)
on 3/3 pt didn't need suppos. H d moderate BM when put on commode. BM when I got to pt at 4pm. "I'm beginning to feel worn."

Consider also: age, immobility ↓ circulation, animal ↓ Shear/friction, incont, 3/2 we fall risk, nutrition, goes to surgery ↑ UTI ↑ UlcER cause more blisters

Dx: (acting) UTI prrbbn pt will Deterrd Spikes the fever, high before chills

How cold she? Incontinence? Could get infected (Foley doesn't foley)

3/3 Neg test ↑ on 2 ↑ TBI
Cont monitoring fecal/urinary ↑ urine + sensory ↑ ↑ ↑ function + 2 ADLS
Needs ADLS
Self ambulate (↑ aspiration)
risk for

Got Tx: confabulation
N LANDING?
1. No sterars Bowel Cleaut prog. (Reg/lat PD)
2. No sterars on diet prog. bowel (Reg/lat Sub) (pt willing)
3. Fluids too dry? will just ↓ goes

STAGE II PRESSURE ULCER
(COCCYX)
- extensive tissue destruction Drainage
- full thickness
- (CLTC 522) (Muscle Bone)
What does stage II mean? Why does she have it? How can we treat?

Foley Cath
Why does she have this?
What are labs (ua)?
How do you care for it?

CULTURE >100,000
SMAR ABET
1+ PROTEIN
1+ BLOOD
+ NITRATE
ESTR
243 WBC
3+ LEUKOCYTE
83 RBC
3+ BACTER, A ADHERES
BLOODY MATRIX TESTING

Ciprofloxacin 500mg BID ordered. Bactericidal - interferes with DNA replication in susceptible gram neg. bacteria

Increased fluids will make urine more dilute + help flush in rectum.

(3) (N)

Dependant drainage. Empty bag regularly keep below bladder level. Wash peri area + meatus BID c soap + H2O.
Also has order for nystatin powder

BOWEL INCONTINENCE
Why does she have it? What can we do? What are realistic goals? How does it feel about this?

TBI - 10Dx
pt admitted from another hosp. 8/m coma blind. Auto accident 1/30. Now RLA stage P treat ploce d 2/13

Dysphagia common with TBI
impaired swallowing
Risk for aspiration

PEG TUBE
Why does she have? How do I know nutrition is OK? How do you give feedings?

1. Upright position
2. Pump set at 45cc/hr Full Strength formula 21 hrs/d.
3. Give 180cc free H2O Q4o
4. Comfeel around tube (it oozes some - need to protect skin)
5. Stop TF 1.0 before meals
6. Constant Supervision during meals

TUBE FEEDING/DIET:
TRIGLYCERIDES

Evaluation: pt ate my 50% of meals but says "I don't want tube feeding anymore"
Goal: ORAL DIET WITH NO ASPIRATION

TYPE 2 D.M.
Dehsrared Insulin this am orally. How is this ordered. Was there an order for Dm x10yrs. Had Dm x? HT 53 WT 199 16q

Giving mixed Insulin:
1. DRAW UP AIR in NPH dose.
2. Inject air into vial + draw dose into Reg dose
3. Inject air in Reg + draw up dose
4. Invert Reg + draw up
5. Carefully withdraw NPH dose to = total.
6. Sub q give

ORDERS:
40 u. NPH Ins. 15u. Reg Ins. BID
Chemstiks q6 Notify md if >200 H t53 U/amc hyper/hyper reactions

CLEAR to CLOUDY

Labs:
Albumin 3.8 (3.4-5.0)
Het: 36-48 (31.0-40)
Hgb 12.3 (12.2-5.4)
RBC 3.42 (4.10)
WBC 11.7 (4-10)
A1a 134 (135-148)
Glucose 151 (70-150)

3/13 glucose = in am 148 @ 5pm gave 40 30

9/10 glucose 203. md said to wait until next am

*very high hyperlipidemia common D/M
on md Simvastin 10mg qd

DIFFERENT POSS RELATED ISSUES - TRAUMA DM, NEUROLOGIC PROBLEMS (CLTC 1219)
PT statd will it just go. Scarred to go.

OTHER THERAPIES OTHER PHYSICAL rehabilities, Speech, OT, PT, Psych. New options Recreation
Speech with OT next

3/5 F D/C'd

OTHER ISSUES PRIOR TO CONS/DL
(DATA her support)
What is her support system? Emotional + socal
Will pt continue self-care?
How reasonable is it? Long term?
Into on pts who need PBLs had

OTHER THERAPISTS MAY HAVE SOME INSIGHT
Will pt need teaching for self? D/C. Can they give her care themselves? Could she need insulin injections?

Bibliography

Adams, M.H., Whitlow, J.G., Stover, L.M. & Johnson, K.W. (1996). Critical thinking as an educational outcome: An evaluation of current tools of measurement. *Nurse Educator, 21* (3), 23–32.

Alexander, M.K. & Giguere, B. (1996). Critical thinking in clinical learning: A holistic perspective. *Holistic Nursing Practice, 10* (3), 15–22.

Alfaro-LeFevre, R. (1998). *Applying nursing process: A step-by-step guide* (4th ed.). Philadelphia: Lippincott.

American Nurses Association. (1980). *Nursing: A social policy statement.* Kansas City: ANA.

American Nurses Association. (1991). *Standards of clinical nursing practice.* Kansas City: ANA.

Andrews, M. (1996). Using reflection to develop clinical expertise. *British Journal of Nursing, 5* (8), 508–513.

Angelo, T.A. & Cross, K.P. (1993). *Classroom assessment techniques: A handbook for college teachers* (2nd ed.). San Francisco: Jossey-Bass.

Baker, C.R. (1996). Reflective learning: A teaching strategy for critical thinking. *Journal of Nursing Education, 36* (1), 19–22.

Bandman, E.L. & Bandman, B. (1988). *Critical thinking in nursing.* East Norwalk, CT: Appleton & Lange.

Becker, H.A. & MacCabe, N. (1994). Indicators of critical thinking, communication, and therapeutic intervention among first-line nursing supervisors. *Nurse Educator, 19*(2), 15–19.

Beeken, J.E., Dale, M.L., Enos, M.F., & Yarbrough, S. (1997). Teaching critical thinking skills to undergraduate nursing students. *Nurse Educator, 22* (3), 37–39.

Begley, S. (1993, June 28). The puzzle of genius: Where do great minds come from and why are there no Einsteins, Freuds or Picassos today? *Newsweek,* 46–50.

Behrens, P.L.J. (1996). The Watson-Glaser critical thinking appriasal and academic performance of diploma school students. *Journal of Nursing Education, 35,* 34–36.

Beitz, J.M. (197). Unleashing the power of memory: The might mnemonic. *Nurse Educator, 22* (2), 25–29.

Belenky, M.F., Clinchy, B.M., Goldberger, N.R., & Tarule, J.M. (1986). *Women's ways of knowing: The development of self, voice, and the mind.* New York: Basic Books.

Benner, P. (1984). *From novice to expert: Power and excellence in nursing practice.* Menlo Park, CA: Addison-Wesley.

Benner, P. & Tanner, C. (1987). Clinical judgement: How expert nurses use intuition. *American Journal of Nursing, 87,* 23–31.

Benner, P., Tanner, C.A., & Chesla, C.A. (1996). *Expertise in nursing practice: Caring, clinical judgement, and ethics.* New York: Springer Publishing Company.

Bevis, E.O. (1993). All in all, it was a pretty good funeral. *Journal of Nursing Education, 32,* 101–105.

Birx, E.C. (1993). Critical thinking and theory-based practice. *Holistic Nursing Practice, 7,* 21–27.

Bowers, B. & McCarthy, D. (1993). Developing analytic thinking skills in early undergraduate education. *Journal of Nursing Education, 32*(3), 106–114.

Brigham, C. (1993). Nursing education and critical thinking: Interplay of content and thinking. *Holistic Nursing Practice, 7* (3), 48–54.

Brookfield, S. (1995). *Becoming a critically reflective teacher.* San Francisco: Jossey-Bass.

Brookfield, S. (1993). On impostorship, cultural suicide, and other dangers: How nurses learn critical thinking. *Journal of Continuing Education in Nursing, 24*(5), 197–205.

Brookfield, S.D. (1987). *Developing critical thinkers.* San Francisco: Jossey-Bass.

Brooks, E.M. & Thomas, S. (1997). The perception and judgment of senior baccalaureate student nurses in clinical decision making. *Advances in Nursing Science, 19* (3), 50–69.

Brooks, K. & Shepherd, J.M. (1992). Professionalism versus general critical thinking abilities of senior nursing students in four types of nursing curricula. *Journal of Professional Nursing, 8* (2), 87–95.

Brown, H.N. & Sorrell, J.M. (1993). Use of clinical journals to enhance critical thinking. *Nurse Educator, 18*(5), 16–19.

Bucknall, T. & Thomas, S. (1997). Nurses' reflections on problems associated with decision-making in critical care settings. *Journal of Advanced Nursing, 25,* 229–237.

Cameron, J. (1992). *The artist's way: A spiritual path to higher creativity.* Los Angeles: Tarcher Perigee.

Carkhuff, M.H. (1996). Reflective learning: Work groups as learning groups. *Journal of Continuing Education in Nursing, 27* (5), 209–214.

Carnevali, D.L. & Thomas, M.D. (1993). *Diagnostic reasoning and treatment decision making in nursing.* Philadelphia: J.B. Lippincott.

Carpenito, L.J. (1997). *Nursing diagnosis: Application to clinical practice* (7th ed.). Philadelphia: Lippincott.

Carroll-Johnson, R.M. (Ed.). (1991). *Classification of nursing diagnoses: Proceedings of the ninth conference of the North American Nursing Diagnosis Association.* Philadelphia: J.B. Lippincott.

Case, B. (1997). *Career planning for nurses.* New York: Delmar Publishers.

Checkley, K. (1997). The first seven . . . and the eighth: A conversation with Howard Gardner. *Educational Leadership, 55* (1), 1–13.

Chinn, P.L. (1989). Nursing patterns of knowing and feminist thought. *Nursing & Health Care, 10,* 71–75.

Chubinski, S. (1996). Creative critical-thinking strategies. *Nurse Educator, 21* (6), 23–27.

Colucciello, M. L. (1997). Critical thinking skills and dispositions of baccalaureate nursing students: A conceptual model for evaluation. *Journal of Professional Nursing, 13* (4), 236–245.

Conger, M.M. & Mezza, I. (1996). Fostering critical thinking in nursing students in the clinical setting. *Nurse Educator, 21* (3), 11–15.

Costa, A.L., Hanson, R., Silver, H.F., & Strong, R.W. (1985). Building a repertoire of strategies. In A.L. Costa (Ed.), *Developing minds: A resource book for teaching thinking* (pp. 141–143). Alexandria, VA: Association for Supervision and Curriculum Development.

Degazon, C.E. & Lunney, M. (1995). Clinical journal: A tool to foster critical thinking for advanced levels of competence. *Clinical Nurse Specialist, 9* (5), 270–274.

Dexter, P., Applegate, M., Backer, J., Claytor, K., Keffer, J., Norton, B. & Ross, B. (1997). A proposed framework for teaching and evaluating critical thinking in nursing. *Journal of Professional Nursing, 13* (3), 160–167.

Diekelmann, N.L. (1992). Learning-as-testing: A Heideggerian hermeneutical analysis of the lived experiences of students and teachers in nursing. *Advances in Nursing Science, 14*(3), 72–83.

Dreyfus, H.L. & Dreyfus, S.E. (1986). *Mind over machine.* New York: Free Press.

Drucker, P.F. (1998). The information revolution. *Forbes ASAP,* August 24, 47–58.

Elliot, D. (1996) Promoting critical thinking in the classroom. *Nurse Educator, 21* (2), 49–52.

Ellis, J.R. & Hartley, C.L. (1992). *Nursing in today's world* (4th ed.). Philadelphia: J.B. Lippincott.

Erikson, E. (1993). *Childhood and society* (2nd ed.). New York: W.W. Norton.

Eyres, S.J., Loustau, A., & Ersek, M. (1992). Ways of knowing among beginning students in nursing. *Journal of Nursing Education, 31*(4), 175–180.

Facione, N.C. (1997). *Critical thinking assessment in nursing education programs: An aggregate data analysis.* Millbrae, CA: California Academic Press.

Facione, N.C., Facione, P.A. & Sanchex, C. A. (1994). Critical thinking disposition as a measure of competent clinical judgement: The development of the California Critical Thinking Disposition Inventory. *Journal of Nursing Education, 33* (8), 345–350.

Facione, N.C. & Facione, P.A. (1996). Assessment design issues for evaluating critical thinking in nursing. *Holistic Nursing Practice, 10* (3), 41–53.

Facione, N.C. & Facione, P.A. (1996). Externalizing the critical thinking in knowledge development and clinical judgment. *Nursing Outlook, 44* (3), 129–136.

Facione, P.A. (1990). *Critical thinking: A statement of expert consensus for purposes of educational assessment and instruction.* The Dephi Report: Research findings and recommendations of the American Philospohical Association, ERIC Doc. No. ED315-423.

Facione, P.A., Sanchez, C.A., Facione, N.C. & Gainen, J. (1995). The disposition toward critical thinking. *Journal of Nursing Education, 44* (1), 1–25.

Facione, P.A., Sanchex, C.A. & Facione, N.C. (1994). *Are students disposed to think?* Millbrae, CA: California Academic Press.

Farrell, M. (1996). Research briefs: Planning for critical outcomes. *Journal of Nursing Education, 35* (6), 278–281.

Fisher, A. (1995). An exploration of an innovative methodological approach for examining nurses' heuristic use in clinical practice. *Scholarly Inquiry for Nursing Practice: An International Journal, 9* (3), 263–376.

Fonteyn, M.E. (1998). *Thinking strategies for nursing practice.* Philadelphia: Lippincott.

Ford, J.S. & Perfetto-McGraph, J. (1994). A model for critical thinking within the context of curriculum as praxis. *Journal of Nursing Education, 33,* 341–344.

Gardner, H. (1983). *Frames of mind: The theory of multiple intelligences* (10th anniversary ed.). New York: Basic Books.

Garrett, M., Schoener, L., & Hood, L. (1996). Debate: A teaching strategy to improve verbal communication and critical-thinking skills. *Nurse Educator, 21* (4), 37–40.

Gebbie, K.M. & Lavin, M.A. (1975). *Classification of nursing diagnoses: Proceedings of the first conference.* St. Louis: C.V. Mosby.

Gehrke, P. (1994). Finding voices through writing. *Nurse Educator, 19*(2), 28–30.

Gendrop, S.C. & Eisenhouer, L.A. (1996). A transactional perspective on critical thinking. *Scholarly Inquiry for Nursing Practice: An International Journal, 10* (4), 329–345.

Gilligan, C. (1993). *In a different voice: Psychological theory and women's development.* Cambridge, MA: Harvard University Press.

Gordon M. (1994). *Nursing diagnosis process and application* (3rd ed.). St. Louis: Mosby.

Gordon, M., Murphy, C.P., Candee, D. & Hiltunen, E. (1994). Clinical judgment: An integrated model. *Advances in Nursing Science, 16* (4), 55–70.

Graham, M.E. (1995). The relationship between critical thinking and how time is structured in the clinical setting for students in a baccalaureate nursing program. *ABNF Journal, 6* (6), 149–157.

Grobe, S.J., Drew, J.A. & Fonteyn, M.E. (1991). A descriptive analysis of experienced nurses' clinical reasoning during a planned task. *Research in Nursing & Health, 11,* 305–314.

Hallett, C.E. (1997). Learning through reflection in the community: The relevance of Schon's theories of coaching to nursing education. *International Journal of Nursing Studies, 34* (2), 103–110.

Hart, L.A. (1983). *Human brain and human learning.* New York: Longman.

Hartley, D. & Aukamp, V. (1994). Critical thinking ability of nurse educators and nursing students. *Journal of Nursing Education, 33* (1), 34–35.

Hartman, D.K. (1993). Critical thinking in psychiatric nursing in the decade of the brain. *Holistic Nursing Practice, 7,* (3), 36–47.

Head, B., Maas, M. & Johnson, M. (January, 1997). Outcomes for home and community nursing in integrated delivery systems. *CARING Magazine,* 50–56.

Heibert, J.L. (1996). Learning circles: A strategy for clinical practicum. *Nurse Educator, 21* (3), 37–42.

Heinrich, K.T. (1992). The intimate dialogue: Journal writing by students. *Nurse Educator, 17* (6), 17–21.

Henry, S.B., Holzemer, W.L., Randel, C., Hsieh, S. & Miller, T.J. (1997). Comparison of Nursing Interventions classification and current procedural terminology codes for categorizing nursing activities. *Image: Journal of Nursing Scholarship, 29* (2), 133–138.

Howenstein, M.A., Bilodeau, K. Brogna, M.J. & Good, G. (1996). Factors associated with critical thinking among nurses. *Journal of Continuing Education in Nursing, 27* (3), 100–103.

Jacobs, P.M., Ott, B., Sullivan, B., Ulrich, Y., & Short, L. (1997). An approach to defining and operationalizing critical thinking. *Journal of Nursing Education, 36* (1), 19–22.

Johnson, M. & Maas, M. (Eds.) (1997). *Nursing outcomes classification (NOC).* St. Louis: Mosby.

Jones, E.A. & Ratcliff, G. (1993). *Critical thinking skills for college students.* University Park, PA: National Center on Postsecondary Teaching, Learning, and Assessment.

Jones, S.A. & Brown, L.N. (1991). Critical thinking: Impact on nursing education. *Journal of Advanced Nursing, 16,* 529–533.

Jones, S.A. & Brown, L.N. (1993). Alternative views on defining critical thinking through the nursing process. *Holistic Nursing Practice, 7,* 71–76.

Kataoka-Yahiro, M. (1994). A critical thinking model for nursing judgment. *Journal of Nursing Education, 33* (8), 351–356.

King, P.M. & Kitchner, K.S. (1994). *Developing reflective judgment.* San Francisco: Jossey-Bass.

Kintgen-Andrews, J. (1991). Critical thinking and nursing education: Perplexities and insights. *Journal of Nursing Education, 30*(4), 152–157.

Kramer, M.K. (1993). Concept clarification and critical thinking: Integrated processes. *Journal of Nursing Education, 32* (9), 406–414.

Kuhn, M.A. (1995). Gaming: A technique that adds spice to learning? *Journal of Continuing Education in Nursing, 26* (1), 35–39.

Lange, L.L., Haak, S.W., Lincoln, N.J., Thompson, C.B., Turner, C.W., Weir, C., Foerster, V., Nilasena, D., & Reeves, R. (1997). Use of Illad to improve diagnostic performances of nurse practitioner students. *Journal of Nursing Education, 36* (1), 36–45.

Lauterback, S.S. & Becker, P.H. (1996). Caring for self: Becoming a self-reflective nurse. *Holistic Nursing Practice, 10* (2), 57–68.

Lee, J.E.M. & Ryan-Wenger, N. (1997). The "Think Aloud" seminar for teaching clinical reasoning: A case study of a child with pharyngitis. *Journal of Pediatric Health Care, 11* (3), 101–110.

Lunney, M. (1990). Accuracy of nursing diagnoses: Concept development. *Nursing Diagnosis, 1* (1), 12–17.

Mahon, S.M., Spies, M.A., Aukamp, V., Barrett, J.T., Figgins, M.J., Meyer, G.A., & Young, V.K. (1997). Presentation of nursing diagnosis content in fundamentals of nursing textbooks. *Nurse Educator, 22* (1), 17–22.

Marrelli, T.M. (1992). *Nursing documentation handbook.* St. Louis: Mosby–Year Book.

Maslow, A. (1970). *Motivation in personality.* New York: Harper & Row.

Maynard, C.A. (1996). Relationship of critical thinking to professional nursing competence. *Journal of Nursing Education, 36,* (1), 12–18.

McCloskey, J. C. & Bulechek, G. M. (Eds.). (1996). *Nursing interventions classification (NIC)* (2nd ed.). St. Louis: Mosby.

McFarland, G.K. & McFarlane, E.A. (1997). *Nursing diagnosis and intervention* (3rd ed.). St. Louis: Mosby.

McGovern, M. & Valiga, T.M. (1997). Promoting the cognitive development of freshman nursing students. *Journal of Nursing Education, 36* (1), 29–35.

McKeachie, W.J. (1986). *Teaching tips: A guidebook for the beginning college teacher* (8th ed.). Lexington, MA: D.C. Heath.

McPeck, J.E. (1990). *Teaching critical thinking.* New York: Routledge.

Middlemiss, M.A. & Van Neste-Kenny, J. (1994). Curriculum revolution: Reflective minds and empowering relationships. *Nursing and Health Care, 15,* 350–353.

Miller, M.A. (1992). Outcomes evaluation: Measuring critical thinking. *Journal of Advanced Nursing, 17,* 1401–1407.

Miller, M.A. & Malcolm, N.S. (1990). Critical thinking in the nursing curriculum. *Nursing and Health Care, 11*(2), 67–73.

Narayan, S.M. & Corcoran-Perry, S. (1997). Line of reasoning as a representation of nurses' clinical decision making. *Research in Nursing and Health, 20* (4), 353–364.

Neill, K.M., Lachat, M.F. & Taylor-Panek, S. (1997). Enhancing critical thinking with case studies and nursing process. *Nurse Educator, 22* (22), 30–32.

Norris, S. (Ed.). (1992). *The generalizability of critical thinking: Multiple perspectives on an educational ideal.* New York: Teachers College Press.

North American Nursing Diagnosis Association. (1996). *NANDA nursing diagnoses: Definitions and classification 1997–1998.* Philadelphia: Author.

North American Nursing Diagnosis Association. (1992). *NANDA nursing diagnoses: Definitions and classification 1992.* Philadelphia: Author.

Northouse, P.G. & Northouse, L.L. (1985). *Health communication: A handbook for health professionals.* Englewood Cliffs, NJ: Prentice-Hall.

Nosich, G.M. (1994). Where to begin? How to design classes to teach for thinking. *Educational Vision: The Magazine for Critical Thinking. 2*(2), 20–21.

Oren, D.E. (1991). *Nursing concepts of practice* (4th ed.). St. Louis: C.V. Mosby.

O'Sullivan, P.S., Blevins-Stephens, W.L., Smith, F.M. & Vaughan-Wrobel, B. (1997). Addressing the National League for Nursing Critical Thinking Outcome. *Nurse Educator, 22* (1), 23–29.

Patton, J.G., Woods, S.J. Agarenzo, T., Brubacker, C., Metcalf, T. & Sherrer, L. (1997). Enhancing the clinical practicum experience through journal writing. *Journal of Nursing Education, 36* (5), 238–240.

Paul, R. (1992). *Critical thinking: What every person needs to survive in a rapidly changing world* (rev. 2nd ed.). Santa Rosa, CA: Foundation for Critical Thinking.

Paul, R.W. & Heaslip, P. (1995). Critical thinking and intuitive nursing practice. *Journal of Advanced Nursing, 22* 40–47.

Percifal, E.G. & Nester, P.A. (1996). The effect of an innovative clinical teaching method on nursing students' knowledge and critical thinking skills. *Journal of Nursing Education, 35* (1), 23–28.

Perkins, D., Jay, E., & Tishman, S. (1993). *Assessing thinking: A framework for measuring critical thinking and problem solving skills at the college level.* Paper prepared for the National Center for Education Statistics.

Perry, W.G. (1970). *Forms of intellectual and ethical development in the college years.* New York: Holt, Rinehart and Winston.

Pesut, D.J. & Herman, J. (1992). Metacognitive skills in diagnostic reasoning: Making the implicit explicit. *Nursing Diagnosis, 3,* 148–154.

Pless, B.S. & Clayton, G.M. (1993). Clarifying the concept of critical thinking in nursing. *Journal of Nursing Education, 32,* (9), 425–428.

Polanyi, M. (1964). The logic of tacit inference. In Grene, M. (Ed.). *Knowing and being: Essays by Michaie Polanyi* (pp. 138–158). Chicago: University of Chicago Press.

Rane-Szostak, D. & Robertson, J.F. (1996). Issues in measuring critical thinking: Meeting the challenge. *Journal of Nursing Education, 35* (1), 5–11.

Rantz, M.J. & LeMone, P. (Eds.). (1997). *Classification of nursing diagnoses: Proceedings of the twelfth conference of the North American Nursing Diagnosis Association.* Glendale, CA: CINAHL Information Systems.

Roberts, C.M., Sucher, K., Perrin, D.G. & Rodriguez, S. (1995). Concept mapping: An effective instructional strategy for diet therapy. Journal of the American Dietetic Association, 95 (8), 908–911.

Romain, D. (1997). *Thinking things through: Critical thinking for decisions you can live with.* Mountain View, CA: Mayfield Publishing Co.

Romer, C.M. (1993). How to outsmart "Murphy." *Journal of Continuing Education in Nursing, 24* (2), 91–92.

Rooda, L.A. (1994). Effects of mind mapping on student achievement in a nursing research course. *Nurse Educator, 19* (6), 25–27.

Roy, C. & Andrews, H.A. (1991). *The Roy adaptation model: A definitive statement.* Norwalk, CT: Appleton & Lange.

Saarmann, L., Freitas, L., Rapps, J., & Riegel, B. (1992). The relationship of education to critical thinking ability and values among nurses: Socialization into professional nursing. *Journal of Professional Nursing, 8*(1), 26–34.

Saba, V.K. & McCormick, K.A. (1996). *Essentials of computers for nurses* (2nd ed.) New York: McGraw-Hill.

Saucier, B.L. (1995). Critical thinking skills of baccalaureate nursing students. *Journal of Professional Nursing, 11* (6) 351–357.

Schon, D.A. (1983). *The reflective practitioner: How professionals think in action.* New York: Basic Books.

Schumacher, J. & Sverson, A. (1996). Building bridges for future practice: An innovative approach to foster critical thinking. *Journal of Nursing Education, 35* (1), 31–33.

Sedlak, C.A. (1997). Critical thinking of beginning baccalaureate nursing students during the first clinical nursing course. *Journal of Nursing Education, 36* (1), 11–18.

Silva, M.C., Sorrell, J.M., & Sorrell, C.D. (1995). From Carper's patterns of knowing to ways of being: An ontological philosophical shift in nursing. *Advances in Nursing Science, 18* (1), 1–13.

Smeltzer, S.C. & Bare, B.G. (1996). *Brunner and Suddarth's textbook of medical-surgical nursing* (8th ed.). Philadelphia: Lippincott.

Tanner, C.A. (1993). More thinking about critical thinking and clinical decision making. *Journal of Nursing Education, 32,* (9), 387.

Tanner, C.A. (1997). Spock would have been a terrible nurse. *Journal of Nursing Education, 36* (1), 3–4.

Tanner, C.A., Padrick, K.P., Westfall, U.E., & Putzier, D.J. (1987). Diagnostic reasoning strategies of nurses and nursing students. *Nursing Research, 36,* 358–363.

Valiga, T.M. & Bruderle, E. (1994). Concepts included in and critical to nursing curricula: An analysis. *Journal of Nursing Education, 33* (3), 118–124.

Vanetzian, E. & Corrigan, B. (1996). "Prep" for class and class activity key to critical thinking. *Nurse Educator, 21* (2), 45–48.

Videbeck, S.L. (1997a). Critical thinking: Prevailing practice in baccalaureate schools of nursing. *Journal of Nursing Education, 36* (1), 5–10.

Videbeck, S.L. (1997b). Critical thinking: A model. *Journal of Nursing Education, 36* (1), 23–28.

Watson, G. & Claser, E. (1964). *Critical thinking appraisal manual.* New York: Harcourt, Brace & World.

White, J. (1995). Patterns of knowing: Review, critique, and update. *Advances in Nursing Science, 17* (4), 73–86.

Whiteside, C. (1997). A model for teaching critical thinking in the clinical setting. *Dimensions of Critical Care Nursing, 16* (3), 152–162.

Wong, F.K.Y., Kember, D., Chung. L.Y.F. & Yan, L. (1995). Assessing the level of student reflection from reflective journals. *Journal of Advanced Nursing, 22,* 48–52.

Woods, J.H. (1993). Affective learning: One door to critical thinking. *Holistic Nursing Practice, 7,* (3), 64–70.

Yura, H. & Walsh, M.B. (Eds.). (1967). *The nursing process: Assessing, planning, implementing, evaluating.* Washington D.C.: Catholic University of America Press.

Yura, H. & Walsh, M.B. (1973). *The nursing process: Assessing, planning, implementing, evaluating* (2nd ed.). New York: Appleton-Century-Crofts.

Yura, H. & Walsh, M.B. (1988). *The nursing process: Assessing, planning, implementing, evaluating* (5th ed.). East Norwalk, CT: Appleton & Lange.

Index

Page numbers followed by f *indicate figures; those followed by* t *indicate tables; those followed by* d *indicate displays.*